ANALYTICAL REPERTORY

OF THE

SYMPTOMS OF THE MIND.

BY

C. HERING, M.D.

" * * * * Some prescriptions
Of rare and proved effects."—*Shakespeare.*

SECOND EDITION.

B. Jain Publishers (P) Ltd.
USA — Europe — India

ANALYTICAL REPERTORYOF THE SYMPTOMS OF MIND

Second Edition
5th Impression: 2014

All rights reserved. No part of this book may be reproduced, stored in a retrieval system or transmitted, in any form or by any means, mechanical, photocopying, recording or otherwise, without any prior written permission of the publisher.

© with the publisher

Published by Kuldeep Jain for
B. JAIN PUBLISHERS (P) LTD.
1921/10, Chuna Mandi, Paharganj, New Delhi 110 055 (INDIA)
Tel.: +91-11-4567 1000   Fax: +91-11-4567 1010
Email: info@bjain.com   Website: **www.bjain.com**

Printed in India by
JJ Imprints Pvt. Ltd.

ISBN: 978-81-319-3220-9

NOTE.

The first edition of the late Dr. C. Hering's well-known work on all mental symptoms observed in connection with bodily conditions being sold, and a demand existing for a second edition, the book has been reprinted, with an appendix of such additions as were found in the venerable author's interleaved copy. A very carefully prepared index, the work of Dr. Levi J. Knerr, adds materially to the value of the book for the busy practitioner.

CHARLES G. RAUE,
CALVIN B. KNERR, } Eds.
CHARLES MOHR.

NOTE.

The first edition of the late Dr. C. Hering's well-known work on all mental symptoms observed in connection with bodily conditions being sold, and a demand existing for a second edition, the book has been reprinted, with an appendix of such additions as were found in the venerable author's interleaved copy. A very carefully prepared index, the work of Dr. Levi J. Knerr, adds materially to the value of the book for the busy practitioner.

Charles G. Raue,
Calvin B. Knerr, Eds.
Charles Mohr

CONTENTS.

	PAGE.
INTRODUCTION	11
HOW TO USE THIS BOOK,	23
THE ARRANGEMENT	26

THE FORTY-EIGHT CHAPTERS.

		PAGE
I.	Mind and Disposition,	29
II.	Sensorium,	29
III.	Headache and Affections of the inner Head,	29
IV.	External Head,	29
V.	Sight and Eyes,	30
VI.	Hearing and Ears,	31
VII.	Smell and Nose,	31
VIII.	Face,	32
IX.	Lower Part of Face,	32
X.	Teeth and Gums,	32
XI.	Taste, Talk, Tongue,	32
XII.	Inner Mouth,	33
XIII.	Palate and Throat,	33
XIV.	Desire for Food and Drink,	33
XV.	Before—During—After Eating and Drinking,	33
XVI.	Gastric Symptoms,	33
XVII.	Epigastric Region,	34
XVIII.	Hypochondriac Regions,	34
XIX.	Abdomen,	34
XX.	Rectum and Anus,	34
XXI.	Urinary Organs,	35
XXII.	Male Functions and Organs,	35
XXIII.	Female Organs,	35
XXIV.	Pregnancy and Parturition,	36
XXV.	Larynx,	37
XXVI.	Respiration,	37
XXVII.	Coughs,	37
XXVIII.	Inner Chest and Lungs,	37
XXIX.	Heart and Circulation,	38
XXX.	Outer Chest,	38
XXXI.	Neck and Back,	38
XXXII.	Upper Limbs,	39
XXXIII.	Lower Limbs,	39
XXXIV.	All the Limbs,	39
XXXV.	Rest—Position—Motion,	39
XXXVI.	Nerves,	41

5

CONTENTS.

	PAGE.
XXXVII. Sleep,	41
XXXVIII. Times of the Day,	42
XXXIX. Relations to Warmth, Air and Water; Wind and Weather; Seasons,	42
XL. Fever,	43
XLI. Changes According to Time,	43
XLII. Relations to Space—Changes According to Space,	44
XLIII. Sensations classified,	44
1.—Increased, Exaggerated Activity,	45
2.—Fixed, *i. e.*, Without Motion,	45
3.—Steady Motion,	46
4.—Motion in Relation to the Dimensions of the Body,	46
5.—Sensation, with a Pulsating, Wavering, Oscillating Motion,	46
6.—Sensation as if the Integrity of the Tissues was Disturbed. Destructive Action,	47
7.—Sensation of Decreased Activity,	47
Index to Chapter Forty-three—Sensations,	48
Conditions and Concomitants of Pain,	50
XLIV. Tissues,	51
XLV. Passive Motions and Touch,	52
XLVI. Skin,	52
XLVII. Stages of Life,	52
XLVIII. Relationship with other Drugs,	52
OUR NOMENCLATURE,	53
ABRIDGEMENT OF NAMES,	56
LIMITATION,	56
LIST OF NAMES AND THEIR ABRIDGEMENTS,	57
NOTES TO THE LIST OF NAMES,	65
NOSODES,	66
REMARKS,	67
ABBREVIATIONS,	67
MARKS AND SIGNS,	67
CONCLUSION,	68
CHAPTER I. MIND AND DISPOSITION,	69
Hahnemann's Organon,	69
BODILY SYMPTOMS CONNECTED WITH THE MIND,	70
1. Ailments from Emotions and Exertions of the Mind.	
Happy Surprise,	71
Complaints after Laughing,	71
Fright and Fear,	72
Shock of Injury,	76
Ailments owing to Fear,	82
After Anxiety,	82
Homesickness, Nostalgia,	84
Love Pangs,	85
Jealousy,	86
Grief and Sorrow,	86
Better in Company and Better when Alone,	87
The Talk of others increases the Sufferings,	90
After Mortification,	90
Vexation,	92

CONTENTS.

	PAGE.
Anger,	95
After Emotions and Excitement,	97
Symptoms appear when Thinking of them,	99
Better when Thinking of Ailments,	100
Better when Thinking about something else,	100
Complaints after Talking, Speaking, Conversing,	101
Headache from Exertions of Mind or Intellectual Work,	102
Other Complaints after Mental Exertion, Over-study, Meditating, etc.	104
Ailings from Overexertion of Mind and Body,	108

II. Mental Concomitants of Bodily Symptoms.

HEAD,	110
According to Locality,	110
According to Sensations,	111
With Headache in general,	112
Headache, with Anxiousness,	113
Headache, with Ill Humor,	114
Headache, with Restlessness,	115
Headache, with Diminished Intellectual Power,	115
Headache, with Deranged Mind,	116
Rush of Blood to the Head,	117
Sensation of Fullness,	117
OUTER HEAD,	118
Movements,	119
Positions,	119
Cold, Heat, Sweat,	119
Bones of the Skull,	120
Scalp,	120
The whole Outer Head,	121
SIGHT,	121
Perverted Vision,	123
EYES,	124
Appearance,	125
Pains,	126
Tears,	126
Weeping,	126
Better after Weeping,	127
Red Eyes and Opthalmia, with Derangement of Mind,	127
HEARING,	128
Noise Unbearable,	129
Subjective Noises,	130
Diminished Sense of Hearing,	130
Earache,	131
Outer Ear,	131
NOSE,	131
Outer Nose,	132
FACE,	133
Features, Countenance,	133
Face Motions,	134
FACE EXTERNAL,	135
Sweat,	136
Redness,	137
Paleness,	138

CONTENTS.

	Page.
Swelling,	140
Skin,	140
JAWS,	140
LIPS,	140
TEETH,	141
TASTE,	142
TALKING,	142
TONGUE,	143
MOUTH,	143
ROOF OF MOUTH AND PALATE,	144
THROAT,	144
THIRST,	146
HUNGER,	146
Diminished Appetite,	147
DESIRES AND AVERSIONS,	147
Before, While, and After Eating and Drinking,	148
Mental States after Eating,	149
GASTRIC SYMPTOMS,	153
Anxiousness, Anxiety, Anguish, with Nausea and Vomituritio,	153
Vomiting and Anxiety,	156
STOMACH SYMPTOMS WITH ANXIETY,	157
Anxiety in Scrobiculum,	158
HYPOCHONDRIAC REGIONS,	159
Præcordial Anxiety,	160
ABDOMINAL COMPLAINTS, WITH ANXIETY AND CONCOMITANTS,	160
Colic, with Anxiety,	162
Colic, with other Mental Concomitants,	163
Other Abdominal Sensations, with Mental Concomitants,	165
Flatulency,	165
Abdominal Diseased States,	165
LOINS,	166
EMISSION OF WIND,	166
LOOSENESS FOLLOWING EMOTION AND EXERTION,	166
Looseness of Bowels, with Mental Concomitants,	167
COSTIVENESS AND CONSTIPATION, WITH MENTAL SYMPTOMS,	169
Mental Complaints Before, During and After Stool,	170
Tenesmus and Involuntary Stool,	171
RECTUM,	172
Anus,	172
UROPOETIC ORGANS,	172
Complaints Before, During and After Urination,	173
SEXUAL DESIRE,	173
Emissions,	174
FEMALE INNER SEXUAL ORGANS,	175
Catamenia too Copious, Menorrhagia,	177
Dysmenorrhœa,	178
Amenorrhœa,	178
Catamenia, with Anxiety, Anguish and Apprehension, Before, During and After,	179
Catamenia, with Mental Concomitants,	179
Leucorrhœa,	182

CONTENTS.

	PAGE.
Outer Parts,	182
Mind Symptoms during Pregnancy,	182
During Parturition,	185
Childbed,	186
Nursing,	186
LARYNX AND WINDPIPE,	187
Voice,	187
Laughing,	189
Sighing,	191
Moaning and Groaning,	192
Weeping, Whining,	194
Crying and Screaming,	198
IN AND EXHALATION,	199
Short Breathing,	199
Slow, Labored, Panting Breathing,	200
Deep Inhalation,	200
Impeded Breathing, with Anxiety and other Concomitants,	201
Threatening Suffocation,	204
COUGH AND MENTAL CONCOMITANTS,	205
PECTORAL ANXIETY,	208
Pain in Chest, with Anxiety,	209
Other Sensations in Chest, with Anxiety,	210
Sensations in Chest, with other Mental Symptoms,	211
ANGUISH IN HEART,	213
Heartache, with Mental Symptoms,	215
Other Sensations about the Heart,	217
Palpitation, with Mental Symptoms,	218
Palpitation, with other Bodily Symptoms and Mental Concomitants,	219
Palpitation from Emotions,	222
Palpitation after Mental Exertions,	223
Rush of Blood to the Heart,	223
Orgasm,	224
Pulse and Mental States,	224
OUTER CHEST,	226
NECK AND BACK,	227
UPPER LIMBS,	228
LOWER LIMBS,	231
ALL THE LIMBS,	233
MOVEMENTS,	235
POSITIONS,	237
SOMNAMBULISM, CLAIRVOYANCE,	239
Ecstasy; Lightness,	239
Excitable, Agitated,	240
Contradictions,	241
RESTLESSNESS,	242
TREMBLING,	244
Starting from Fright,	246
CONVULSIONS; EPILEPTIC AND OTHER SPASMS,	247
MIND AND BODY WEAK, FEEBLE AND RELAXED,	249
Weakness, with other Mental Concomitants,	251
Weakness and Anxiety,	252
Weakness and Ill Humor,	253

CONTENTS.

	PAGE.
SLEEP,	257
Sleepiness,	257
Before Sleep,	259
Exaltation and Delirium before Sleep,	261
Sleeplessness, with Exaltation,	262
Sleeplessness, with anxiety,	263
Slumber,	265
Sleep and Anxiety,	267
Other Mental Complaints at Night,	270
On Awakening or being Woke,	273
When Awaking in the Morning,	277
After Loss of Sleep,	279
After Sleep,	280
TIMES OF DAY,	281
Morning,	281
Forenoon,	284
Noon,	285
All Day,	286
Afternoon,	287
Evening,	291
WARMTH,	298
SEASONS,	302
CHILL, HEAT, SWEAT,	303
Feelings,	303
Anxiety,	306
Other unpleasant Feelings,	313
Feelings and Conations,	314
Actions,	316
Desires,	317
Aversions,	317
Exaltations,	317
Restlessness,	318
Intellect,	321
Reproductions,	323
PERIODICITIES, ATTACKS OR SPELLS,	324
Worse during the Phases of the Moon,	325
SIDES,	325
Peculiar Sensations, with Mental Symptoms,	327
Oversensitiveness to Pain,	328
TISSUES,	330
TOUCH,	331
Passive Motions,	332
SKIN,	333
TEMPERAMENTS AND CONSTITUTIONS,	334
Children,	336
Women and Old People,	343
OTHER DRUGS,	344

INTRODUCTION.

The following work has been the result of an endeavor to collect and unite in one book the facts developed by our school from our provings, through practice. This has been done without excluding, through arbitrary notions, any useful remarks from trustworthy observers. The scatterings of our books and journals, together with a great deal that has hitherto remained unpublished, has here been condensed into the smallest compass, in such an order and form, as to facilitate as much as possible, the selection of *the* remedy for a given case. The intention being, to enable the practitioner to review the whole subject at a glance, as it were, and with rapidity find the curative medicine, even in apparently difficult cases. The arrangement as well as the style of printing, has the one object especially in view, viz.: to make it as easy as possible for the eye, and through the eye, for the mind to find what is looked for.

A somewhat similar work were those monographs of some of our medicines, which have been published during the last few years, at first as an appendix to our journals, then as a separate volume. The attempt was there made, to collect under each drug all that had become known about its effects; arranging it in such manner as to bring it before the eyes of the reader in a *comparable form*, thus enabling every thinking reader, to make a satisfactory abstract for personal use.

Such readers can easily compare the manner in which each drug acts upon, and influences each organ and part of the body, both as regards the nature, kind, and degree of such action. They can compare the peculiar sensations or kinds of affection; may follow up the different functions of our organism in their various connections;

may find all the modalities of the various symptoms, or changes observed in them, as brought about by or related to, external influences, or by the connection of different functions; finally the concomitants, and the groups, as they appear together: yet during the whole, with a constant view to the general character of the drug. Of course this cannot be done without a proper physiological and pathological training; *never* can be done without *real* study —*i. e.*, with great exertion of the mind. Hence, there are some who prefer to have it done for them; some who prefer the "mummed to the crumbed," while others prefer to do the chewing themselves.

Although, as before remarked, the present work bears some similarity to the Materia Medica, yet the mental process is of different character; for while the *Materia Medica* requires a constant *synthesis* in the mind of the reader, a constant action of the mind aiming at that which is general in the numerous single observations as recorded in the symptoms; the *therapeutical work* requires a constant *analysis*.

The main object being, to render in every case such assistance to the practitioner, that the selection of a proper remedy may be facilitated, this work necessarily becomes a *Digest*, containing the most essential results of our provings, and at the same time the results of our practice. Thus has been collected, not only that which was observed as appearing, but also that disappearing after the use of a drug. Clinical reports coming from reliable parties, must be received as bona fide; and we must likewise assume that the drug is (with more or less certainty) the cause of what followed its administration. Our Materia Medica has already been used by many, who have not shunned *labor* in their work of healing the sick. Another score of years will enable us to separate the wheat from the tares.

Being well aware that these two kind of symptoms, viz.: those produced and those cured, are essentially different, we still have, after long and matured consideration, decided to give both without marks of distinction. The marking of such different origin, should always be done with the utmost care in the monograph of the Materia Medica; it should there be considered as a matter of the highest importance, never to mix indiscriminately, symptoms *reported as cured* (not having been observed on the healthy), with the symptoms *produced* by the drug.

Hahnemann's warning must never be forgotten, see Chronic Diseases, Vol. 2, second edition, note to Alumina.

Hahnemann was right, when he advised us not to be ruled by former cures, but always by the symptoms produced.

If we should ever have a complete collection of all our important proved medicines printed, with all their symptoms arranged comparably, then our therapeutic advice may be given with differential marks. Until then, it is no doubt much better to have every searcher for similarity led by the degree markings, according to the plan of Bönninghausen. Perplexity instead of lucidness would be developed through the combination of the differential and degree marks. Every one following the advice hereafter given, under the heading "How to use this work", will be enabled to *decide* on the remedy, in most cases, and, in the shortest time; such choice being mostly governed, by the symptoms coming from the provings. Thus much for the class of symptoms employed in this work. Next let us look at the arrangement. The headings throughout are either: organs, or, parts of the body, general symptoms, altered functions, sensations, leading modalities, groups of symptoms, or names of diseases. One or more such prominent statement, will be found in every individual case of sickness, for which the work may be consulted. In each such division, the eye of the reader will fall on a list of names of medicines, at the margin. This arrangement is an entirely new one and affords great relief to the eyes, as the motion from above downwards is accomplished with less fatigue and with more certainty, than the necessary repetition of the linear motion, required in the common arrangement.

Such marginal lists are collections of the names of all drugs, known to deserve remembrance with regard to what is given in the heading. Distinguishing marks are placed to the remedies, indicative of their value or importance in relation to the subject embraced in the heading.

Under the heading of *an organ*, or, *part of the body*, the principal medicines affecting the part or organ, are mentioned in the mar ginal list, being there marked according to their importance. This has been done, principally according to Bönninghausen, and without the least intention of favoring a revival of the old erroneous notion of "specifics for organs." Since Dioscorides, this doctrine has, from time to time, been intruded on the profession, only to be again discarded as untenable. Some few years ago it again appeared among us as a monstrosity, called Organopathy.

In this department there are many additions not easily found in the common repertories, for instance, Ear-lobe, Throat pit, Cœcal region, Os coccygis, Thumb and several others. Such localities are in some cases very significant, and frequently may decide the choice.

Under the head of *General Symptoms, i. e.* such according to which, alone, it would be impossible to base a correct prescription, there will be found at the margin of the page a list of medicines with the marks indicative of their grades of value. In the text adjoining, the different shades of variation will be given according to the uniform rule: that all similar sensation and feelings must be placed near each other; provers as well as patients, may have used different words in endeavoring to express the same sensation. After this we have the connections, then the modalities and concomitants, of such a symptom or altered function.

The different *modalities* also have their pages, where in a condensed review all can be found that our school knows in relation to each. Not only is a list of remedies given at the margin, but also an analysis on the page. For instance, of all drugs in which warmth or heat has been observed to aggravate or ameliorate—the text will specify, as clearly as possible, the function affected; or, the sensation is given in particular. Thus, we find, burning pain in ulcers, ameliorated by heat under Arsen., but aggravated under Secale, etc. For the majority of beginners, those headings formed by the *names of* "*diseases,*" or such pathological names as are used to designate groups of symptoms which have been frequently observed in combination, will be found of the greatest importance. The most common of such names have always been preferred, and have been used in the most comprehensive manner, being employed only for the purpose of arranging under them what has been reported in our literature, as individual experience in such or such "disease." In some instances remedies have been mentioned, from which we have no clinical record, the similarity which they bear to certain "diseases," as established by our provings, rendering them however, worthy of notice, thus we have mentioned, Fluor. ac. in Typhoid fevers, Tabacum in Angina Pectoris, etc. Here it may be well to say a few words in explanation. It is by no means a disregard of pathology when Hahnemann advises, always to give the remedy according to the symptoms in each case, and not according to the *names* of diseases. Still, nothing was more abhorrent to the old schools! They called it an attempt to destroy all medical science; consequently a majority of the converts to homœopathy have been over-anxious to appear as real scientific men, and were more or less governed by the old error, "that *diseases* could be cured by *specifics*." These pathological names of diseases are mere abstracts. Hahnemann, according to the strict method which he rigorously followed during his life, wanted us to look to the reality; to the real sick individual; to take an image of all the symptoms and compare such a picture of the one reality with the other, that is, with the real symptoms of a drug. All the homœopathic practitioners who go by names (Bæhr, Kafka, and many others), repeatedly complain of their want of success, and in dangerous cases they frequently feel *their* "absolute necessity" of falling back into the crudities, barbarisms and follies of the old school, viz., massive doses, the knife, caustics, ice, etc., etc. All who follow Hahnemann's advice are much more successful, though, of course, never pretending, as slander says, to be "infallible."

The collections of remedies under the head of names of diseases have been made with the view of aiding individualization. Where the practitioner finds the symptoms of his case do not exactly correspond with any here given, he ought to go farther and select the exact counterpart, in case such can be found, even though it never had been given in the disease (according to name) before. Our lists of remedies given under the head of the name of a disease have thus increased each year; where fifty years ago we had two or three, we now have, perhaps, ten or twenty times as many.

Bönninghausen's works, especially his repertory, have been made free use of throughout, because he was the only practitioner who entered all his corroborations and all successfully cured symptoms in his case books; and that, too, during more than two scores of years. He states in the preface, that use was made of the symptoms from provings, and the symptoms cured—"what is offered in the Materia Medica Pura" and "the results of practice after careful examination" have to be "made use of together," to "afford the means of judging of the value of each symptom, completing the imperfect ones among them, and filling up the numerous vacancies, which the practitioner at every moment meets with." Bönninghausen's Repertory has been made, as it were, the basis of this Analytical Therapeutics, and all that could possibly be of any use has been given, especially in the margins, but none without additions. Many of the additions or alterations were made by Bönninghausen himself, in the copy used by him in his practice. Dr. Dunham, during his stay with Bönninghausen, was allowed to copy the author's own marks, corroborations and additions, which had been made from his practice, during more than ten years. Dr. Dunham with his well known liberality left his copy long enough in Philadelphia to be compared and carefully copied.

The English translation by Stapf has many errors in the names, and was reprinted here with all of them. The errors in the language were partly corrected by Okie, and many more by Hempel; Laurie's translation was made from the French, of Roth, in Paris, and though somewhat better in the arrangement, was not free from errors, and had besides many omissions.

Bönninghausen's pathological mistakes, as for instance the confounding of pale blood and bright blood, quick pulse and frequent pulse, etc., have been corrected; and a great many of his unnecessary repetitions avoided by the new arrangement.

It was a great mistake, of Bönninghausen, to separate the conditions, as if every one of them could have a general applicability. He mentions a case in his preface, where there was an *aggravation after shaving*; this is one of the combined and of course most important "conditions" observed by Adams, a prover of Carbo animalis, a hyperæsthesia of the nerves of the skin on the cheeks, around the mouth, and on the chin. This aggravation had led a friend of Bönninghausen's to give Carb. an. to a consumptive patient with "the most decided and lasting effect," for a disagreeable smoothness of the teeth, worse every time he shaved. But this *does not* give us the right to generalize it into "worse after shaving." Both of these *different* symptoms are within the sphere of the so-called fifth pair of nerves, or trigeminus. In several cases where the same aggravation was a leading symptom, this limitation seemed to be corroborated. It is worthy of notice, that it is not stated whether the prover was shaving himself, or was being shaved by a barber. The position of the head in the latter case, or the standing position in the former, might also have some influence.

In Bönninghausen's repertory we find a paragraph, "getting worse in the dark." Here the cause may be either *mental*, as from fear; or, the *eyes may want light*. According to the repertory, it is impossible to say with which of the ten drugs named, (to which we now have ten more according to Dunham's copy), it is the one, or the other, or both. With "getting better in the dark" the inquiry as to cause, becomes still more important, seventy-three drugs are mentioned, mostly such as affect the eyes.

To illustrate this, we will compare the Pathogenetic Cyclopœdia, London, 1850, pp. 42. We find among the mental symptoms as "aggravated by the dark": Berber., fear, things appear too large; Lycop., frightened when a door will not open; Rhus tox., suicidal tendency in the twilight; Valer., fear of being injured by others; to these we may add: Phosphor., depression in the dark; and from Jahr's Mental Diseases translated by Galloway, 1857, Calc. acet., afraid of darkness; Carb. veg., delirium worse in the dark; Pulsat., dread of darkness; Stramon., sorrowfulness in the dark.

All these remedies, *except the Rhus tox.*, have also aggravation of eye symptoms in the dark. It would be an assumption, not at all allowable, to generalize this modality, by supposing that Rhus tox. must also have the eye symptoms aggravated in the dark The modalities are not convertible from one part or function to another in every case, though in many they may correspond. This fact may be illustrated by the Stramon., which has a very remarkable desire for bright light, and symptoms of mind and body better in the light; yet it has just the reverse with the eye symptoms, which are worse from either natural, or artificial light.

In Bönninghausen's repertory we find entire lists of remedies, under what to him appeared to be convertible terms; this is altogether wrong. Symptoms will not bear such turning; they are not like stockings, to be turned inside out, for easy adjustment. Not every symptom "better in the dark," gets "worse in the light;" nor is every one "worse in the light," "better in the dark."

This use of lists of remedies, under apparently opposite conditions, must be misleading. True, most symptoms depending on bright light, abate in the dark, but this widely differs from a real amelioration in the dark; as the one may be very striking without the other existing. This will appear plainly, if we consult Berridge's repertory, we there find one hundred and fifty-seven drugs with "aggravation from light;" ninety-two from natural light, fifteen only from artificial light, and fifty from either. According to the same excellent repertory, only seven of the one hundred and fifty-seven have "amelioration in the dark." Of thirty-one drugs having symptoms "worse in the dark," only five have symptoms "better in the light."

While making use of Bönninghausen's most valuable work, we have endeavored as far as possible, to rectify such reversed lists, according to the Materia Medica; but until access to his case books can be had, a *complete* revision will be almost impossible.

The greatest stress is laid, in the following work, on the entire *abolishment of the alphabetical arrangement*, for in fact nothing in the whole book has been arranged alphabetically, except the names of the drugs, and even there we trust it will be abandoned by the next generation. All our, many, repertories have suffered under this most miserable of all "orders," taking up our time and wasting it by increasing the difficulties. It is true that Hahnemann added to his first collection (his "Fragmenta" of 1805), an index where every word could be found; but it was altogether out of proportion, and could only have been a help in this very first beginning. The text, in large type spaciously printed, filled 268 pages; the index in small type, condensedly printed, filled 469 pages. The number of em's, according to the printers measure, in the first part, was 203,680, while in the second part, we find 597,506; thus we find it requires nearly three times as much space. A repertory, according to this plan at the present time, would require as many folios as the Acta Sanctorum (still unfinished) with its fifty-seven volumes. As soon as Hahnemann (1811) made it a rule to arrange each drug according to the adopted schema, this great step forward brought us to the necessity of adopting the same order in the repertory. Most of the various works of this kind have partially done so. Some adopted even a loose rule; they arranged arbitrarily, according to notions, as far as they could without difficulty, but with the first obstacle they fell back on the alphabet as their sheet-anchor.

The different words used by the provers to indicate what was frequently the same, or at least a very similar symptom, separated such observations, and placed them remote from each other, to the greatest torment of the reader; or if different expressions were arbitrarily bundled together, we had to select as it were from heaps, that which is wanted; while frequently the only result is more confusion, and we are finally left like one lost in the woods.

We should always find words of similar import placed near together. The British Cypher Repertory adopted to a certain extent this arrangement by similars. Roth, in his translation of Bönninghausen, avoided the alphabetical *disorder* as far as he could, but it was never done consistently or thoroughly.

The cumbersome alphabetical order can only be abolished by following a natural arrangement, one which every reader can learn as readily as an alphabet; as necessary to the thorough understanding of this work, as the alphabet or a dictionary to the study of the Hebrew, Greek, or any oriental language. It would be of immense advantage if we could agree upon and adopt a uniform arrangement in all our books. Hahnemann's arrangement is for us a kind of alphabet. Following this order, all the symptoms of each medicine in his Materia Medica were arranged, partially according to the parts of the human body, and partially arbitrarily.

It was framed, after Hahnemann had collected symptoms for twenty years; with each new volume of his Materia Medica, and with each new edition from 1811 to 1839, he endeavored to improve it. Much has been said against it, but the whole opposition supposed abstracts and theories to be realities, not understanding the strict induction method of Hahnemann, a method through which all natural sciences have made their progress; they could not comprehend the absolute necessity of taking hold of the closest observation of the single phenomena, individual symptoms, both as related to the prover, as well as to the sick. In such a new field of research, where, unavoidably, every observer is surrounded by uncertainties, nothing could be gained by theorizing or soaring into the clouds of opinions. The facts had first to be collected, one by one, and then arranged in some way, that they might be applied again and again, until the probabilities increased, and a scientific certainty was within reach. Every one who tried to follow Hahnemann's advice, had the satisfaction of seeing the sick getting well; but, the opposition, instead of walking in this plain common-sense way, did but cry, science! Science was in danger! Of course, old mouldy doctrines were; but we are working for a new science. To be sure, old time honored yet worthless rules and superstitions had to be abandoned; this they would not do. There was not one among them, who had even the most remote idea of what real science is! They were like the man who ploughed his field and sowed crumbs of bread, expecting a harvest of fresh baked loaves. They could not see, that, as in all other natural sciences, so to, we had, first, to collect observations; then make the application of such facts; then compare results; then sift and sort them; and finally bring them in order, that we might arrive at a standard deserving the name of science. This is the way to winnow, and is the only way! Our half-homœopaths, Anti-Hahnemannians, over-anxious to be considered scientific men, raised a terrible hue and cry about such "heaps of symptoms," "orderless complexes," "manufactured for mechanical use." They invented all kinds of nick-names, yet they could not prevent the growth and further development of our Materia Medica, and the return to Hahnemann's way and arrangement. All this bustling noise is over, but most of our practitioners have ever since remained dependent only on the extracts, thus impeding progress.

After Bönninghausen had with great success published a kind of short repertory, our industrious Jahr followed in the newly opened way. Bönninghausen had rather arbitrarily not only left out some of the later provings, but even slandered them, from 1835 to 1846, by frequently comparing them with Fickel's counterfeit proving of Osmium. Yet afterwards adding one by one, as his time allowed him to enter their symptoms into his book. In 1846 he had added some formerly omitted, viz., Borax, Wahle's Kreosote, and later Fluor. ac., Merc. subl. and Apis; while he still would not acknowledge the master proving of Berberis, and many others of much greater importance, than several which he had carefully given a place to throughout his repertory.

Jahr followed his smaller work with a larger one. He carried out the most unwise idea of mending Hahnemann's arrangement by cutting off a portion from the end of each remedy, and placing it at the beginning. Thus commencing each medicine with the hodge podge, of so-called generalities. (See C. Hg's Materia Medica, Vol. I., Introduction, pp. VIII., IX.) When this large work of Jahr was translated here, Hahnemann's order was restored. The same has likewise been followed in Lippe's Text-Book.

Hahnemann's arrangement is also the basis of the following work. All the modalities, conditions and concomitants have been placed next to the function they belong to.

Hahnemann in his later editions finally placed the mental symptoms first; thus he adopted as a rule, first inner symptoms, then outer ones. This order we have now uniformly preserved throughout the whole work; functions of each organ are placed first, then the bodily symptoms. According to the same rule the symptoms of the whole body have been classified, as will be fully explained in the introduction to the arrangement.

Objections have been made, that too much is given. This may be the case for some. In the composition of a symphony like Beethoven's, there is much more given than can be understood by all, yet that does not detract from the merits of the work, but rather reflects against the intelligence of the reader. Yet our pages are not so restricted as the score to a symphony. Every beginner may learn from the most crowded pages some valuable fact; let him but rest his eyes and mind on the most distinguished remedies; after becoming acquainted with these, a farther survey will be quite readily made, till the whole will be at his command.

Objections have also been made, that, what is given is not enough. Here at once the pleading will be "*Guilty.*" Yet by extenuation we will say, every possible exertion has been made to get at least the most essential. During the last forty years, by preference, work has been bestowed on the Materia Medica. Much has been placed in the drug monographs; what was arranged could be used, but what yet remained in an unarranged condition, could not be at present made useful.

If the arduous labor bestowed for years upon this work should render efficient aid to all who are earnestly trying to heal the sick, if it should enable them to select in most cases, entrusted to their care, the proper drug, the author will be richly repaid for all his exertions. Yet, at the same time, he hopes that it will gradually lead some beginners into the right way of the true Hahnemannian school: *always to individualize.*

May it be one of the fruits of this work, that the detrimental and most unscientific alphabetical order shall be more and more abandoned, as it renders our researches not only very difficult, but also impedes and hinders all true study, all real progress. May it help to introduce, gradually, a uniform arrangement; may it lead to uniform terminology, especially with regard to the names of our drugs, and a uniform adoption of abridgements. As no one in such matters can presume to dictate, the majority must and will decide.

HOW TO USE THIS BOOK.

RULE I. Examine *as many cases as possible:* according to Hahnemann's advice, Organon, Paragraph 83, etc., that is:—
  a Let the patients or friends tell their own story, without interrupting them.
  b Write it down in separate symptoms.
  c Complete it by questions and observations with regard to every function.
  d Never ask a question which must be answered Yes or No. Consider yourself a tyro if you do it!
  e Inquire with regard to every single symptom, about place, time, kind of sensation, modalities, and connections.

This done, Hahnemann says, *the most important has been accomplished.*

RULE II. Arrange the symptoms according to their importance. The beginner should do this in writing; the more practiced by underlining or extracting; the sufficiently experienced and skillful may do it in his mind, as we do in mental calculations. Certain symptoms of a case may appear to have great importance, according to the opinion of the sufferer; this, however, should not be regarded in all cases. The physiological rank, according to the organs affected or the functions altered, is more worthy of consideration. It is very often in contradiction with the patient's view.

The pathological and therapeutical rank-order are of the greatest importance, but the last, we may say, is above all.

Every doctor is asked: What is the matter? Can it be cured? How long will it take? He is therefore under the necessity on this account, if for no other, to make not only a diagnosis, but also a prognosis. Easy as both are in most cases, just that uncertain are they in many others. The most learned are compelled to acknowledge the utter impossibility of arriving at a certainty.* Of these doubts and uncertainties we are freed, through the doctrines given us by Hahnemann.

And as regards the greater or lesser importance of the single symptoms, the tables have turned; what is of the highest importance in diagnosing, holds but a minor position in a diagnosis of the drug. Here we decide in all cases by symptoms, which in pathology are scarcely mentioned, nearly always being considered of not the slightest importance. Hence the Anti-Hahnemannians call them useless, or even foolishly term them "moonshine."

We have to bring the symptoms of the sick into an entirely new and generally different order. We must look for such distinguishing symptoms as mark this individual case from other cases of the same "disease" by name. Having thus searched out, we must then arrange them according to their importance, that we may look for a drug characterized by the same symptoms. If possible, we ought to find a drug having the symptoms of the case in the same order of rank.† The diagnostic symptoms, pathologically speaking, are very seldom symptoms diagnosticating between similar drugs; the symptoms less diagnostic, pathologically, being those which give the shades of difference between the many remedies having a general resemblance to the disease in question. We have only to add, as a rule for arranging the symptoms of the sick, that *ætiological peculiarities have always a very high rank* with us, even so far, that in most cases the last medicine employed, allopathically or homœopathically, forms the main indication for the next choice.

In all chronic and lingering cases, the symptoms appearing last, even though they may appear insignificant, are always the most important in regard to the selection of a drug; the oldest are the least important; all symptoms between have to be arranged according to the order of their appearance. *Only such patients remain well and are really cured, who have been rid of their symptoms in the reverse order of their development.*

* See Pamphlet against Organopathy, pp. 10, 11. Note by Raue.
† See Stapf's Archives, 1832, Vol. 11, No. 3, p. 92.

In all zymotic diseases we have, as in other epidemics, to sum up all the symptoms of as many cases as we can examine properly, and concentrate their symptoms into one image, from which to select that remedy really "specific" to the zymosis. Further, we have in all zymotic diseases, or contagious epidemics, an additional rule to bear in mind, viz., take the most characteristic symptoms at the invasion, at the height of the disease, and lastly during the decline of the disease; that is, during the recovery. These three points have to be "covered" by the characteristics of the drug. We may find in this way a preventive, "prophylactic," or a medicine, which, if it cannot prevent altogether, will make all cases lighter and more readily curable.

According to this rule, Sulphur was found to correspond better than any other medicine to Asiatic Cholera of 1849, and Carbo vegetabilis to Yellow Fever of 1855.

After deciding upon the leading symptoms of a case, three of which at least we ought to have (Lectures in Allentown, 1835), we can refer to such pages or chapters in this work as are devoted to them; there the concomitant conditions may be examined into, and the closest similarity with one or another drug may be confirmed. Next to this the pages, or chapter, with the pathological names nearest to the case, may be consulted. Very often the practitioner may find that he has omitted some questions, the answer to which he must, if possible, obtain, in order that he may complete his image of the sick.

The greater the number of drugs which are to be found under the same heading, the more ought the beginner to be convinced that he cannot select the medicine looked for out of so many by the similarity of such a symptom as is named in the heading. Not even if several peculiarities are known which, however, happen to have been produced by nearly all the drugs proven. For instance, *vertigo* does not indicate any medicine, even if it comes on while walking in the open air or with a tendency to fall, or with nausea and vomiting.

In all important cases the monographs should be consulted, and last though not least the "Materia Medica."

THE ARRANGEMENT.

Hahnemann published his order of arrangement first in his Materia Medica in 1811; improved it in 1822, and again in 1830. He observed the same in his Chronic Diseases as the main rule, but not without making several modifications, especially in the second edition of the anti-psoric remedies; the fifth part of which, published in 1839, is the last we have from him.

The same order has been observed as the main rule in the following work, making only such modifications as were necessary to render it consistent and uniform throughout. Such consistency in the whole, followed also in all the parts, enables the mind to find the way through the thickets of endless varying symptoms. Only the comprehension of general principles, ruling through the whole in every part, can make it possible to become well versed in and able to set one's self right anywhere.

Since, Hahnemann, in his second, 1835, edition of the Chronic Diseases, adopted what Hartlaub had already done in 1826, viz., to place the symptoms of the mind (and mood) before the head symptoms. Commencing with the mind, he adopted as a general principle, inner symptoms first, outer afterwards. He followed the same rule with the head, commencing with the inner symptoms,—the sensorial—the aches and pains, giving the symptoms of the outer head afterwards. But he could not find the time to carry out this order with all the other parts of the body, senses, etc. In this present work this has been done throughout; the functional symptoms always first, the organic afterwards.

With regard to the *functions* the order has been kept as strictly as possible, giving all symptoms with an increase of action first, next morbid alterations and last decrease or lessening of the functions.

From the very first, Hahnemann, according to his inductive philosophy and the strict method he always observed, commenced with the parts and followed them by the whole. The parts of the body, the organs and their functions, he arranged mainly from above downwards, commencing thus with the head and ending with the lower limbs; while observing this as the main rule, he, however, made another subdivision, and after the head and the senses, he went from the mouth down through all the organs, sustaining the individual, the nutritive organs; then the organs keeping up the species—sexual organs. After this, he began a second series from above downwards, viz., respiration, circulation and motion, organs of connection with the outer world; from the larynx to the lungs and heart; from the outer chest, neck and back, to the upper limbs, lower limbs and all the limbs. Thus far we follow Hahnemann; from here on the method of arrangement which Hahnemann inaugurated has been still farther developed; thus we have next the symptoms of the limbs and of the whole body. The influence of motion, rest, and of different positions. The next chapter contains all symptoms depending on the action of the nerves: over-excitement, convulsions, weakness, lameness. Sleep, the great restorer of the nerve force, is placed in the next part, where will also be found the symptoms before, during and after sleep. In this chapter the symptoms occurring during the night have been inserted. In the next chapter the symptoms are put which appear at the various times of the day.

All symptoms relating to heat and cold, in doors and out of doors, are placed in the next chapter, together with the influences of wind and weather. A new chapter contains all symptoms of chills, fever and sweat; what has been observed with regard to intermittent fever and other periodical diseases. This leads to a review of all periodical symptoms and then the relation to time and space naturally follows. A general idea of the different kinds of sensations is next given, because peculiar sensations indicate the effects upon particular tissues; the next chapter is taken up—even before Hausmann—with what we know in relation to tissues as regards their treatment.

As the skin, according to the rule from within outwards, is the last of the organs, the influence of touch and pressure is here inserted; also the effect of all other passive motions, concussions and hurts; a review of our surgical treatment is added in the same chapter.

Skin and eruptions would be the last, were it not for an important class of observations to be added in a chapter containing the result of observations with regard to age, sex, constitution, and so-called temperament. The chemical action of drugs—the antidotes; the relation to other drugs; the rules by which to be guided to the best order in which drugs should follow each other, conclude the work.

After having considered all this, the reader will find no difficulty in comprehending our arrangement, keeping in mind the main rules:

I. Inner symptoms and functions first, outer and organic changes afterwards.

II. First increased functional activity, then altered, then decreased.

III. First the parts, then the whole body.

IV. First the upper parts, then the lower.

V. All modalities placed to the related function.

In a few instances some deviations from the main rules have been made, just as was done by Hahnemann (Arzml I., pp. 8, 9, 3d edition) in case of symptoms which might be looked for in connection or combination with others, or where they form a kind of transition.

Symptoms are arranged according to the organ or part of the body in which they appear, not where they originate; for instance, motions or positions of the head are placed to the outer head, not to the neck, the muscles of which cause the position or motion.

The use of the book, particularly the first chapter, will accomplish the rest.

According to the principles and rules laid down in the foregoing, the symptoms, their groups, and the names of diseases, have been arranged and divided in forty-eight parts.

Each part will have at the beginning a key to the special order if necessary, and an index at the end if it is considered an advantage to the reader.

THE FORTY-EIGHT CHAPTERS.

I. MIND AND DISPOSITION.

A collection and arrangement of all the symptoms observed by our school. as regards the mind and the disposition, was made nearly a score of years ago by Dr. C. G. RAUE, who, being now engaged with his forthcoming Psychology, cannot complete it at present, by adding all the later observations.

Dr. E. W. Berridge says, p. xiii. in the Preface to his Complete Repertory, Diseases of the Eyes, 1873: "The volume on the Head (second edition), *including the mental group*, is being prepared," and will, we hope, soon appear. In the meantime, the place may be filled by an entirely new collection of all the mind symptoms, appearing under certain conditions or as concomitants with bodily symptoms.

Practitioners will find this chapter of great use, and at the same time it will make every student familiar with the plan of the arrangement.

II. SENSORIUM.

Oversensitiveness and irritability of the brain and senses, noises, apparent motions or movements; other unpainful sensations.
Vertigo with all its concomitants and conditions.
Dullness, heaviness, cloudiness, apathetic state, unconsciousness.
Fainting spells.
Asphyxia.

III. HEADACHE AND AFFECTIONS OF THE INNER HEAD.

According to locality, intensity and periodicity—kinds of sensation according to the arrangement adopted in part 43.
Conditions and concomitants of headache.
Affections of inner tissues, cold and heat, inflammation and other organic changes in brain diseases.

IV. EXTERNAL HEAD.

Sensations according to locality.
Cold, heat, sweat.
Skull, bones, periosteum.
Movements and positions of head and concomitants.
Scalp, hair, eruptions.

V. SIGHT AND EYES.

Perception increased, as morbid desire for light; also shunning light and symptoms caused by light.
Perverted—in regard to light, colors, size, form, etc.
Decreased—from dimness to blindness.
Symptoms after using the eyes.
Modalities in general.

Eyeball, consisting of nervous apparatus, viz., optic nerve, retina, together with the vitreous body and lens.
Vascular apparatus and fluids, together with the choroid and iris.
Fibrous part, viz., sclerotica, together with the cornea.
Next to the main function, viz., sight, we have that of nutrition— this may be either increased, congestion to inflammation, perverted, as in hypertrophy and malformation, or decreased, as in atrophy or destructive ulceration.

We then have the supporting parts surrounding the eye, viz., bones, muscles and fat. Their united function being *motion and position;* this may be either increased, perverted or decreased.
In close proximity to the supporting parts we have the lubricating apparatus, consisting of the lachrymal glands and ducts, together with the mucous membrane and conjunctiva. The united function is to sustain the proper relation of moisture and temperature between the inner and outer parts; this may also be increased, perverted or decreased.

External protectors: Lids with the meibomian glands, lashes and eyebrows.
Symptoms caused by touch or pressure; hurts and lesions; other symptoms around the eyes.
Appearances or expressions of the Eyes have been placed to the Face, Chapter 8.

VI. HEARING AND EARS.

HEARING.—Increased sense of hearing—as acute sensitiveness to sounds, etc.
Perverted—subjective noises, etc.
Decreased—dullness to deafness.
INNER EAR.—Unpainful sensations—numbness to itching.
Earache; kind of pain with regard to space and time.
Connections, conditions and concomitants.
Otitis.   Tympanitis.   Concomitants.
Cerumen.   Otorrhœa.
Eustachian tube.
Polypi, fungi, etc.   Caries.   Ulcers, etc.
EXTERNAL EAR.—Meatus and orifice.
Concha, tragus and anti-tragus; helix and anti-helix; dorsum.
The whole ear; auricle, earlobe.
Around the ear—in front, behind, above, below.
Parotids.
Review of the conditions and concomitants.

VII. SMELL AND NOSE.

SMELL.—Increased sense of smell; dislike to particular odors; aggravation from certain odors.
Perverted sense of smell
Decreased, lost.
INNER NOSE.—Unpainful sensations—from want of feeling to itching; painful sensations.
Bones of the nose.
Epistaxis—conditions and concomitants.
Sensation of dryness; dryness.
NASAL SPEECH AND SOUNDS FROM THE NOSE WHEN BREATHING.
Sneezing—conditions and concomitants.
Coryza dry, fluent, obstruction—conditions and concomitants.
Soreness, eruptions, ulcerations, scabs.
Ozœna.   Polypus.
Choanæ.
OUTER NOSE.—Pains; locality; root, wings, angles, tip.

Motions of the alæ.
Coldness, heat, sweat.
Color—pale, red, blue, etc.
Itching eruptions—cancer.
Around the nose.
Recapitulation of localities and modalities.

VIII. FACE.

EXPRESSION OF EYES AND COUNTENANCE.—Unpainful sensations.
Faceache, conditions and concomitants.
Muscular conditions.
Expression and appearance; complexion.
Cold, hot, pale, red, blue, etc.; sweat.
Puffed, swollen, itching; eruptions, ulcers, etc.
ARTICULATION OF THE JAWS.—Lockjaw; cracking, relaxation, luxation.

IX. LOWER PART OF FACE.

LOWER JAW.—Sensations, pains, bones.
OUTER MOUTH.—Lips, upper; lower; angles of the mouth; around the mouth.
Pains, motions, warmth, color, eruption.
CHIN.
SUBMAXILLARY GLANDS.

X. TEETH AND GUMS.

TEETH.—Incisors, canines, bicuspids, molars; upper, lower; carious teeth.
SENSATIONS AND PAINS.—Toothache; appearance and conditions of the teeth.
DENTITION.—First, second; wisdom teeth.
GUMS.—Sensations, pains, color, bleeding, scurvy, ulcers, fistula, conditions and concomitants.

XI. TASTE, TALK, TONGUE.

TASTE.—Sense of taste increased, perverted, decreased.
TALK.—Mobility of the tongue increased, perverted, decreased.
TONGUE.—Sensations, pains, organic changes, furred, eruptions.
Ranula, sublingual glands.

XII. INNER MOUTH.

SENSATIONS, pains, dryness, humidity.
SALIVA; mucus.
ODOR, perceived by the sick, or only by others.
COLOR; eruptions, etc.
Conditions and concomitants.

XIII. PALATE AND THROAT.

HARD PALATE, soft palate, velum palate; uvula; tonsils; fauces; pharynx.
SWALLOWING.
Condition and concomitants.
ŒSOPHAGUS.—Sensations and pains.
Inflammation, ulcerations, and other diseased states.

XIV. DESIRE FOR FOOD AND DRINK.

APPETITE.—Increased; canine hunger.
Dainty; capricious, etc.
Perverted; decreased; lost. Conditions and concomitants.
THIRST.—Increased; changed or perverted; decreased.
Conditions and concomitants.
DESIRES, or longing for peculiar things.
DISLIKES, or aversion to peculiar things.

XV. BEFORE—DURING—AFTER EATING AND DRINKING.

PECULIAR THINGS agree or ameliorate, disagree or aggravate. Complaints caused by them.
Comparative tables with former. Index to both.
SYMPTOMS appearing shortly before eating or drinking; during the act, or sooner or later after it.

XVI. GASTRIC SYMPTOMS.

HICCOUGH.
ERUCTATIONS, or belching; heartburn; waterbrash; regurgitation, gulping up.
LOATHING—nausea, gagging, vomituritio, vomiting.
Conditions and ameliorations, aggravations and concomitants.

XVII. EPIGASTRIC REGION.

SENSATIONS in scrobiculum and in region of stomach; pains, swellings, etc.
INFLAMMATIONS and other organic diseases.
External symptoms and appearance of infra-xiphoid regions.

XVIII. HYPOCHONDRIAC REGIONS.

SYMPTOMS of the diaphragm.
REGION OF LIVER.—Sensations, pains, diseases.
REGION OF SPLEEN.—Sensations, pains, diseases.
BOTH HYPOCHONDRIA.—Sensations, pains, diseases.
EXTERNAL SYMPTOMS.—Appearance; itching; eruptions.

XIX. ABDOMEN.

UMBILICAL and lumbar regions.
HYPOGASTRIC and inguinal regions.
SENSATIONS AND PAINS.
COLDNESS, heat, inflammation, and other conditions.
NOISES, flatulence, distention, swelling, glandular swelling, dropsy, tumors.
OUTER WALL; muscular motions, itching, eruptions.
LOINS; groins, hernia, boils.

XX. RECTUM AND ANUS.

EMISSIONS OF WIND.
STOOLS—too loose, and corresponding states.
STOOLS—color, odor, substance.
STOOLS—looseness and costiveness in alternation.
STOOLS—constipation.
Complaints before, during and after stool.
RECTUM.—Urging, tenesmus, pains, dysentery, involuntary discharges.
Prolapsus of the rectum; hæmorrhoids.
ANUS. Perinæum.

Connected anal and urinary symptoms.

XXI. URINARY ORGANS.

KIDNEYS AND URETERS.—Sensations, pains, diseases.
BLADDER.—Sensations, pains, diseases.
URETHRA.—Compare sexual parts.
DESIRE TO URINATE; urging.
DISCHARGE OF URINE; copious, frequent, scanty, seldom.
Stream according to form.
Passage free, interrupted; by drops; involuntary.
RETENTION OF URINE.—No secretion of urine.
Complaints before, during and after urination.
Urine according to quality; sediment.
Diabetes mellitus. Hæmaturia. Albuminuria.
GRAVEL.—Calculi in the kidneys; ureters; bladder.

XXII. MALE FUNCTIONS AND ORGANS.

SEXUAL DESIRE—conditions and concomitants.
Sexual power—erections, impotence.
COITION.—Seminal emissions; before, during and after coition.
Complaints after sexual excess; after masturbation.
Involuntary seminal emissions.
TESTICLES.—Spermatic cords.
Prostate glands and discharge of prostatic fluid.
PENIS.—Glans; prepuce.
SCROTUM.—Sensations, cold, heat, sweat; dropsy; eruptions.
All the male genitals.
Diseases, principally of the genital parts: Orchitis; hydrocele; chronic swelling; prostatitis; strictures; blennorrhœa; gonorrhœa; sycosis; syphilis; chancre; buboes.
Bone diseases.
Mercurial diseases.

XXIII. FEMALE ORGANS.

Increased desire; nymphomania; inability; sterility; complaints during or after coition.
OVARIES, uterus; sensations, position.

CATAMENIA sooner than four weeks, at irregular times; later than four weeks; increased, suppressed, too profuse, altered, decreased, scanty, protracted, longer than half a week, too short, less than three days, symptoms appearing instead of the menses. *Complaints before, at the beginning, during and after menses.*

Menses appear too early in life; delay of the first catamenia; sufferings with the development; menses continue too late in life; too early cessation.

Symptoms with the climaxis.

UTERINE HÆMORRHAGES; metrorrhagia. See Menorrhagia or Parturition.

CHARACTER OF CATAMENIA.—Bright red, light color, clotted, brown, dark; acrid, offensive smelling, viscid, membranous.

LEUCORRHŒA.—Watery, milky, mucous, viscid, thick, purulent, mild, itching, acrid, burning; yellow, red, bloody, brown, green; offensive smelling.

Complaints before, during and after leucorrhœa. Conditions and concomitants.

VAGINA.—Labia minora, labia majora, clitoris.

GENITALS PROPER.—Pubes, mons veneris, outer parts, around the organs.

XXIV. PREGNANCY AND PARTURITION.

COMPLAINTS AFTER CONCEPTION AND DURING PREGNANCY.—The first term, middle term and last month.

Abortion.—Moles.

LABOR PAINS.—Forerunners; pains too severe; spasmodic; ineffectual; too weak; cessation of pains; afterbirth; afterpains.

COMPLAINTS IN CHILDBED.

Lochia—abundant, bloody, putrid, cessation of them.

COMPLAINTS WHILE NURSING.

The milk is increased, running, bad, decreased, suppressed.

MAMMÆ.—Sore nipples, tumors, abscesses, scars, scirrhosities and cancer.

Infants at the breast.

XXV. LARYNX.

Voice.—Hoarseness; aphonia; complaints from singing; weakness of voice.

Complaints from talking; loud reading.

Catarrh.—Sensations, pains; roughness.

Collection of mucus; hemming and hawking; hacking cough.

THROATPIT, or supra sternal region; sensitiveness to touch.

LARYNGITIS.—Laryngismus stridulus; œdema glottidis; spasm of the glottis; croup; paralysis of vocal cords. Ulcers: catarrhal, diphtheritic, tubercular, variolar, typhoid, syphilitic and carcinomatous; tuberculosis, perichondritis, stenosis; new growths; papilloma; polypi; cancers.

TRACHEA AND BRONCHIAL TUBES.—Sensations, pains, secretions, inflammation.

Thyroid Gland.—Supraclavicular region and external throat.

XXVI. RESPIRATION.

Rythm and character. Conditions and concomitants. Also the constriction and spasms interfering with breathing.

NOTE.—The different respiratory actions with their connections have been placed in the following chapters: Weeping, to that of the mind, 1, or eyes, 5. Sneezing and blowing the nose, 7. Speaking to the tongue, 11. Gurgling to the throat, 13. Hiccough to gastrics, 16. Hemming, reading loud, public speaking and singing to the larynx, 25. Laughing, sighing and sobbing to this chapter, 26. Coughing to the next, 27; and gaping to sleep, 37.

XXVII. COUGH.

Location of exciting cause to cough; character of cough.

Conditions and concomitants.

Complaints before, during and after cough.

Diseases in which the cough is the most prominent symptom.

XXVIII. INNER CHEST AND LUNGS.

Upper part, lower part, right, left, front and back portions.

Painless sensations—tightness; constriction; spasms   See Chapt. 26.

Painful sensations, as drawing, tearing, stitching.

Cold, warmth, heat; congestion; throbbing, beating; œdema; suppuration; pleuritis.

Inflammation; hydrothorax; pneumonia; pneumothorax; atelectasis.
Emphysema; compression; induration; collapse.
Empyema; gangrene.
Hæmorrhage; tuberculisation; cancer; melanic deposit.

XXIX. HEART AND CIRCULATION.

Sensations and pains in the region of the heart.
Congestion.
PALPITATION OF HEART.—Basedow's disease.
Perverted action; cardiac tremor.
Angina pectoris; endocarditis; myocarditis; fatty degeneration; hypertrophy; dilatation; atrophy; pericarditis; hydropericardium; pneumopericardium; cardiac asthma; valvular changes; aneurism.
PULSE.—Increase; alteration; cessation.
Endarteritis; atheroma.

XXX. OUTER CHEST.

Pit of throat. See Larynx, Chapter 25.
CLAVICLES.—Sternum; ensiform or xiphoid cartilage.
SENSATIONS, pains; cold, heat; eruptions.
Mammæ. See Chapter 24.

XXXI. NECK AND BACK.

Supraclavicular region and thyroid gland. See Chapt. 25.
Position of head. See Chapt. 4.
NAPE OF NECK, back of the neck; ligamentum nuchæ.
Sensations, pains; stiffness; complaints on turning the neck.
GLANDS OF THE NECK AND SIDES OF THROAT.
Scapulæ. See Arms, Chapt. 32.
REGION BETWEEN THE SHOULDERS.
BACK.—Region of kidneys. See Chapt. 21.
LOINS.—Lumbar regions. Comp. Chapt. 19.
SACRUM.—Small of back; sacral region.
OS COCCYGIS.
SPINAL DISEASES.—Tabes dorsalis; curvatures.

XXXII. UPPER LIMBS.

Scapula, shoulders, shoulder-joint; axilla.

UPPER ARM.—Elbow-joint, point of elbow, bend of elbow, forearm, wrist, hand, back of hand; metacarpal region; palm of hand, thumbs, joints, fingers; between the fingers, the tips, nails.

THE WHOLE ARM.—Bones of upper limbs and arm-joints.

Worse retracting shoulders, better bending them backwards.

Worse moving Arms; worse working with the hands, sewing, knitting, etc.

ERUPTIONS.—Tetters; warts.

XXXIII. LOWER LIMBS.

HIP-JOINTS, buttocks, nates. Comp. lumbar region.

THIGHS.—Front; back, inner side, outer side.

KNEE-JOINTS.—Patella, hollow of the knee.

LEGS.—Tibia, fibula, calves.

TENDO ACHILLIS.—Heel, ankle, joint of foot, dorsum of the foot, instep, foot soles.

TOES.—Big toe, toe-joints, balls of toes, toe tips, toe nails; corns.

THE BONES.—The joints; the whole of lower limbs.

XXXIV. ALL THE LIMBS.

Upper and lower; arms and legs; hands and feet. Comparison.

Sensation of lightness; stretching, bending and stretching.

Twisting, etc. See Chapt. 36.

Pains compared. Rheumatic and gouty pains.

Contortion.—Limbs drawn crooked.

Joints.—Stiffness; lameness; paralysis.

Coldness.—Upper, lower; hands and feet; heat; sweat.

Parched state of palms of hands and soles of feet.

Itchings. Eruptions. Comp. Chapt. 47.

XXXV. REST—POSITION—MOTION.

REST.—While at rest, complaints appear or are aggravated, lessened or disappear.

Inclination to lie down.

On lying down; after assuming the lying posture; while in a lying posture; while lying in bed. See Chapt. 37.

Worse or better from certain positions while lying, as head high or low, body horizontal, bent or crooked; on back, sides, painful and unpainful; on the belly. Position in sleep. See Chapt. 37. Right or left. See Chapt. 42.

Worse or better lying on a hard place. Comp. Chapt. 45.

Worse from an uncomfortable position in lying; from leaning on or toward one side or backwards, etc.; from crossing the legs; letting the legs hang down; from holding the part bent; while couching, kneeling, etc.

Inclination to sit down.

On—after—while assuming the sitting posture.

Position as upright, erect, bent, stooped.

On rising from a seat; after, etc. When rising from lying to sitting; on rising from bed; after rising from bed.

From stretching out a limb; from stretching and bending.

While standing, bending backwards, forwards, stooping a long while, doubling up the body; continued flexion.

MOTIONS.—Bending forwards, backwards, inwards, outwards, right, left, sideways.

Stretching the limb, drawing it towards the body, then retraction of the affected limb.

Worse while taking off the boots.

From lifting the arm; the affected limbs; raising a limb; from overlifting.

While bending or turning a part; the affected part.

From changing position, turning around, or when turning in bed.

WALKING.—On starting to walk; while walking; when walking quickly; walking on level ground; from stepping sideways.

From running, dancing, leaping.

Ascending.—A height; from mounting a horse; going up stairs.

From descending; going down stairs.

MOTION.—Desire to move; on beginning to move; during motion; from continued motion; after moving; from motion of the affected part; from a false movement; from exertion of the body; from fatigue.

Taking hold of things; turning at a lathe; playing instruments and other handiwork. See Upper Limbs.

XXXVI. NERVES.

Comfortable feeling; sensation of vigor; bodily irritability too great; excitement; mobility too great; bodily restlessness; sensation of inward trembling; sensation of anxiousness in the body.

HYPOCHONDRIA AND HYSTERIA.

TREMBLING—Startings, jerkings, spasms, chorea, epilepsy, tetanus, catalepsy.

Attacks of indisposition, malaise, nervous weakness, sensation of fatigue, lassitude of body, weakness, difficulty in supporting the body, tendency to fall.

Paralytic weakness.—Want of bodily irritability; single parts "go to sleep;" motion difficult; immobility of affected parts; lameness; paralysis.

XXXVII. SLEEP.

SLEEPINESS.—In the morning, forenoon, during the day, afternoon, evening. Gaping; desire for sleep and other concomitants.

Drowsiness, with inability to fall asleep.

SLEEPLESSNESS.—Before or after midnight; complaints causing it.

Complaints from sleeplessness; loss of sleep; night watching; complaints from night revelling.

SLEEP.—Anxious, restless; sound, deep, sonorous; too long in the morning; somnolency; coma; coma vigil.

POSITION IN SLEEP.—Head bent forward, turned sideways, bent backwards; low.

Hands above head, under the head, on the abdomen, lying on the back, on one side, on the belly, legs stretched, drawn up, one flexed, the other extended, crossed knees, spread apart, bent. Sitting posture.

CONCOMITANTS.—Complaints before falling asleep; on falling asleep; during the first sleep; during sleep.

Better while slumbering; while half asleep; during sleep; after sleep.

Falling asleep late; inability to get asleep; to get asleep again after being awakened; complaints preventing sleep; frequent waking during the night.

Sleep too short; awaking too early; too long; awaking too late.

Refreshing and unrefreshing sleep; worn after sleep; after a long sleep; after a siesta; complaints on awakening.

DREAMS.

XXXVIII. TIMES OF THE DAY.

Night. See Chapt. 37.

TABLE OF THE HOURS OF THE NIGHT.

MORNING.—Towards it; after sunrise; morning hours; forenoon.

NOON.

All day. Table of the hours of the day.

AFTERNOON.—After sunset; in the evening twilight.

EVENING.—Before midnight; after midnight.

Aggravations; remissions and comparisons.

XXXIX. RELATIONS TO WARMTH, AIR AND WATER; WIND AND WEATHER; SEASONS.

WARMTH.—Better or worse from it; from heat in the sun; sunburn; sunstroke.

From getting warm, overheated, near the fire, the warm stove. Burns, see Lesions, Chapt. 45.

From being covered, wrapped up warmly; getting warm in bed; in featherbeds.

Warm air; getting warm in the open air, in a warm room.

AIR.—Open air, out doors; walking in the open air; inclination, aversion to it.

Indoors, in a room, in a room full of people; in arched places, cellar-rooms; damp air, evening air.

WIND.—From uncovering; after undressing the whole body or part of it; the head.

Walking in the wind; against the wind; from a draught.

N.B.—North wind or polar wind in Rio Janeiro the south wind or cold wind; south wind or tropic wind in Brazil the north wind or warm wind. East wind in Europe the land wind; here the sea wind, or damp wind. West wind in Europe the sea wind; here the land wind or dry wind.

WATER.—From water and washing; wetting the affected part; wet dressing.
Getting wet through; while sweating; getting head wet; feet.
Aversion to washing; worse or better from washing; from washing the face; bathing face.
Complaints from bathing; in cold water; in the sea.
COLD.—Disposition to catch cold; after exposure to cold, of the head, of the feet.
In the cold; going into cold air; in cold air; cold or dry air; getting cold, chilled through single parts; taking hold of cold things.
Frostbitten parts, see Lesions, Chapt. 45.
CHANGE OF TEMPERATURE; of weather.
Weather calm, clear; dry; windy; before or during a thunderstorm; in snowy air; in foggy weather; cloudy; damp; wet.
SEASONS.—In the spring; in the summer; in autumn; in winter.

XL. FEVER.

COLD SENSATIONS.—Coldness, crawl, shiver, shudder.
Chill and rigor comparably arranged; sweat same way.
HEAT.—Sweat relieving; checked sweat; dry skin.
COLD SWEAT, or sweat in stages compared.
Combinations and successions.
CONDITIONS AND CONCOMITANTS.—Before, with and after the fever stages.
REMITTENT.—Intermittent from *quotidian* to *quartan;* postponing; anticipating.
Typhoid; nervous; putrid. Comatose and sweating sickness.
Yellow fever. Plague, etc.

XLI. CHANGES ACCORDING TO TIME.

In attacks periodically; in groups.
Intermitting in severity.
Appearing quickly and vanishing quickly.
Appearing quickly and decreasing slowly.
Increasing slowly and decreasing quickly.

Increasing slowly and decreasing slowly.
Alternating same hours or days. Different groups of symptoms.
Interstitial.—Interrupted spells; returning again; new symptoms arising when earlier ones cease.
Every day at the same hour.
Every day about the same time; earlier, (*Hydrog.*); later, (*Oxyg.*).
Every other day.
Every week. Septimani. Every two weeks. Every four weeks.
Every two or three months.
Every new moon; increase; full; decrease.
Every year at the same time, same day, same season.

XLII. RELATIONS TO SPACE—CHANGES ACCORDING TO SPACE.

MOVING.—From in out; from out in.
From up down, descending; from down up, ascending.
From right to left; from left to right.
From front to back; from back to front; oblique.
Changing place, by shifting about. Metastasis.
STANDING.—Inner organs, internal parts. Outer organs, external parts.
Anterior body. Posterior body.
On the right side; left side; one sided.
Upper right and lower left. Upper left and lower right.
Upper half, upper body; lower half, lower body.
PECULIAR PARTS OR PLACES.—Angles or corners of eyes, nose, mouth, etc.; points or tips of ears, nose, etc.; crossings of tubular organs; angles of tubular organs.

XLIII. SENSATIONS CLASSIFIED.

Explanation of the arrangement into seven classes.—The different expression in each class.—Index.—Conditions and concomitants.

That all the different sensations may be brought into a comprehensible order, the general rule for functions may be applied; as all abnormal sensations are the result of some one or more functions developed, either into greater activity, or depressed and rendered less active, or perverted, that is to say, changed from the normal action, not only in quantity and quality, but also in kind.

THE ARRANGEMENT. 45

The morbid increase or exaggeration of functional activity, forms our *first* class; its opposite decreased functional activity, the *seventh* (our last) class. The large number of sensations remaining between these two extremes we again subdivide, separating all such as are fixed as regards place, *i. e.*, without motion, *second* class, from those which are apparently moving. Again, from among those sensations which convey to the mind some more or less clear idea of motion, we separate all such in which the perception is as of a destructive action, or in other words, sensations as if the integrity of the tissues would be, or had been imperiously affected; these form the *sixth* class.

The remaining sensations apparently moving, are subdivided into three classes: a, steady motions *third* class; β, such as have a relation to *space*, *i. e.*, have motion inward, outward, upward, or downward *fourth* class; γ, such as have a relation to time, *i. e.*, where distinct repetitions, either pulsating, wavering or oscillating, are perceived, these form the *fifth* class. The subjoined schema will give a clear idea of the classes:

```
A ⎡   Increased, exaggerated activity.                                       1
  ⎢ a ⎡ Fixed, i. e. without motion.                                         2
  ⎢   ⎢         ⎡ a. Steady motion.                                          3
B ⎨ b ⎨ Moving  ⎨ β. Steady motion in relation to space.                     4
  ⎢   ⎣         ⎣ γ. Pulsating, wavering, oscillating motions.               5
  ⎢ c ⎣ Destructive action, as if the integrity of the tissues was disturbed. 6
C ⎣   Decreased activity.                                                    7
```

1.—INCREASED, EXAGGERATED ACTIVITY.

Comfortable feeling; feeling of ease.
Feeling of lightness; sense of being lifted up, floating, flying.
Mobility too great; pliant; flexibility.
Dexterity; inclined to dance.
Nervous excitement; fidgety; beside himself.
Irritability too great; susceptibility; sensitiveness.
Cannot bear the pressure of clothing; aching all over.

2.—FIXED, *i. e.*, WITHOUT MOTION.

Sensation as of a foreign body, like dust, in inner parts; spiderwebs (cobwebs); as from a hair, a thread, a loose piece of skin, of a lid, of a valve, a lump, a ball, a plug, a wedge.

Sensation of obstruction, fullness, bloatedness, swelling, tightness, pressure, like a band as from an iron clamp, a load, (inner or outer parts), as if inner parts were grown together; roughness.

Sensation as if becoming larger, of being larger; becoming smaller, being smaller; of emptiness, hollowness, as if parts became dilated, expanded; as if covered with fur.

Other illusions of feeling.

3.—STEADY MOTION.

Sensation as of wind blowing; blowing upon a part; sensation like cold or hot streams; running in limbs, like a mouse; sensation as of something living; sensation like a spring; sensation of being lifted up, of rising up.

Tension; tenseness.

Pecking, picking; pinching; nipping, clawing; squeezing, grasping; griping, cramping pain, cramp-like.

Twitching, jerking, starting.

Urging, forcing, thronging.

Straining, like tenesmus.

Bearing down; forcing; labor-like.

Drawing, dragging, tugging, as if pulled (by the hair, etc.).

Cutting, lancinating, chopping.

Tearing, rending.

Stitching, shooting.

4.—MOTION IN RELATION TO THE DIMENSIONS OF THE BODY.

In, out; pressure; boring; stitching; tearing; torn out.

Out, in; pressure; contracting.

Pressing together; twisting; contracting; screwing; pinching.

Pressing asunder; expansive; bursting; thronging; rending.

Upward, downward, as of something drawn down; moving crossways.

Real motions changing in space. See Chapt. 42.
Affection of inner or outer organs. See Chapt. 44.

5.—SENSATIONS WITH A PULSATING, WAVERING, OSCILLATING MOTION.

Quivering, trembling, shaking, crepitating, crackling, cracking, buzzing, humming, whirring, droning, vibrating, turning, twisting, writhing, wringing, whirling, rolling.

Pulsating, beating, knocking, hammering, blows, shocks.

Bubbling, gurgling, fluctuation, undulating, wave-like; water striking against, etc.; motion; moving up and down.

Penetrating, boring, digging, rooting.

Titillation, formication, creeping, crawling, tickling, tingling, as if "asleep."

Itching, prickling, pungent feeling, gnawing, scraping, scratching.

6.—SENSATIONS AS IF THE INTEGRITY OF THE TISSUES WAS DISTURBED. DESTRUCTIVE ACTION.

Sensation as from lying on a hard place; from a painful pressure; suggillation; contusion; from a concussion; as if broken; as from spraining; as if torn; as of rending, torn asunder.

Pain as if ulcerated; from subcutaneous ulceration; from internal festering; as if sore, raw, chapped; as of skin peeling off, smarting.

Gnawing, corrosive, corroding; burning; as from being burned; as from a hot iron running through.

7.—SENSATIONS OF DECREASED ACTIVITY.

Debility, weakness, lassitude, fatigue.

Laxness of body or joints (not of bowels); difficulty in supporting the body; weakness, as if lame; sensation in parts, as if paralyzed; inclination to lie down; aversion to exertion or work; motion more difficult; stiffness of limbs; inflexibility of body; immobility; sensation as if parts were grown together.

As if too heavy in parts or whole body; unwieldiness of the body.

Pains dull, obtuse, paralytic, benumbing.

Sensation of emptiness, hollowness.

Sensation as if being drawn downwards; as of falling down in inner parts; as if inner parts were falling out.

Numbness, (as if "asleep"). See also Tingling.

Torpid feeling; insensibility; unpainfulness; sensation as if wooden: as if covered with fur.

Sensation of dryness.

Sensation of softness of hard parts.

Uncomfortable feeling, or sensation of discomfort; sensation of illness.

Sensation of exhaustion; of fainting.

INDEX TO CHAPTER FORTY-THREE—SENSATIONS.

a, above or upper part of page; b, below; c, centre.

Class 1 is on p. 45 b; Class 2, pp. 45 b, and 46 a; Class 3, p. 46 a, c; Class 4, p. 46 c, b; Class 5, pp. 46 b, and 47 a; Class 6, p. 47 c; Class 7, p. 47 b.

Aching all over,	1 b	Crawling,	5 a
Aching in parts. See pressure.		Creeping,	5 a
Activity,	1 b	Crepitating,	5 b
Asleep, as if (tingling),	5 a	Crossways,	4 b
" " (numb),	7 b	Cutting,	3 c
Asunder, pressing,	4 b	Dancing, inclined to,	1 b
Aversion to exertion or work,	7 b	Debility,	7 b
Ball, as from a,	2 b	Destructive action,	6 a
Band around, like a,	2 a	Dexterity,	1 b
Bearing down,	3 c	Difficult motion,	7 b
Beating,	5 b	Difficulty in supporting body,	7 b
Becoming larger, as if,	2 a	Digging,	5 a
Becoming smaller, as if,	2 a	Discomfort, sensation of,	7 b
Benumbing pains,	7 b	Disturbed, as if parts became,	2 a
Beside himself,	1 b	Downward motion,	4 b
Bloatedness,	2 a	Drawing,	3 c
Blowing upon a part,	3 c	Drawn down, as if,	4 b
Blows,	5 b	Drawn downward, sensation,	7 b
Boring—in, out,	4 b	Droning,	5 b
Boring, penetrating,	5 a	Dryness, sensation of,	7 b
Broken, as if,	6 c	Dull pains,	7 b
Bubbling,	5 a	Dust in inner parts,	2 b
Burned, as from being,	6 c	Easy feeling,	1 b
Burning,	6 c	Emptiness, sensation of,	2 a
Bursting,	4 b	Emptiness, hollow,	7 b
Buzzing,	5 b	Exaggerated activity,	1 b
Cannot bear pressure of clothing,	1 b	Exertion, aversion to,	7 b
Chapped, as if,	6 c	Excitement, nervous,	1 b
Chapping,	3 c	Exhaustion,	7 b
Clamp, as from an iron,	2 a	Expanding, as if,	2 a
Clawing,	3 c	Expansive, pressing,	4 b
Clothing pressure, cannot bear it,	1 b	Fainting, sensation of,	7 b
Cobweb, as from a,	2 b	Falling down in inner parts,	7 b
Cold streams,	3 c	Falling out, as if inner parts,	7 b
Comfortable,	1 b	Fatigue,	7 b
Concussion, from a,	6 c	Feeling comfortable,	1 b
Contracting,	4 b	Feeling of ease,	1 b
Contusion,	6 c	Feelings, illusions of,	2 a
Corroding, corrosive,	6 c	Feelings of lightness,	1 b
Covered with tar, as if,	2 a, 7 b	Festering, internal, as from,	6 c
Cracking,	5 b	Fidgety,	1 b
Crackling,	5 b	Fixed sensations,	2 b
Cramping, cramp-like,	3 c	Flexibility,	1 b

THE ARRANGEMENT. 49

Floating,	1 b	Lying, on a hard place, as from,	6 c
Fluctuation,	5 a	Mobility too great,	1 b
Flying,	1 b	Motion in relation to dimensions	
Forcing,	3 c	of the body,	4 b
Foreign body,	2 b	Motion, up and down,	5 a
Formication,	5 a	Motion more difficult,	7 b
Fullness, sensation of,	2 a	Mouse, running like it,	3 c
Fur, as if covered with,	2 a, 7 b	Nervous excitement,	1 b
Gnawing,	5 a, 6 c	Nipping,	3 c
Grasping,	3 c	Numbness,	7 b
Griping,	3 c	Obstruction, sensation of,	2 a
Grown together, as if,	2 a	Obtuse pain,	7 b
" " parts, as if,	7 b	Oscillating,	5 b
Gurgling,	5 a	Out—in,	4 b
Hair, as from a,	2 b	Paralytic pains,	7 b
Hair, as if pulled by,	3 c	Paralysed sensation in parts,	7 b
Hammering,	5 b	Parts as if grown together,	7 b
Hard place, as from lying on a,	6 c	Pecking,	3 c
Heavy, as if too, parts or whole,	7 b	Peeling off, as of skin,	6 c
Hollowness, sensation of,	2 a, 7 b	Penetrating, boring,	5 a
Hot iron running through, as if a,	6 c	Picking,	3 c
Hot streams,	3 c	Piece of skin, loose, as if,	2 b
Humming,	5 b	Pinching (steady pinch),	3 c
Illness, sensation of,	7 b	Pinching together,	4 b
Illusions of feeling,	2 a	Pliant,	1 b
Immobility,	7 b	Plug, as from a,	2 b
Inclination to lie down,	7 b	Pressing asunder,	4 b
Inclined to dance,	1 b	Pressing together,	4 b
Increased activity,	1 b	Pressure,	2 a
Inflexibility of body,	7 b	Pressure in out or out in,	4 b
In or out,	4 b	Pressure of clothing unbearable,	1 b
Inner parts, as if grown together,	2 a, 7 b	Pressure, as if from a painful,	6 c
Insensibility,	7 b	Prickling,	5 a
Integrity disturbed,	6 a	Pulled, as if,	3 c
Iron clamp, as from a,	2 a	Pulsating,	5 b
Irritability too great,	1 b	Pulsations,	5 a
Itching,	5 a	Pungent feeling,	5 a
Jerking,	3 c	Quivering,	5 b
Knocking,	5 b	Raw, as if,	6 c
Labor-like,	3 c	Rending,	3 c
Lancinating,	3 c	Rending asunder,	4 b, 6 c
Large, as if being,	2 a	Rising up, sensation of,	3 c
Larger, as if becoming,	2 a	Rolling,	5 b
Lassitude,	7 b	Rooting,	5 a
Laxness,	7 b	Roughness,	2 a
Lid, as of a,	2 b	Running in limbs like a mouse,	3 c
Lifted up, sensation, flying,	1 b	Scraping,	5 a
Lifted up, rising,	3 c	Scratching,	5 a
Lie down, inclination to,	7 b	Screwing together,	4 b
Light feeling,	1 b	Sense of being lifted up,	1 b
Living, as of something,	3 c	Sensitiveness,	1 b
Load, from a,	2 a	Shaking motion,	5 a
Lump, as from a,	2 b	Shocks,	

4

50 THE ARRANGEMENT.

Shooting,	3 c	Tingling,	5 a
Smarting,	6 c	Titillation,	5 a
Smaller, as if being,	2 a	Torn out,	4 b
" as if becoming,	2 a	" asunder,	6 c
Softness of hard parts,	7 b	Torpid feeling,	7 b
Something living, as of,	3 c	Trembling motion,	5 b
Sore, as if,	6 c	Tugging,	3 c
Spraining, as from,	6 c	Turning,	5 b
Spider-web, as from,	2 b	Twisting together,	4 b
Spring, like a,	3 c	Twisting,	5 b
Squeezing,	3 c	Twitching,	3 c
Starting,	3 c	Ulcerated, as if,	6 c
Stiffness of limbs,	7 b	Ulceration, as from subcutaneous,	6 c
Stitching,	3 c	Uncomfort,	7 b
" in, out,	4 b	Undulating,	5 a
Straining,	3 c	Unpainfulness,	7 b
Streams, cold or hot,	3 c	Upward motion,	4 b
Subcutaneous ulceration, as from,	6 c	Urging,	3 c
Suggillation,	6 c	Unwieldiness of body,	7 b
Supporting body, difficult,	7 b	Valve, as from a,	2 b
Susceptibility,	1 b	Vibrating,	5 b
Swollen,	2 a	Water, striking against,	5 a
Tearing,	3 c	Wave-like,	5 a
" in, out,	4 b	Wavering,	5 b
Tenesmus, like,	3 c	Weakness,	7 b
Tenseness,	3 c	" as if lame,	7 b
Tension,	3 c	Wedge, as from a,	2 b
Thronging,	3 c	Whirling, whirring,	5 b
" asunder,	4 b	Wind blowing, as of,	3 c
Thread, as from a,	2 b	Wooden, sensation as if,	7 b
Tickling,	5 a	Work, aversion to,	7 b
Tightness,	2 a	Wringing, writhing,	5 b

CONDITIONS AND CONCOMITANTS OF PAIN.

Oppression; restlessness; anxiety; fear; want of confidence; fretfulness; mental depression; discontent; quarreling, scolding, swearing; weeping, moaning, sighing; over sensitiveness; driven to despair; hopeless; delirium; madness, rage; sensitive to touch; great debility.

PAINS, alternating with chill, with pain in heart, with mental and bodily symptoms.

Disturbed circulation; fainting; formication; coldness; rigor; wants to be covered; heat, sweat; nausea; thirst; weakness; drowsiness; convulsive shocks; trembling; dyspnœa; difficult breathing; unconsciousness.

Has to lie down, keep quiet; driven out of bed; immobility; numbness; swellings.

XLIV. TISSUES.

In treating of the tissues, we will give as an introduction what is known about that form of matter to which all tissues are ultimately reducible, and from which it might be said all are more or less remotely created, viz.: first, the gaseous state. This part will comprise the exhalations and odors emanating from the various organs. Next to the gaseous state, the fluids will be considered; and first among these, those with floating cells, viz.: lymph and blood. Then the fluid secretions and excretions—wasted or worn out elements of the body.

The vessels for the conveyance of the tissue-forming fluids will be next in order. Then the tissues proper, of which the first to be spoken of will be the serous membranes, as the regulators of circulation. The glands will come next; these have, however, in many instances been treated of under their specific names, at the appropriate place with the parts of the body. Thus here only a resumè of sensations and conditions of general applicability will be found. The mucous membranes will close this, the first series of the tissues, i. e., those tending to the nourishment and protection of life.

The second series comprises the motory apparatus: 1, bones, cartilages and joints; 2, muscles; 3, tendons; 4, ligaments; 5, fascia, adding 6, cellular tissues; after which 7, skin, following in the separate chapters 45 and 46. After the morbid affections of each tissue treated in this chapter, the diseases consisting in the affection of such tissues will be treated of. The following table gives the chapters in which here, as elsewhere, these constitutional affections may be looked for:

		In other chapters of the work.	*In chapter* 44. Number.
1.	Brain, spinal marrow,	2, 3 and 31	—
2.	Nerves,	36	—
3.	Muscles,	35	8
4.	Blood, lymph,	29	2
5.	Vessels,	29	3
6.	Serous membranes,	—	4
7.	Bones, cartilages,	—	7
8.	Joints,	—	7
9.	Glands,	—	5
10.	Mucous membranes,	—	6
11.	Cellular tissues,	—	9
12.	Skin,	45 and 46	10

XLV. PASSIVE MOTIONS AND TOUCH.

Passive motions up or down, sideways, forwards or backwards, of a part or the whole body; riding in carriage, cars, on horseback, on board of ship.

Pressure, touch, complaints from; the part of the body being acted on is passive, therefore this rubric is incorporated with this chapter.

Mechanical injuries; wounds in general; comprising the whole homœopathic surgery.

XLVI. SKIN.

First sensations unpainful, then painful; next the temperature, and then the contractibility, humidity and elasticity; then eruptive states, tumors, ulcers, etc., and finally warts, corns, followed by the appendages of the skin, viz., nails and hair.

XLVII. STAGES OF LIFE.

Stages of life. Constitutions, diathesis, dyscrasias.

XLVIII. RELATIONSHIP WITH OTHER DRUGS.

Antidotes.—1. To the effects of massive doses.
2. To the effects of molecular doses.
3. To the lasting effects, changes of constitution, superinduced by the drug; chronic effects; dyscrasia.
4. To the sudden acute attacks of disease to which the chronic poisoned are predisposed.

After the antidotes are mentioned the drugs to which each individual drug is an antidote.

Drugs following well.—Complementary drugs.

Drugs disagreeing; inimical.

The arrangement of drugs in this chapter is according to their natural relationship.

OUR NOMENCLATURE.

Hahnemann, after his first work on Materia Medica (1807), has changed the names of some of his drugs; in this as in all other things, showing a willingness to correct and improve. For the chemicals he adopted, with but few exceptions, the most common and best known names, such as were preferred by the chemistry of his time. He never could agree fully with the ruling doctrine of Lavoisier, and considered it his duty to enter a protest. *Chronic Diseases*, 1839, Vol. 5, *Silic.*, p. 240. The frequent alterations proposed by the French and English chemists, he did not and could not adopt; after new names came in fashion, he named the newly proved in conformity with the older terminology.

In the first edition of his Chronic Diseases (1828, Vol. 2, p. 275), it had escaped his notice, that the scriba named the medicine next to the Magnesia carbonica, Murias magnesiæ; in the second edition (1838, Vol. 4, p. 178), this was corrected and called Magnesia muriatica.

The plants he named according to Linnæus, or the botanical works of his time, rarely deviating from the rule. In 1807 he had Helleborus niger as *Melampodium*, a name it had in the older drug shops, in order to distinguish it from the Veratrum album, treated in the same work. Melampodium was the name given by the Greek to the plant which Linnæus had called Helleborus niger. But with the Greek Helleborus signified another plant now called Veratrum. The frequent mistakes made by physicians and apothecaries, particularly as they did not, like Hahnemann, collect those roots themselves, induced him to adopt the older name. In 1817 in his Materia Medica, he dropped this distinction, because the same name had been used elsewhere for an altogether different herb.

Most medical plants then in the pharmacopœia had a name used in the shops and the pharmacies; some for ages past. Linnæus, introducing his generic and specific names, applied some of the most common to signify a genus, and many others he added as names of a species. Hahnemann already in his first work adopted either the name of the genus, *f. i.:* Aconitum, Arnica, etc.; or of the species: Belladonna, Camphora, etc., or for very good reasons preferred the name which the drug had in the shops, Copaiva, Ipecacuanha, Opium, etc. Some homœopathicians thought it better to give in all cases the preference to the old shop names, and in some of the books of our school, names like Napellus, Cynapium, Lappa, Sphondylium, Lupulus, etc., made their appearance. The majority disapproving of them, they have disappeared from our later works. With the new provings in later times, the last botanical name was generally preferred.

When in 1835 and 1836 the first attempt was made to translate homœopathic Materia Medica from the German into the English language, Jahr's Manual was chosen and published in 1838 at Allentown, Pa. The nomenclature of the U. S. Dispensary was therein adopted. The chemical substances under their latest chemical name; plants under their latest botanical; animals according to their latest zöological. But this was unanimously disapproved of by the increasing number of new converts. The majority of these, the Americans who learned German in order to use the literature of our school, and the many Germans who were spreading homœopathy, all preferred the customary nomenclature of the German school. In this they were perfectly right.

The chemical and botanical nomenclature has, since 1835, changed so frequently, that our alphabetical lists in the repertories would have had to undergo great alterations with almost every new edition.

To establish as much uniformity as can be gained, the American Institute nominated a committee and received their report. This nomenclature, adopted by the Institute at their twenty-second annual meeting, Boston, 1869, has been followed with but few deviations, which will be explained and justified, for no one has a right to decide arbitrarily. Still there is a great confusion in our books. There is no better guide in coming out of it than to admit the principles and rules of a master-mind like that of James D. Dana, who in his Mineralogy, 1868, cleared the way through a horrible heap of names. Never was a problem more satisfactorily solved than his; bringing light and order out of the confused mass of names in the mineralogical works prior to that time. We can use many of his wise decisions, and do well to adopt the following: Page xxx., Dana says: "In order then that the acquired uniformity may be attained, changes should be made in existing names only when it can be done without great inconvenience." "Science should not only have a system of nomenclature, but should also stand by it." "Names which are part of general literature must remain unaltered." "The law of priority has the same claim to recognition as in other natural sciences." "In some cases it may be set aside;" "ignorance or carelessness should not be allowed to give perpetuity to its blunders under any law of priority."

Relative to the law of priority with us we may remark, first: We may alter a name to avoid mistakes by confounding it with others, *f. i.:* Carburetum sulphuris instead of the older Alcohol sulphuris.

Second. It should not be used to keep bad names alive.

Third. When the name was put forth without a proving, it may be changed.

Fourth. If the original prover prefers to introduce a better name, it may be done.

In some points it may be excusable to differ with Dana, viz., in reference to the rule given by him, page xxxii.: "In the transfer of Greek words into Latin or English, the K becomes C." This would then have to be done also with the names from the Arabic and other languages. The rule should be, *all name words taken into our language from the Romans, or Latin authors, we write as we have taken them, even if the original was the Greek; but what has been taken from the Greek direct, as Kreosot, or from the Arabic, as Kali, or from the German, as Kobalt, should retain the K.*

As we only give a name to secure identity, we follow Dana in another of his rules, and adopt the most correct popular name by preference, rather than the latest chemical or botanical, as the latter is frequently either unknown, or liable to change.

ABRIDGEMENT OF NAMES.

According to the main rule of this whole work—to enable the eye to bring to the mind with "rapidity, certainty and ease" what is given in print—the abridgement of names had to be made different from any other similar work.

The rule will be to make the abridgements, in general, two syllables in length. The exception to this rule is where abridgements of two syllables through slight clerical or typographical errors may be mistaken one for another, three syllables may be given, or the name may be given in full.

Errors have been very frequent in such single syllable abbreviations, as Ang., Arg.; Arg., Arn.; Bell., Hell.; Bar., Bor.; Bor., Bov.; and many others. Again some abridgements are ambiguous, as Crot. may be either Crotalus or Croton tiglion; Cocc. for Coccionella or Coccus cacti.

The cases in which even two syllables are not sufficient are such as the following: Anac., Anag.; Asaf., Asar.; Cinnam., Cinnab., etc., and ought to be distinguished by a third syllable, at least in the margin list or in some other way.

LIMITATION.

Drugs of which we possess neither provings nor sufficient clinical observations, have been omitted. Hahnemann's valuable observations relative to the effects and uses of the *magnet*, as well as what others have collected in regard to galvanism and electricity as remedial agents, have been set aside for a separate department, in which these, together with the use of sunlight, blue light, heat, cold, air and water, may be treated.

The many medicinal springs, their analyses, provings and uses, together with the sea water, also require a separate work.

The reception of many drugs from the animal kingdom as well as a number of nosodes (morbid productions) will no doubt meet with opposition, like unto that against the Sepia in 1820, and later the Lachesis; yet in spite of all the objections offered, these same drugs are becoming daily more useful.

LIST OF NAMES AND THEIR ABRIDGEMENTS.

Such as only have been mentioned are not marked; I means somewhat proved; II more proved; I used; II used often; II very often; III polychrests.

Acal. Acalypha indica.
II Acet. ac. Aceticum acidum.
Achillea. See Millefol.
I Acon. lyc. Aconitum lycoctonum.
III Acon. Aconitum Stœrkianum.
II Act. rac. Actæa racemosa vulgo Cimicifuga; radix.*
II Act. spic. Actæa spicata.
I Adam. Adamas, the diamond.
I Aesc. glab. Aesculus glabra.
II Aesc. hipp. Aesculus hippocastanum.
Aeth. sulph. Aether sulphuricum.
II Aethus. Aethusa cynapium.
II Agar. Agaricus muscarius.
II Agn. cast. Agnus castus.
I Ailanth. Ailanthus glandulosa.
II Alcohol. Alcohol.
Alc. sulph. See Carb. sulph.
I Alet. far. Aletris farinosa.
All. cep. See Cepa.
II All. sat. Allium sativum.
Aln. rub. Alnus rubra.
II Alœs. Aloe soccotrina.
Alth. off. Althæa officinalis.
II Al. p. s. Aluminæ and potassæ sulphas; common alum.
II Alum. Alumina, the oxide; also the metal.
Aman. See Agar. musc.
II Ambra. Ambra grisea; one of the nosodes.
II Amm. gum. Ammoniacum gummi; Dorema A.
I Amm. benz. Ammonium benzoicum.
I Amm. brom. Ammonium bromatum.
II Amm. carb. Ammonium carbonicum.
Amm. jod. Ammonium jodidum.
II Amm. mur. Ammonium muriaticum; chloridum. Sal ammoniac.
Amm. phosph. Ammonium phosphoricum.
Amp. quin. Ampelopsis quinquefolia.
I Amph. ver. Amphisbæna vermicularis, Mure.
Amygd. Amygdala amara.
II Anac. Anacardium occidentale.
I Anagal. Anagallis arvensis.
Anem. Anemone nemorosa.
II Ananth. Anantherum muricatum.

II Angust. Angustura, s. Galipea.
Anis. Pimpinella anisum.
Anis. stell. See Illicium.
Anten. Antennaria margarita.
Anth. nob. Anthemis nobilis.
I Anthrac. Anthracinum; anthraxin; one of the nosodes.
Anthrakok. Anthrakokali; a mixture.
Ant. tox. Antiaris toxicaria.
III Ant. crud. Antimonium crudum.
II Ant. tart. Antimonium tartaricum.
Antirrh. lin. Antirhinum linaria.
I Aph. chen. Aphis chenopodii glauc.
III Apis. Virus apis mellificæ.
II Ap. mell. Apium tinctura.
I Ap. grav. Apium graveolens.
I Apoc. andr. Apocynum androsæmifolium.
I Apoc. can. Apocynum cannabinum.
Aquil. Aquilegia vulgaris.
I Aral. rac. Aralia racemosa.
Aranea. See Diadema.
Aran. scin. Aranea scinencia.
I Arct. lap. Arctium lappa.
II Argent. Argentum, the metal.
II Arg. nitr. Argentum nitricum.
I Arist. clem. Aristolochia clematitis.
I Arist. mil. Aristolochia milhomens.
Arist. virg. Aristolochia virginica; s. Serpentaria.
I Armor. Cochlearia armoracea.
II Arnic. Arnica montana; radix.
III Arsen. Arsenicum album, the oxide.
Ars. bis. See Realgar.
Ars. cit. See Auripigm.
II Ars. hydr. Arsenicum hydrogenisatum.
II Ars. jod. Arsenicum jodatum.
II Ars. met. Arsenicum, the metal.
Ars. rubr. See Realgar.
Ars. trisulph. See Auripigm.
Art. vulg. Artemisia vulgaris.
Arum it. Arum italicum.
I Arum mac. Arum maculatum.
I Arum triph. Arum triphyllum.
II Arund. maur. Arundo mauritanica.
II Asaf. Ferula asafœtida.
Asar. can. Asarum canadense.

|| Asar. eup. Asarum europæum.
| Askal. Askalabotes lævis.
 Ascl. inc. Asclepias incarnata.
|| Ascl. syr. Asclepias syriaca.
| Ascl. tub. Asclepias tuberosa.
|| Asim. tr. Asimina triloba.
 Assac. See Hura brasiliensis.
|| Astac. fluv. Astacus fluviatilis.
|| Aspar. Asparagus officinalis.
 Asp. od. Asperula odorata.
|| Ast. rub. Asterias rubens.
| Atham. ores. Athamanta oreoselinum.
 Atr. olid. Atriplex olida.
|| Atrop. Atropinum.
 Atrop. sulph. Atropinum sulphuricum.
 Aurip. Auripigmentum; arsenicum trisulphuratum.
|| Aurum. Aurum, the metal.
 Aur. mur. Aurum muriaticum.
|| Badiag. Badiaga; Spongia fluviatilis.
|| Baptis. Baptisia tinctoria.
|| Barb. ov. Cyprinus barbus, the roe.
 Bar. cren. Barosma crenata.
|| Bar. ac. Baryta acetica.
|| Baryt. Baryta carbonica and acetica.
| Bar. mur. Baryta muriatica.
 Bals. cop. See Copaifera.
 Bals. per. See Peruvianum.
||| Bellad. Atropa belladonna; radix.
 Bell. bacc. Belladonnæ baccæ.
| Bell. per. Bellis perennis.
|| Benz. ac. Benzoicum acidum; Flores Benzoes.
 Benz. of Amm. See Amm. benz.
|| Berber. Berberis vulgaris.
|| Bism. nitr. Bismuthum subnitricum.
| Blatt. am. Blatta americana; Mure.
|| Bol. lar. Boletus laricis; Polyporus.
 Bol. pin. Boletus pini; Pinicola.
 Bol. sat. Boletus satanas.
|| Borax. Borax; Natrun boracicum.
 Bounafa. Ferula glauca.
|| Bovist. Lycoperdum Bovista.
 Branc. urs. See Heracleum.
 Brom. of Lith. See Lithium.
 Brom. of Pot. See Kali brom.
|| Bromum. Bromum.
 Bruc. ant. See Nux vom. cortex.
||| Bryon. Bryonia alba.
 Buchu. See Barosma crenata.

|| Buf. cin. Bufo cinereus; s. vulgaris.
| Buf. sah. Bufo sahytiensis. Mure.
 Buxus. Buxus communis.
|| Cactus. Cactus grandiflorus.
 Cadmium. See Kadmium.
|| Cahinc. Chiococca racemosa.
 Cajup. Melaleuca cajuputi.
|| Calab. Calabar; Physostigma venenosum.
|| Calad. Caladium seguinum or Dieffenbachia seguinum.
 Calam. Acorus calamus.
|| Calc. ac. Calcarea acetica.
| Calc. ars. Calcarea arsenica.
| Calc. carb. Calcarea carbonica.
| Calc. caust. Calcarea caustica, calcium oxide.
| Calc. fluor. Calcarea fluorica.
 Calc. mur. Calcarea muriatica, chlorata.
|| Calc jod. Calcarea jodata.
 Calc. hypoph. Calcarea hypophosphorica.
||| Calc. ostr. Calcarea ostrearum.*
|| Calc. phosph. m. Calcarea phosphorica mixta.
|| Calc. phosph. b. Calcarea phosphorica basica.
 Calc. sil. See Wollastonit. Tabashir.
 Calc. sulph. See Hepar s. c.
| Calc. sulph. Calcarea sulphurica; Gypsum.
| Calend. Calendula officinalis; flores.
| Calth. pal. Caltha pulustris.
|| Camphor. Camphora officinarum.
 Camph. brom. Camphorae bromidum.
 Cancer. See Astacus.
| Cann. ang. Canna angustifolia; Mure.
 Canchal. See Chironia.
|| Cann. ind. Cannabis indica; Hashish. Mure and Philal. Prover's Society.
|| Cann. sat. Cannabis sativa.
|| Canthar. Cantharides; Meloe vesicatoria; Lytta.
|| Capsic. Capsicum annuum; the berries.
|| Carb. an. Carbo animalis; corium taurinum ustum.
||| Carb. veg. Carbo vegetabilis. See *
|| Carb. ac. Carbolicum acidum.
|| Carb. sulph. Carburetum sulphuris; s. Alcohol sulphuris.

LIST OF NAMES AND THEIR ABRIDGEMENTS.

| Card. ben. Carduus benedictus; Cnicus.
| Card. mar. Carduus marianus; Silybum M.
| Cascar. Cascarilla; Croton eluteria.
Cast. vesc. Castanea vesca.
| Castor. Castoreum muscovitum; Sibiricum.
|| Cast. equ. Castor equorum, the residuum of the thumbnail of horses.
| Cauloph. Caulophyllum thalictroides.
||| Caustic. Causticum Hahnemanni.*
Ceanoth. Ceanothus americanus.
Cedron. Cedron; Simaba.
|| Cepa. Allium cepa.
Cer. virg. Cérasus virginica.
Cerium. Cerium oxydum.
Cer. oxal. Cerium oxalicum.
| Cerv. bras. Cervus brasiliensis; (skin) Mure.
||| Chamom. Matricaria chamomilla; flores.
|| Chelid. Chelidonium majus.
Chel. glab. Chelone glabra.
| Chen. ant. Chenopodium anthelminticum.
Chen. glauc. See Aphis.
| Chim. mac. Chimaphila maculata.
|| Chim. umb. Chimaphila umbellata.
China. See Cinch. off.
| Chinin. Chininum purum.
|| Chin. sulph. Chininum sulphuricum.
Chin. ars. Chininum arsenicosum.
Chioc. See Cahinca.
Chir. chil. Chironia chilensis; Canchalagua.
| Chloral. Chloral hydratum.
| Chlorof. Chloroformium.
| Chlorum. Chlorum.
| Chrom. ac. Chromicum acidum.
|| Cicut. Cicuta virosa.
|| Cimex. Cimex lectularius.
Cimicifuga. See Actæa racemosa.
|| Cina. Cina, Artemisia judaica; s. Vahliana.
|| Cinch. off. Cinchona officinalis or Peruvian bark.*
|| Cinch. sulph. Cinchoninum sulphuricum.
|| Cinnab. Cinnabaris, Merc. bisulphuretum rubrum.
Cinnam. Cinnamomum zeylanicum.

|| Cist. can. Cistus canadensis, s. Helianthemum.
Citr. ac. Citrinum acidum.
Citr. med. Citrus medica.
|| Clemat. Clematis erecta.
Cobalt. See Kobaltum.
|| Coca. Erythroxylon coca.
| Coccion. Coccionella septempunctata.
|| Coccul. Cocculus indicus, Menispermum.
|| Cocc. cact. Coccus cacti, Cochineal.
Cochlearia. See Armoracia.
| Codein. Codeinum.
|| Coffea. Coffea arabica.
Coff. tost. Coffea tosta.
|| Colchic. Colchicum autumnale.
| Collin. Collinsonia canadensis.
|| Coloc. Cucumis colocynthis
| Comoc. Comocladia dentata.
Condur. Condurango.
|| Conium. Conium maculatum.
Convolv. Convolvulus arvensis.
| Con. duart. Convolvulus duartinus; Mure.
| Copaiv. Balsamum Copaivum from Copaifera multijuga.
|| Corall. Corallia rubra.
Cor. sat. Coriandrum sativum.
| Corn. circ. Cornus circinata.
| Corn. flor. Cornus florida.
| Corn. ser. Cornus sericea.
Coryd. f. Corydalis formosa.
|| Cotyl. Cotyledon umbilicus.
Creosot. See Kreosot.
| Crocus. Crocus sativus.
| Crotal. Crotalus horridus.
|| Crot. cas. Crotalus cascavella; Mure.
Crot. eleut. See Cascarilla.
|| Crot. tigl. Croton tiglium.
|| Cubeb. Cubeba officinalis.
|| Cuprum. Cuprum, the metal.
| Cupr. ac. Cuprum aceticum.
|| Cupr. ars. Cuprum arsenicosum.
Cupr. sulph. Cuprum sulphuricum.
Curcas. See Jatropha.
|| Cyclam. Cyclamen europæum.
Cynap. See Aethusa.
Cynoglos. Cynoglossum officinale.
| Cypriped. Cypripedium pubescens.
Cytis. Cytisus laburnum.
Daphne. See Mezereum.
|| Daphn. ind. Daphne indica.

Dat. arb.	Datura arborea.
Dauc. car.	Daucus carota.
Delph. amaz.	Delphinus amazonicus; (skin) Mure.
Diad.	Diadema, Aranea d. Epeira.
Dict. alb.	Dictamnus albus.
Diefenbachia.	See Caladium.
Digit.	Digitalis purpurea.
Diosc. vill.	Dioscorea villosa.
Dips. sylv.	Dipsacus sylvestris.
Dirc. pal.	Dirca palustris.
Dolich.	Dolichos pruriens.
Doryph.	Doryphora decemlineata.
Dracont.	See Pothos.
Droser.	Drosera rotundifolia.
Dryob.	See Camphora.
Dulcam.	Solanum Dulcamara.
Elais guin.	Elais guiniensis; (fruit) Mure.
Elaps cor.	Elaps corallinus; Mure.
Elat.	Momordica Elaterium.
Epig. rep.	Epigæa repens.
Equis.	Equisetum hyemale.
Erecthit.	Erecthitis hieracifolia.
Ergot.	See Secale cornutum.
Eriger.	Erigeron canadense.
Erv. Ervil.	Ervum Ervilia.
Eryng. aqu.	Eryngium aquaticum.
Erythox.	See Coca.
Eserine.	See Calabar.
Euc. glob.	Eucalyptus globulus.
Eugenia.	See Jambos.
Eupat. arom.	Eupatorium aromaticum.
Eupat. perf.	Eupatorium perfoliatum.
Eupat. purp.	Eupatorium purpureum.
Euph. am.	Euphorbia amygdaloides.
Euph. cor.	Euphorbia coronata.
Euph. hyp.	Euphorbia hypericifolia.
Euph. vill.	Euphorbia villosa; s. Sylvestris.
Euphorb.	Euphorbium officinarum.
Eupion.	Eupion.
Euphras.	Euphrasia officinalis.
Euspongia.	See Spongia.
Eriod.	Eriodendrum anfractuosum.
Eryng. aqu.	Eryngium aquaticum.
Ervon. atrop.	Evonymus atropurpureus.
Evon. eur.	Evonymus europæus.
Fagopyr.	Fagopyrum esculentum.
Fel taur.	Fel tauri.
Fel vulp.	Fel vulpis.
Ferrum.	Ferrum, the metal.
Ferr. ac	Ferrum aceticum.
Ferr. brom.	Ferrum bromicum.
Ferr. carb.	Ferrum carbonicum.
Ferr. mur.	Ferrum muriaticum; F chloratum, F. sesquichloridum.
Ferr. iod.	Ferrum iodatum.
Ferr. lact.	Ferrum lacticum.
Ferr. mag.	Ferrum magneticum.
Ferr. phosph.	Ferrum phosphoricum.
Ferr. sulph.	Ferrum sulphuricum.
Filix mas.	Aspidium Filix-mas.
Fluor. ac.	Fluoricum acidum.
Formica.	Formica rufa.
Form. spir.	Formicarum spiritus.
Form. ac.	Formicicum acidum.
Frag. vesc.	Fragaria vesca.
Fras. car.	Frasera carolinensis.
Fusc. vesic.	Fuscus vesiculosa.
Gadus.	Gadus morrhua (Vertebra).
Galipea.	See Angustura.
Galium.	Galium aparine.
Gall. ac.	Gallicum acidum.
Gambog.	Gambogia. Gummi gutti.
Gelsem.	Gelsemium sempervirens; s. nitidum.
Gen. tinct.	Genista tinctoria.
Gent. cruc.	Gentiana cruciata.
Gent. lut.	Gentiana lutea.
Geran. mac.	Geranium maculatum.
Gill. trif.	Gillenia trifoliata.
Ginseng.	Panax quinquefolium.
Glonoinum.	Nitro-glycerinum.
Gnaph. pol.	Gnaphalium polycephalum.
Goss. herb.	Gossypium herbaceum.
Gran. cort.	Granatorum cortex; Punica granatorum.
Graphit.	Graphites.
Gratiola.	Gratiola officinalis.
Guaco.	Mikania guaco.
Guan. austr.	Guano australis; Mure.
Guaiac.	Guaiacum officinale.
Guaræa.	Guaræa trichloides.
Gummi gutt.	See Gambogia.
Gymnocl.	Gymnocladus canadensis.
Hamam.	Hamamelis virginica.
Hæmatox.	Hæmatoxylum campechianum.
Hed. pul.	Hedeoma pulegioides.
Hed. ild.	Hedysarum ildefonsianum; Mure.

HELIANTH. Helianthus annuus.
HEKLA. Siliceous ashes of the last years. Dr. Holcombe.
HELIOTROP. Heliotropium peruvianum.
HELL. FŒT. Helleborus fœtidus.
❙❙ HELLEB. Helleborus niger.
❙❙ HELON. DIOIC. Helonias dioica.
❙❙❙ HEPAR S. C. Hepar sulphuris calcareum, Hahnemanni.
❙ HEPAR S. K. Hepar sulphuris kalicum.
❙ HEPAT. TRIL. Hepatica triloba.
❙ HERAC. SPHOND. Heracleum sphondylium.
❙❙ HIPPOM. Hippomanes.*
❙❙ HUM. LUP. Humulus lupulus.
❙❙ HURA BRAS. Hura brasiliensis; Assacu, Mure.
❙❙ HYDRAST. Hydrastis canadensis.
❙ HYDR. AC. Hydrocyanicum acidum.
HYDROC. Hydrocotyle asiatica.
HYL. ARA. Hyla arborea.
HYDROPH. Hydrophobinum; one of the nosodes.
❙❙ HYOSC. Hyoscyamus niger.
❙❙ HYPER. Hypericum perforatum.
❙ IACEA. Viola tricolor.
❙❙ IBER. AM. Iberis amara.
❙❙ IGNAT. Ignatia amara.
ILEX. Ilex quinquefolium.
❙ ILL. AN. Illicium anisatum, Franz and Mure.
❙❙ INDIGO. Indigo.
INUL. DYS. Inula dysenterica.
INUL. HELEN. Inula Helenium.
IODUM. Iodium.
IPEC. Cephaëlis Ipecacuanha.
IRIDIUM. Iridium, the metal.
❙❙ IRIS VERS. Iris versicolor, the root.
❙ IRIS FŒT. Iris fœtidisima, the root.
❙❙ JACAR. Jacaranda caroba, Bignonia caroba; Mure.
JALAP. Convolvulus jalapa.
JAMBOS. Eugenia Jambos, the seed.*
❙ JAN. MAN. Janipha manihot; Mure.
❙❙ JATROPH. Jatropha curcas, the seed.
❙ JUGL. CIN. Juglans cinerea.
❙❙ JUGL. REG. Juglans regia.
JUNC. EFF. Juncus effusus.
JUNC. PIL. Juncus pilosus.
KADMIUM. Kadmium, the metal.
KADM. SULPH. Kadmium sulphuricum.

KALI AC. Kali aceticum.
❙❙ KALI BICHR. Kali bichromicum.
❙❙ KALI BROM. Kali bromium.
❙❙ KALI CARB. Kali carbonicum.
KALI CHLOR. Kali chloricum.
❙ KALI CYAN. Kali cyanicum.
KALI HYPER. Kali hypermanganicum.
❙❙ KALI HYDR. Kali hydriodicum.
❙ KALI MUR. Kali muriaticum, Kali chloratum; Schüssler.
KALI NITR. See Nitrum.
❙ KALI PHOSPH. Kali phosphoricum; Schüssler.
❙ KALI SULPH. Kali sulphuricum; Schüssler.
❙❙ KALMIA. Kalmia latifolia.
KAMEELA. See Rottlera.
❙ KAOLIN. Kaolinite, Dana.
❙ KINO. Kino; from the shops, either African or East Indian.
❙❙ KOBALT. Kobaltum, the metal.
KOUSSO. Hagenia Abyssinica.
KRAMERIA. See Ratanhia.
❙❙ KREOSOT. Kreosotum Reichenbachii.*
❙❙ LAC CANIN. Lac caninum; Swan.
LAC. OVILL. Lac ovillum; Jenichen.
❙ LAC VACC. Lac vaccinum defloratum; Swan.
LACERT. Lacerta viridis.
❙❙ LACHES. Trigonocephalus Lachesis.
❙❙ LACHNANTH. Lachnanthes tinctoria.
LACT. AC. Acidum lacticum.
LACTUC. SAT. Lacctuca sativa.
❙❙ LACTUC. VIR. Lactucca virosa.
❙ LAMIUM. Lamium album.
LAP. ALB. Lapis albus; Grauvogl's great medicine.
❙❙ LAUROC. Laurocerasus; Prunus L.
LAVA. See Hecla.
❙❙ LEDUM. Ledum palustre.
LEONTODON. See Taraxacum.
❙❙ LEPID. BON. Lepidium bonariense; Mure.
❙ LEPTAND. Leptandra Virginica.
❙❙ LIL. TIGR. Lilium tigrinum.
❙❙ LITHIUM CARB. Lithium carbonicum.
LITH. BROM. Lithium bromicum.
LITH. MUR. Lithium muriaticum.
❙ LOBEL. CARD. Lobelia cardinalis.
❙❙ LOBEL. COER. Lobelia coerulea, vulga syphilitica.

‖ Lobel. infl. Lobelia inflata.
Lobel. long. Lobelia longiflora.
Loli jm. Lolium temulentum.
Lycoperdon. See Bovista.
Lycopersicum. See Solanum.
‖ Lycop. Lycopodium clavatum.
‖ Lyc. virg. Lycopus Virginicus.
Macrotis. See Actea.
‖ Magn. carb. Magnesia carbonica.
‖ Magn. mur. Magnesia muriatica.
‖ Magn. phosph. Magnesia phosphorica; Schüssler.
‖ Magn. sulph. Magnesia sulphurica.
Magnol. glauc. Magnolia glauca.
Majoran. Majorana hortensis.
Malva rot. Malva rotundifolia.
‖ Mancin. Hippomane mancinella; Drs. Bute and Mure.
Mangan. ox. Manganum binoxydum.
‖ Mangan. acet. Manganum aceticum.
Mangan. carb. Manganum carbonicum.
‖ Mar. ver. Teucrium Marum verum.
Matico. Piper angustifolium.
Medorrhoin. One of the nosodes.
Melaleuca. See Cajuput.
‖ Melast. ack. Melastoma ackermani; Mure.
Melc. sale. Honey triturated in salt, a very effectual preparation of Dr. Jeanes.
Melilot. Melilotus vulgaris.
Meloe maj. Meloe majalis.
‖ Menisp. can. Menispermum canadense.
Menth. pip. Mentha piperita.
‖ Menyanth. Menyanthes trifoliata.
‖ Mephit. Mephitis putorius.
‖ Merc. perenn. Mercurialis perennis.
Merc. sol. See Mercurius.
‖ Mercur. Mercurius, the metal.
Merc. ac. Mercurius aceticus.
‖ Merc. cyan. Mercurius cyanatus.
Merc. dulc. Mercurius dulcis, calomel.
Merc. iod. flav. Mercurius iodatus flavus, protiodide.
Merc. iod. rub. Mercurius iodatus ruber, biniodide.
Merc. præc. alb. Mercurius præcipitatus albus.
Merc. sol. H. Mercurius solubilis Hahnemanni.

Merc. sublim. Mercurius sublimatus, corrosivus.
Merc. sulphuret. See Cinnabaris.
Merc. sulph. nig. Æthiop. mineralis.
Merc. sulph. See Turpeth.
Mercur. vivus. See Mercurius.
‖ Mezer. Mezereum; Daphne M.
‖ Millef. Millefolium; Achillea M.
‖ Mitch. rep. Mitchella repens.
‖ Mimos. hum. Mimosa humilis; Mure.
Molybd. ac. Molybdænicum acidum.
Momord. bals. Momordica balsamina.
Monard. punct. Monarda punctata.
Monotrop. Monotropa uniflora.
Morph. Morphine.
Morph. ac. Morphium aceticum.
Morph. mur. Morphium muriaticum.
Morph. sulph. Morphium sulphuricum.
Moschus. M. moschiferus.
Murex p. Murex purpurea.
Mur. ac. Muriaticum acidum.
‖ Murure. Murure leite; Mure.
‖ Mygale. Lasiodora Cubana.
‖ Myr. cerif. Myrica cerifera.
‖ Myrist. seb. Myristica sebifera; Mure.
Myroxylon. See Peru balsam.
‖ Myrtus. Myrtus communis.
‖ Nabal. alb. Nabalus albus; Prenanthes serpentaria.
‖ Naja tr. Naja tripudians.
Napellus. See Aconitum.
Narc. ac. Narcotinum aceticum.
Natr. borac. See Borax.
‖ Natr. carb. Natrum carbonicum.
‖ Natr. mur. Natrum muriaticum.
‖ Natr. nitr. Natrum nitricum.
‖ Natr. phosph. Natrum phosphoricum; Schüssler.
‖ Natr. sulph. Natrum sulphuricum.
Necros. cuspid. See Momordica balsamina.
‖ Niccol. Niccolum, the metal.
‖ Nicc. carb. Niccolum carbonicum.
Nicc. sulph. Niccolum sulphuricum.
Nicot. Nicotinum.
‖ Nitr. sp. d. Spiritus nitri dulcis.
‖ Nitr. ac. Nitri acidum.
Nitro-glycerin. See Glonoin.
‖ Nitro muriatic acidum.
‖ Nitrum. Kali nitricum.

LIST OF NAMES AND THEIR ABRIDGEMENTS.

| Nuphar. Nuphar luteum.
| Nux juglandis. See Juglans.
|| Nux mosch. Myristica Nux moschata.
|| Nux vom. Strychnos Nux vomica, seed.
| Nuc. vom. cort. Nucis vomicæ cortex.*
Nymph. od. Nymphæa odorata.
Nymph. lut. Nymphæa lutea.
Ocim. c. Ocimum canum; Mure.
Œnanth. cr. Œnanthe crocata.
Œnoth. b. Œnothera biennis.
|| Oleand. Nerium Oleander.
| Ol. anim. Oleum animale Dippelii.
|| Ol. jec. Oleum jecoris aselli.
| Onisc. Oniscus asellus.
Onon. spin. Ononis spinosa.
|| Opium. Papaver somniferum.
Opopon. Pastinaca Opoponax.
| Origan. Origanum vulgare.
Orobanch. Orobanche Virginiana.
Orpiment. See Auripigment.
|| Ostr. virg. Ostrya Virginica.
|| Osmium. Osmium, the metal.
|| Ox. ac. Oxalicum acidum.
|| Oxygen. Oxygenum.
| Ozon. Ozon.
| Pæon. off. Pæonia officinalis.
| Pallad. Palladium, the metal.
| Pan. bras. Panacea brasiliensis; Mure.
Panax. See Ginseng.
Pareir. Pareira brava; Cissampelos.
|| Paris. Paris quadrifolia.
Patchouli. See Plectranthus.
|| Paull. pinn. Paullinia pinnata; Mure.
Paull. sorb. Paullinia sorbilis; Guarana.
|| Pedic. Pediculus capitis; Mure.
| Peruv. bals. Peruvianum balsamum.
| Petiv. tetr. Petiveria tetrandra; Mure.
| Petrol. Petroleum.
Petrosel. Petroselinum, Apium petr.
Phelland. Phellandrium aquaticum.
|| Phosphor. Phosphorus, the common transparent variety.
|| Phosph. ac. Phosphoricum acidum.
Phosph. ruber. Phosphorus ruber, the amorphous variety.
Physostigma. See Calabar.

|| Phytol. dec. Phytolacca decandra.
Pin. sylv. Pinus sylvestris.
|| Piper nigr. Piper nigrum.
|| Plant. maj. Plantago major, Pl. latifolia.
||| Platin. Platinum, the metal.
|| Plectranth. Plectranthus fruticosa; Patchouli.
Plumb. litt. Plumbago littoralis; Mure.
Plumbum. Plumbum, the metal.
Plumb. jod. Plumbum jodatum.
|| Plumb. ac. Plumbum aceticum.
|| Podoph. Podophyllum peltatum.
Polyporus officin. See Boletus.
Polyp. pinicula. See Boletus.
| Polyg. punc. Polygonum punctatum.
| Pop. trem. Populus tremuloides.
| Poth. fœt. Pothos fœtidus; Symplocarpus fœtidus.
Prun. pad. Prunus padus.
|| Prun. spin. Prunus spinosa.
|| Psorin. Psorinum; C. Hg. One of the nosodes.
|| Ptel. trif. Ptelea trifoliata.
Pulm. vulp. The fox lung in trituration.*
||| Pulsat. Pulsatilla; Anemone pratensis.
|| Pulsat. nut. Pulsatilla nutalliana.
Pyrola. See Chimaphila.
Quassia. Picræna excelsa.
Rana. See Bufo.
|| Ran. bulb. Ranunculus bulbosus.
| Ran. scel. Ranunculus sceleratus.
|| Raphan. Raphanus æstivus niger.
| Ratanh. Ratanhia, Krameria triandra.
Realg. Realgar, arsenicum bisulphuretum.
Resin. itu. Resina itu; Mure.
|| Rheum. Rheum palmatum, rhabarbarum.
Rhodium. Rhodium, the metal.
| Rhodod. Rhododendron chrysanthum.
Rhus glab. Rhus glabra.
|| Rhus rad. Rhus radicans.
||| Rhus tox. Rhus toxicodendron.
|| Rhus ven. Rhus venenata or Vernix.
Ricin. Ricinus communis.
|| Robin. Robinia pseudacacca.
Rottler. Rottlera tinctoria.

RUBIA. Rubia tinctorum.
‖ RUMEX. Rumex crispus.
‖ RUTA. Ruta graveolens.
‖ SABAD. Veratrum sabadilla.
‖ SABINA. Juniperus Sabina.
‖ SACCH. OFF. Saccharum officinale.
SALIX. Salix alba.
‖ SAMBUC. Sambucus nigra; flor.
| SAMB. CORT. Samb. nigr. cortex.
SAMB. EBUL. Sambucus ebulus.
‖ SANGUIN. Sanguinaria canadensis.
SANTAL. OL. Santali oleum.
| SANTON. Santonium.
‖ SAPO DOMEST. The pure soda soap.
‖ SARRACEN. Sarracenia purpurea.
‖ SARSAP. Sarsaparilla; Smilax officinalis.
SASSAFRAS. Sass. officinalis.
SCILLA. See Squilla.
SCOLOPEND. Scolopendrum morsitaus.
SCROF. NOD. Scrofularia nodosa.
SCUT. LAT. Scutellaria lateriflor.
| SEC. CORN. Secale cornutum; Ergot; one of the nosodes.
| SEDINHA. Sedinha; Mure.
SEDUM ACR. Sedum acre.
| SELEN. Selenium.
SEMP. TECT. Sempervivum tectorum.
| SENEC. AUR. Senecio aureus.
‖ SENEG. Polygala Senega.
SENNA. Cassia Senna.
‖ SEPIA. The poison of the Mediterranean cuttle fish.
SERICUM. The silk from the common silk worm.
SERPENTARIA. See Aristolochia.
‖ SILIC. Silicea, oxyde of Silicium.
‖ SIL. AQU. Aqua Silicata.
SILPH. LACIN. Silphium laciniatum.
‖ SINAP. ALB. Sinàpis alba.
| SINAP. NIGR. Sinàpis nigra.
| SMARAGDUS. The emerald.
| SOLANUM ARREBENTA. Mure.
| SOL. TUB. ÆGROT. Solanum tuberosum ægrotans; Mure; one of the nosodes.
SOLAN. LYCOP. Solanum lycopersicum.
SOL. MAM. Solanum mammosum.
‖ SOL. NIGR. Solanum nigrum.
| SOL. OLER. Solanum oleraceum; Mure.
SOLIDAG. V. Solidago virga-aurea.
SPART. SCOP. Spartium scoparium; Cytisus S.

| SPIGEL. Spigelia anthelmia.
SPIG. MARYL. Spigelia Marylandica.
SPIGGUR. Spiggurus martini; a bristl of Hystrix subspinosus; Mure.
SRIRIT. NITRI DULC. See Nitri sp. d.
‖ SPONGIA. Spongia marina tosta; Eu spongia.
SPONGIA PALUSTRIS. See Badiaga.
‖ SQUILLA. Squilla maritima; Scilla.
| STACHYS BETONICA.
‖ STANNUM. Stannum, the metal.
| STAPHIS. Delphinium Staphisagria.
STERCUL. ACUM. Sterculia acuminata
STIBIUM. See Antimonium.
‖ STICTA PULM. Sticta pulmonaria.
| STILLING. SYLV. Stillingia sylvatica.
| STRAMON. Datura Stramonium.
‖ STRONTIAN. Strontia carbonica.
STRYCHNIA. Strychninum.
SUCCIN. AC. Succinicum acidum.
‖ SULPHUR. Sulphur sublimatum; Hah nemann.
| SULPH. AC. Sulphuricum acidum.
SULPH. ÆTH. Æther sulphuricus.
SULPH. PRÆC. Lac sulphuris.
‖ SUMBUL. A root from Asia; als called Jatamansi.
‖ SYMPHYT. Symphytum officinale.
SYPHILIN. One of the nosodes.
| TABAC. Tabacum; Nicotiana T.
TABASHEER.*
| TANAC. Tanacetum vulgare.
‖ TARAX. Leontodon Taraxacum.
‖ TARANTUL. Tarantula hispanica.
| TART. AC. Tartaricum acidum.
TART. EMET. See Ant. tart.
| TAX. BACC. Taxus baccata.
| TELLUR. Tellurium, the metal.
‖ TEREBINTH. Terebinthinæ oleum.
THALLIUM, the metal.
TEUCRIUM. See Marum verum.
THLASPI. Thlaspi bursi pastoris.
| THEA. Thea Chinensis.
| THERID. Theridion curassavicum.
‖ THROMBID. Thrombidium muscæ d mesticæ.
‖ THUYA. Thuya occidentalis.
‖ TILIA. Tilia Europæa.
‖ TINCT. ACRIS. Tinctura acris si kali, Hahnemanni.
‖ TONGO. Dipterix odorata.
| TRADESC. DIUR. Tradescantia di retica; Mure.

TRIFOL. PRAT. Trifolium pratense.
TRILL. PEND. Trillium pendulum.
TRIOST. PERF. Triosteum perfoliatum.
I I TURPETHUM. Mercurius sulphuricus.
TUSSIL. FAR. Tussilago farfara.
TUSSID. PET. Tussilago petasites.
ULM. CAMP. Ulmus campestris.
ULM. FLAVA. Ulmus flava.
UPAS TIEUTE. An arrow poison.
I I URAN. NITR. Uranium nitricum.
URT. DIOCC. Urtica dioica.
I I URT. UR. Urtica urens.
I USTIL. Ustilago maidis.
UVA URSA. Arctostaphylos Uva ursi.
VACCININUM. One of the nosodes.
I I VALERIAN. Valeriana officinalis.
VARIOLINUM. One of the nosodes.
I I VERATR. Veratrum album.
I I VER. VIR. Veratrum viride.
I I VERBASC. Verbascum thapsus.
VERBENA. Verbena officinalis.
VERB HAST. Verbena hastata.
VERON. BECC. Beccabunge.

VESPA. Crabro.
VIBURN. OPUL. Viburnum opulus.
VIBURN. PR. Viburnum prunifolium.
I VINCA MIN. Vinca minor.
I I VIOL. OD. Viola odorata.
I VIOL. TRIC. Viola tricolor; Jacea.
VIP. TORV. Vipera torva or redi.
VITEX. See Agnus castus.
I VISCUM ALBUM.
I VULPIS HEPAR. Tincture of the liver of the European fox.*
WOLLAST. Wollastonite; tabular spar.*
I I XANTH. FRAX. Xanthoxylum fraxineum.
I XIPHOS. Xiphosuræ sanguis; Limulus.
I I ZINCUM. Zincum, the metal.
ZINC. AC. Zincum aceticum.
I ZINC. OX. Zincum oxydatum.
ZINC. PHOSPH. Zincum phosphoricum.
ZINC. VAL. Zincum valerianicum.
I I ZINGIBER. Zingiber officinale.
ZIZIA AUR. Zizia aurea; Smyrnium aureum.

NOTES TO THE LIST OF NAMES.

Actæa racemosa.—There are seven reasons for rejecting the name *Cimicifuga:*

1. It was a genus split off from *Actæa* during the time when the fashion of dividing old genera prevailed. There is no necessity for, nor the least advantage in such a new genus. Who, but a hair-splitter, would care about a few capsules standing singly or not? The whole appearance of the plant is like *Actæa spicata.* Darwinism will soon do away with such new genera.

2. It is a very badly made name; all new composites in the Latin are against the genius of this language.

3. It is nearly always pronounced by gardeners, by the apothecary boys and eclectic doctors in such a way as to shock a scholar, viz.: *Cimicifúga.*

4. The only right pronunciation being *Cimicifugá*, which sounds horribly to every musical ear.

5. The name is a falsehood, as bed-bugs do not run at sight of the root, and have not been driven out of a single bedstead by it. The Persian powder does it.

6. We have a right to give our medicines a more proper name when botanists have adopted a bad one. Hence we say *Lobelia coerulea* instead of *Syphilitica,* another lie, and *Rhus venenata* instead of the mistaken *Vernix,* etc.

7. It was known by the good old name before, was proved by Helbig and applied by Rückert long before it was taken here out of the dirty shops of the eclectics.

Calcarea ostrearum Hahnemanni is not a carbonate of lime like some rocks or what chemists could prepare, but an animalized preparation of nature; besides that it contains traces of phosphate of lime, and what else we do not know. The similarity of Hahnemann's proving of *Calcarea acetica* with it depends altogether on his preparation; he dissolved oyster-shells in vinegar.

Carbo vegetabilis.—Dr. Caspari, the first prover, used the wood of the *Fagus sylvatica;* Hahnemann preferred the *Betula alba*. Where the symptoms differ, the *Carbo fagi* is marked by an f.

Causticum.—Hahnemann's preparations are neither *Potassæ hydras*, nor *Caustic potash*, nor *Kali oxidum*, nor *Calcarea caustica*, but something which the chemists do not yet know, but we do. We know how to prepare it and what to cure with it.

Cinchona officinalis.—It is unworthy of men of science to give the Peruvian bark a name synonymous with that of a country which had nothing at all to do with it, and synonymous with that of porcelain. Such errors should never be perpetuated.

Hippomanes.—This old famous *Aphrodisiacum* of the Greek authors is taken from the colt, a meconium deposit out of the amniotic fluid, and contains *Calcarea oxalica*.

Jambos instead of *Eugenia iambos* is a rather arbitrary change, but it is made by the first and only prover, and he has his good reasons and wishes to be pardoned.

Kreosot.—To "improve" it into *Kreass*. shows ignorance of the rules of the Greek language. See H. Gross, Comp. Mat. Med., *Calcarea* and *Kreosot*. compared.

Nucis vomicæ cortex.—Since it has been decided beyond all doubts, by scientific men in Great Britain, fully able to judge, that the so-called "*Angustura falsa*" or "*spuria*" is the bark of the strychnos nux vomica tree, we should never use any name but the right one. The name *Brucea antidysenterica* is still worse; it was given by an ignorant druggist. In Bönninghausen's Repertory several symptoms have to be stricken out which do not belong to the real *Angustura*.

Pulmo vulpis.—An old and famous remedy, mentioned already by Paulus Aegineta and Avicenna. It was first recommended in our school in 1847, by Dr. J. F. Hermann, and mentioned and used by Grauvogl (Part I., p. 170).

Tabasheer.—*Silicea calami indici*, the silicious deposit in the knots of the bamboo, obtained by the favor of Mahenda lál Sircár, M.D., in Calcutta.

Vulpis hepar.—See *Pulmo vulpis*.

Wollastonite.—Crystals of tabular spar from Willsborough, N. Y., forming the sides of a large vein of garnet, traversing gneis, a natural combination of calcarea and silica. Has been triturated, proved and used since 1851 by C. Hg., and especially by Dr. Neidhard.

NOSODES

Is the general term given to the alcoholic extracts of morbid productions, foolishly called isopathic remedies. The most useful and fully proved are *Hydrophobinum* and *Psorinum*.

To these nosodes belong the *Ustilago maidis*, the *Secale cornutum*, the fungus of potatoes, the ambra of the pot-fish, the *Anthracin*, the *Vaccinin*, *Variolin* and *Medrorrhoin*, etc.

The sneering remarks of Trinks and others in 1826 against *Sepia*, and the ignorant opposition to *Lachesis* have sunken into oblivion during the succeeding score of years. All the condemning remarks against the *Hydrophobinum* and *Psorinum* will meet the same fate. We can afford to wait.

REMARKS.

Some remarks about the translation of certain words from the German Materia Medica.

East wind in the midst of Europe means a dry land wind, not like our East but more like our West wind.

West wind in Europe is the moist wind like our East. Therefore we use but "dry" or "damp" wind.

In Rio Janeiro or New Holland, the same reversion has to take place with regard to the North and South wind of this hemisphere. Hence it is given as "cold" or "warm" wind.

Bread in Germany means rye bread.

Bread and butter means sandwiches.

The German "Suppe" is not soup, but means all dishes taken with the spoon.

"Gurken" does not mean pickles, but either the raw cucumber or such as have undergone the vinous fermentation.

"Branntwein" is not our brandy, but means whisky.

With regard to names for the parts of body, different functions and the expressions for the numerous feelings and sensations, great care has been taken to avoid the palpable errors of some of the former translators.

We may expect a comparative glossary of all these words from Dr. Korndœrfer, which would be a great help to our school, as it would aid us in using for all the different feelings, as well as for the phenomena, the word nearest adapted.

ABBREVIATIONS.

Authors are only quoted when a distinction from others seems to be required. H., means Hahnemann; B., Bönninghausen; B.R., Bönninghausen's Repertory. Quotations have been given, but exceptionally.

Many cases used have never been printed before; but to all additions sent in by letter during the publication of this work, the name of the observer will be added.

Model cures have the name, if known; N.N., means Nomen Nescio.

Names of drugs are abridged throughout by the same rules given in the introduction, but sometimes, in the text, may have been shortened to save space; of course only when the margin list makes a mistake impossible, for instance *Crot.* in the text can only mean *Crotalus* if this is contained in the list and not *Croton tiglion* if this is not in the list.

MARKS AND SIGNS.

In the *margin lists* the four degrees of Bönninghausen have been distinguished by the following marks:

    I Observed on the healthy.
    II Observed often and repeatedly.
    I Applied successfully with the sick.
    II Applied very often and repeatedly.

In most margin lists the I has been omitted and appears only when it seems necessary to make a distinction from others of less value.

Sometimes intermediate or higher degrees are signified by ∥ or ∭.

Observing practitioners will often have opportunity to make additional marks of distinction, with a red or blue pencil, to the margin lists.

Other abbreviations and signs added to some of the margin lists are always explained at the head.

The margin lists ought to contain the names of all the medicines mentioned in the text; if some have been overlooked, they may be added with the pencil.

Not all the names given in the margin lists are contained in the text. Sometimes nothing more than the name is known. In all such cases diagnostic observations are very desirable.

---

r. and l., right and left side, refers to what was mentioned before or relates to the medicine following, thus it stands between the symptom and the medicine.

r. to l. or l. to r. signifies the symptoms observed *on the healthy* going from r. to l. or vice versa. If an * is added, it signifies that the symptoms went from one side to the other *with the sick* and is supposed to have been cured by the named medicine.

C.C.C., conditions, connections and concomitants.

The initials of the words in the headings are sometimes given in the text instead of the whole word.

— stands for the beginning of last paragraph, distinguished by black type.

> lessened or ameliorated by what follows.

< increased or aggravated by what follows.

a.m.m. indicates: and many more.

S. See or compare.

CONCLUSION.

All those who complain of it being too much for them, all who say "no man's brain is large enough to hold it," we refer to the pamphlet "The Last Events of 1867," Boericke, Philadelphia, pp. 20, 21, where a glance is given at the astronomer's, chemist's, botanist's and zoologist's overwhelming riches and the advice: "Look to the brain of a Dana or a Leidy, containing not only this, but a great deal more besides."

If we never learn to unite all of these symptoms, we never can arrive by careful induction at *characteristics*, which is the true Hahnemannian way.

Chapter I.

MIND AND DISPOSITION.

According to the reasons given in the schedule of the arrangement, only such symptoms of the mind can be given in this edition of Analytic Therapeutics, as have been observed *in connection with bodily symptoms*.

Every real follower of Hahnemann ought to know what he said in his Organon, from the first to the fifth editions, about the importance of the *mind symptoms*, and it is given here as an introduction, being translated by Dr. Conrad Wesselhœft. Let us all hear our great master!

HAHNEMANN'S ORGANON, FIFTH AND LAST EDITION.

§ 88. If, in his voluntary statements, the patient neglects to mention certain parts, or functions of the body, *or his state of mind*, the physician should request him to recall his observations concerning those parts, functions, or his mental and sensorial condition; but the inquiry should be pursued without putting leading questions, so that the respondent may be obliged to make special unbiased statements.

N. B. The physician should ask for example: What is your frame of mind, your moods or your power of memory.

§ 208. Next to this the physician should not overlook the patient's state of mind and temperament (Gemuethszustand), to notice if it inclines to prevent the cure; or, whether it might be necessary to direct, to favor or to modify his mental condition.

§ 211. This is true to such an extent, that the state of the patients mind and temperament (Gemuethszustand) is often of most decisive importance in the homœopathic* selection of a remedy, since it is a sign possessing a distinct peculiarity, that should least of all escape the accurate observation of the physician.

§ 212. This change of the condition of mind and disposition—the chief ingredient of all diseases—has been especially regarded by the Creator of all healing powers; for there is not a single potent medicinal substance in the world, that does not possess the power of altering perceptibly the mental state and mood of a healthy person trying the drug; indeed, *each drug affects the mind in a different manner*.

§ 213. Hence the cure would be unnatural, that is, unhomœopathic, unless we noted also the symptomatic changes of mind and temperament, occurring in every case even of acute disease, and unless there is selected from our remedies a morbific potency, which, next to the similitude of its other symptoms to those of the disease, is also capable of producing, by itself, a similar state of mind or disposition.

N. B. Thus Aconitum Napellus will rarely or *never* produce a rapid or permanent cure in a patient of calm and complacent disposition, as little as Nux vomica will affect a mild phlegmatic, or Pulsatilla a happy, cheerful but obstinate temperament; or as little as Ignatia proves efficacious in an unchangeable state of mind, inclined neither to fright or to grief.

---

* It should be noticed that Hahnemann calls the *selection* of a remedy "homœopathic"; denoting that the *method involves the principle*, though the remedy may not.   C. W.

§ 253. The condition of the mind and general behaviour of the patient are to be counted among the most certain and intelligible signs (not visible to every one) of a slight beginning of improvement or of aggravation in all diseases, especially the acute ones. The signs of incipient improvement, however slight, are: an increased sensation of comfort; greater tranquillity and freedom of mind, and heightened courage—the patient experiences, as it were, a return of naturalness. The signs of aggravation, however slight, are the opposite of the foregoing: an embarrassed, helpless state of mind and disposition, where the behaviour, attitude and actions of the patient appeal to our sympathy—a condition readily seen and appreciated by a careful observer, but not to be described in so many words.

BODILY SYMPTOMS CONNECTED WITH THE MIND.

I. Ailments from Emotions and from Exertions of the Mind.

Happy surprise. Complaints after laughing. Fright and fear. Shock of injury. Ailments the result of fear. Anxiety   Local anxiety.

Homesickness. Love pangs. Jealousy. Grief and sorrow.

Better in company or better when alone. Will not be looked at, dislikes to be spoken to. Worse from friendly persuasion, from talking of others.

Mortification. Vexation. Anger.

Emotions in general.

Worse when thinking about his condition. Better when thinking about something else.

Complaints after speaking. Complaints from thinking or meditating.

Ailings from over-exertion of mind and body.

II. Mental Concomitants of bodily Symptoms.

Head, eyes, ears, etc.

BODILY SYMPTOMS CONNECTED WITH THE MIND.

I. Ailments from Emotions and Exertions of the Mind.

HAPPY SURPRISE.
Freudige Ueberraschung.

I Acon.
Aloes.
II Coffea.
II Cinch. off.
I Coca.
Crocus.
I Cyclam.
I Gelsem.
Hyosc.
Kali carb.
Laches.
Mercur.
Natr. carb.
I Opium.
I Pulsat.
I Scutellar.

Excessive joy: **I***Acon.*, *Caustic.*, **II** *Coffea*, *Crocus*, *Cyclam.*, *Natr. carb.*, **I** *Opium*, **I** *Pulsat.*

Startled or struck by it: trembling, crying, weeping, sobbing or fainting away, even apparent death; particularly children and women: *Coffea.*

Stunned by it, laughing and crying: *Hyosc.*; talkative, with sudden changing of the subject: *Laches.*

Merry madness, with headache, blindness or pale face: *Crocus.*

Fainting: *Acon.*, *Coffea.*

Headache after mental exhilaration: *Coca*, *Coffea*; glowing red cheeks: *Mercur.*; following such or other excitement: *Scutellar.*

After it mouth was suddenly filled with bright blood: *Cinchon.*

Gagging or vomituritio: *Kali carb.*; diarrhœa: *Acon.*, *Gelsem.*

Metritis: *Coffea.*

Weeping, coughing, trembling: *Acon.*, *Mercur.*

Chilly, as of chills running over him: **I I** *Gelsem.*; shivering, flitting sensation: *Acon.*, **I** *Kali carb.*

Unusually excited by joyous news towards evening: *Aloes.*

NOTE.—If *Nitrite of amyl*, which has a sweet fruit-like odor, be inhaled, exactly the same condition results as from sudden emotions, so that one can, by diffusing a little of its vapor through a room, flush every cheek with crimson and quicken every pulse. Hence Roth recommends it as homœopathic to the effects of emotions. (*British Quarterly*.)

COMPLAINTS AFTER LAUGHING.

Mind. Easily depressed: *Formica.*

Sadness: *Phosphor.*; as if her body were borne upon wings: *Thuya.*

Headache: *Ars. met.*, *Crocus*, *Iris vers.*, *Phosphor.*, *Tongo*, *Zincum*, *Zingib.*; throbbing: *Lycop.*; beating in the head, most after sitting long: *Phosphor.*; deep shooting, right side: *Tongo.*

MIND AND DISPOSITION.

‖ Acon.	
׀ Angust.	Head internally hot, confused and heavy: *Therid.*
׀ Argent.	Tearing in right side of occiput: *Zincum.*
׀ Arsen.	**Eyes.** Obscuration of sight, dilatation of pupils: *Crocus.*
׀׀ Aurum.	
׀ Bellad.	Shedding tears: *Formica;* weeping: *Lycop.*
‖ Borax.	**Ear.** Drawing stitch from stomach into the ear: *Mangan.*
Bryon.	
׀׀ Carb. veg.	**Face.** Heat and redness of cheeks: *Veratr.*
׀׀ Cinch. off.	Paleness: *Crocus;* stiff jaws: *Formica;* jerking stitches from lower jaw to region above the temple: *Mangan.*
׀ Coloc.	
׀ Conium.	
Crocus.	
Cuprum.	Toothache in upper molar, afternoon: *Tongo.*
Droser.	**Abdomen.** Stitches around the ribs in the left side: *Acon.;* right side of abdomen like a fine jerking: *Kali carb.;* digging and rooting around the navel, also when exhaling: *Coloc.*
Formica.	
Hepar.	
׀׀ Kali carb.	
Laches.	
׀ Lauroc.	Pain in belly: *Conium;* digging, rooting colic: *Coloc.;* sore pain, also with coughing: *Arsen.*
Lycop.	
׀ Mangan.	
׀ Mezer.	Aching pressure in the region of the hernia: *Sepia.*
׀ Mur. ac.	
׀ Natr. mur.	Stitches in mamma: *Lauroc.*
Nitr. ac.	**Chest.** Slime in windpipe and cough: *Argent.*
Nux mosch.	
׀ Nux vom.	Asthma: *Arsen., Aurum, Cuprum.*
‖ Phosphor.	Dyspnœa: ׀Arsen., Aurum, Cuprum, ׀׀Laches., Lycop., Plumbum.*
Platin.	
׀ Plumbum.	
Sepia.	Cough: ׀Argent., Arsen., Bryon., Cinch. off., Cuprum, Drosera, ׀Laches., Kali carb., Mur. ac., Nitr. ac., ׀Phosphor., ׀Stannum, Zincum.*
׀ Stannum.	
Veratr.	
׀ Zincum.	

Pressing, like from a piece of wood, in left side of chest: *Plumbum;* stitch: *Mezer.;* pressing: *Platin.;* pain: *Lauroc., Lycop., Mezer., Mur. ac., Plumbum,* ׀׀*Stannum.*

Limbs. Hot hands: *Veratr.;* weakness of muscles of arms and hands: *Carb. veg.*

Relaxation: *Calc. ostr., Conium;* great debility, prostration, collapse, *Crocus.*

Does not sleep: *Veratr.*

Worse in open air: *Nux mosch.*

Stitches in the ulcer: *Hepar s. c.*

FRIGHT AND FEAR.
Schreck.

Fright. Every little surprise frightens him; trembling and glowing red cheeks: *Mercur.*

With fear and anxiety. See margin list.

With vexation: ׀׀*Acon.,* ׀*Bellad.,* ׀׀*Calc. ostr.,* ׀*Coccul.,* ׀׀*Cuprum,* ׀*Gelsem.,* ׀׀*Ignat.,* ׀׀*Natr. carb.,* ׀*Nux vom.,* ׀*Opium,* ׀׀*Petrol.,* ׀*Phosphor.,* ׀*Platin.,* ׀*Pulsat.,* ׀*Sambuc.,* ׀*Sepia,* ׀׀*Sulphur,* ׀*Zincum.*

For other emotions following, see their respective pages.

Terror: *Gelsem., Nux vom., Opium, Silic., Verat.*

FRIGHT AND FEAR. 73

|| Acon.
| Anac.
|| Apis.
|| Arnic.
|| Arsen.
| Aurum.
|| Bellad.
|| Bryon.
| Calc. ostr.
| Carb. veg.
| Caustic.
|| Chamom.
| Cicuta.
Coccul.
| Coffea.
|| Cuprum.
|| Gelsem.
|| Glonoin.
| Graphit.
| Hepar.
| Hyosc.
|| Ignat.
|| Laches.
| Lauroc.
|| Lycop.
|| Mercur.
Mur. ac.
Natr. carb.
|| Natr. mur.
| Nux mosch.
| Nux vom.
|| Opium.
Petrol.
|| Phosph.
|| Platin.
|| Pulsat.
| Rhus tox.
|| Sambuc.
|| Secale.
| Sepia.
| Silic.
| Spongia.
| Stannum.
|| Stramon.
| Sulphur.
|| Veratr.
| Verbasc.
|| Zincum.

After sudden noises, as if thunder-struck, unconscious, convulsions, twitching around mouth; hot, red face, feces pass involuntarily: *Opium;* incessant screaming after a heavy thunderclap: *Gelsem.;* often cries without a cause: *Rhus tox.*

After fright: Soon *Opium,* later *Acon.;* fear remaining: *Mercur., Natr. mur., Bellad.,* I *Verat.;* fear: | *Opium, Sambuc.;* fear and anger: *Acon.;* fear and anxiety: *Lycop.;* sorrow: *Ignat.*

Long remaining anxiousness: *Bellad., Laches., Mercur., Sambuc., Silic.*

— and weakness, cannot sleep from frightful visions, night full of complaints, wants to go out doors, far away: *Mercur.*

—, timidity and nightly complaints: *Mercur.*

— and loss of reason, frightful visions, wants to run away, rush of blood to head, headache rising from the neck up, widened pupils: *Bellad.*

Mind. Insanity: *Bellad., Laches., Mercur., Platin., Stramon.* Raving madness: *Bellad., Stramon.;* loss of reason, talks confusedly as if insane, pain going through the neck up into the head, widened pupils, red burning hot face, or pale and moist, nose dry, neck and throat sore to the touch, fears things he sees: *Bellad.;* talking, preaching, telling stories, greatest sensitiveness of throat or other parts to the touch even of light clothing: *Laches.;* often cries out without a cause: *Rhus tox.;* maniacal notions, starting in sleep, laughing in sleep, convulsions in sleep, spasmodic cough: *Hyosc.;* insanity with laughable jests: *Bellad.;* loss of reason, things appear smaller, sadness in the evening or haughtiness, things appear larger: *Platin.;* delirium with fearful visions: *Bellad., Sambuc.;* delusions of the imagination: *Bellad.;* imagines people find fault with her: *Rhus tox.*

Indifference or contempt of others; fear of the near approach of death, very sad; mostly in the evening: *Platin.*

Melancholy: *Stramon.*

Horror, full of apprehensions, lamed: *Natr. mur.*

Fearful imaginations, particularly at night; cannot bear the warmth of bed; wants to run away, travel; quarrels with family; complaints about others: *Mercur.*

Despair of eternal salvation of soul: *Stramon.;* crying, howling and getting beside himself: *Coffea.*

Children weep, move arms and hands about: *Sambuc.;* very much dejected and lachrymose, particularly in the evening: *Platin.;* pride and contempt of others: *Platin.;* discontent, complains of everything, the whole world: *Mercur.*

Disposition to quarrel: *Mercur.;* to escape in the night: *Bellad., Mercur., Hyosc.*

Sensorium. Over-sensitiveness of the organs of the senses: *Coffea.*

Unconsciousness: *Opium;* stupor: *Bellad.;* stupor with internal heat: *Opium.*

Fainting: *Acon., Coffea;* apparent death, neither pulse nor breathing perceptible, after a pain in heart from fright with grief: *Laches.*

Head. Rush of blood to the head: *Opium*, later: *Acon.*, still later: *Bellad.*; beating in temple if head is in a low position: I *Rhus tox.*; heat in it: *Bellad.*; heat with stupor: *Opium;* hot with twitching about the mouth: *Opium;* pain in the forehead: *Opium;* heavy feeling: *Rhus tox.*

Pain passes into the head through the nape of the neck: *Bellad.*; stitches in the left side of head: *Cicuta.*

Eyes. Objects around him appear smaller: *Platin.*

Eyes dim, shunning the light: *Rhus tox.*

Cannot see, twitches and starts: *Opium, Glonoin.*; loss of sight, relaxed, sinking together, deadly pale: *Glonoin.*; enlarged pupils: *Bellad.*; and darkening of sight: *Opium;* squinting and rolling of the eyes: *Hyosc.*

Nose. Dryness of the nose: *Bellad.*; fluent coryza: *Mercur.*

Face. Red: *Platin.*; and burning: *Bellad., Opium;* glowing red cheeks: *Mercur.*

After trouble a glowing heat rises in the right cheek; it swells and turns bluish red for two hours, followed by restlessness and shaking chill: *Mercur.*

Red, turns deadly pale in sitting up: *Acon.*; red in bed, getting up instantly pale: *Veratr.*

Bluish, bloated with snoring: *Opium;* with wheezing: *Sambuc.*

Changing pale and red, rising headache, loses sight, sinking, relaxed, twitching, fingers or toes spread out: *Glonoin.*; twitching around the mouth: *Glonoin., Opium;* foam at the mouth: *Hyosc.*

Mouth. Offensive breath and saliva: *Merc.*

When swallowing danger of choking, cramp in the throat: *Bellad.*

Stomach. Aversion to food: *Platin.*

No thirst: *Pulsat.*

Weak digestion and continual hunger: *Mercur.*

Complaints from eating fat food: *Pulsat;* sour eructations, vomiting: *Opium.*

Stitches in pit of stomach: *Rhus tox.*; — after it suffocating sensation: *Sambuc.*; and gastric complaints: *Acon.*

Abdomen. Heaviness in abdomen with long-lasting anxiety: *Mercur.*

Stitches from abdomen up to the chest: *Chamom.*; motions in bowels: *Rhus tox.*

Diarrhœa: *Opium, Gelsem., Veratr.*; returning with every new fear: *Acon.*; returning at twilight: *Pulsat.*; often at night, painless, much wind: *Ignat.*; with tenesmus: *Mercur.*; outer coldness, inner heat without thirst: *Pulsat.*; involuntary escape of stool: *Opium;* after it very cold: *Rhus tox.*; with icy coldness of the body: *Veratr.*; retention of stool: *Bellad.*

Urine. Frequent and great discharge: *Sambuc.*

Involuntary escape of urine and stool: *Hyosc.*

Retention: *Bellad., Opium.*

Sexual Organs. Metritis: *Opium;* catamenia too soon and too copious: *Platin.*; too late and too weak: *Pulsat.*; to prevent suppression: *Acon.*

Amenorrhœa: *Acon., Lycop.*; displacement of uterus: *Opium.*

During pregnancy diarrhœa: *Opium;* hemorrhage: *Secale.*

Threatened abortion: *Acon., Gelsem., Opium.*

Suppression of labor pains: *Opium;* of lochia: *Ignat., Opium.*
Chorea returning in child-bed: *Stramon.;* spasms: *Secale.*
Chest. Pain in the larynx when touched: *Bellad.*
Wheezing breathing: *Sambuc.*
Takes his breath away and fills him with great fear: *Opium.*
Suffocation with anxiety: *Opium;* after vomiting coughing: *Sambuc.;* with violent pains in stomach and scrobiculum: *Acon.*
Convulsive choking spells in the night, with crying and grasping about: *Sambuc.;* struggle for breath, points to pit of stomach; after Opium: *Acon.;* suffocation after vomiting or some coughing, bluish puffed-up face, anxious trembling and whining, gasping, heat without thirst: *Sambuc.*
Bluish face in morning: *Opium;* ice-cold chest: *Veratr.;* loses breath with even a little cough: *Sambuc.*
Dry spasmodic cough: *Bellad.;* in the night: *Hyosc.*
Whooping cough: *Acon., Ignat., Stramon.*
Coughs when lying down, with stitches in pit of stomach: *Rhus tox.;* ebullitions of blood with trembling of limbs: *Sambuc.*
Trembling of the heart, palpitation: *Nux mosch.,* violent and anxious: *Bellad.,* most in the evening and when sitting: *Pulsat.*

Back and Limbs. Stiff: *Ignat.;* children move arms and hands about and weep: *Sambuc.;* stitching in the elbow-joint, later on a place rubbed open on the foot: *Phosphor.;* knocking of knees: *Cinnab., Mercur.*
Spreading the fingers: *Glonoin.;* swelling of the feet in evening: *Pulsat.*
Trembling and twitching of the limbs: *Opium.*
Tearing pain at night: *Mercur.*
Aching in arms and legs, the limbs very languid; sleepy: *Calc. phosph.*
Limbs become numb and torpid: *Opium.*
Heaviness and lameness of the limbs: *Bellad.;* lameness of left arm and foot, disappearing over night: *Stramon.;* worse when the body is at rest: *Pulsat.*
Twitchings. With anxiety: *Veratr.;* loss of consciousness: *Opium;* wild thrashing about with hands and feet: *Hyosc.;* coldness: *Opium, Veratr.,* around the mouth: *Opium;* starting, with stiff back: *Ignat.;* chorea: *Stramon.*
Convulsions: *Bellad., Hyosc., Ignat., Opium,* ❙*Stramon., Sulphur;* with a loud scream: *Opium;*— and head hot: *Opium,* then *Bellad.;* red face: *Opium, Bellad.;* pale face: *Ignat.;* twitchings in face: *Opium;* froth on mouth: *Hyosc.;* involuntary stools: *Veratr.;* trembling: *Opium;* laughing in sleep: *Hyosc.;* coldness: *Veratr., Opium;* copious sweat: *Opium, Bellad.*
Convulsions of children, with starts: *Opium;* in sleep: ❙*Ignat.*
Tonic spasms, the whole body stiff: *Opium;* epileptic attacks: *Cuprum, Hyosc., Stramon.,* ❙*Sulphur.*
Trembling: ❙*Coffea., Glonoin., Ignat., Mercur., Opium;* — and difficult breathing: *Glonoin., Ignat., Opium;* after slight exertions: *Mercur.*
Debility. Weakness: *Coffea, Mercur., Opium;* after slight exertions: *Mercur.;* with cold sweat: *Opium;* fainting: *Opium;* lasting very long: *Laches.*
Sleep. Prevented by fearful visions: *Mercur.;* goes to sleep late in the evening, and is restless during the night: *Pulsat.;* stupor-like somnolence with

snoring: *Opium;* coma vigil., *Hyosc.;* snoring: *Opium;* wheezing: *Sambuc.;* laughing: *Hyosc.;* starting: *Hyosc.;* worse at night, anxiety and other complaints: *Mercur.;* worse in the evening: *Bellad., Pulsat.*

Warmth. Worse in bed: *Mercur.;* in a warm room: *Pulsat.;* better in open air: *Pulsat.*

Chill. Chilly hands and feet: *Rhus tox.;* chilliness, as if having been drenched with cold water: *Mercur.;* external coldness of body, and inner heat: *Pulsat.;* alternating attacks of chill, heat and sweat, for 24 hours: *Lycop.;* heat without thirst: *Sambuc., Pulsat.;* inflammatory fever: *Acon.*

Pains. Unbearable, as if driving to distraction: *Coffea.*

An ulcer on the hand appeared after Lachesis, was aggravated by fright and cured by *Silic.*

Genteel, timid and lachrymose disposition: *Pulsat.*

If a sudden fright interrupts the good effects of other medicines: *Laches.*

MODEL CURES.

A little girl was accidentally wounded by a pistol. *Her mother* suffered mental shock, paleness and faintness, especially on attempting to sit up; great concern for the result. Relieved after a dose of *Acon.*⁶—J. C. MORGAN.

A young lady had seen the residence of her lover struck by lightning. At the approach of another thunderstorm, she was greatly distressed, with apprehensive feeling. After a dose of *Gelsem.*¹ᵐ she forgot all about it and disregarded the storm.—J. C. MORGAN.

After fright—heavy feeling in the forehead. A week later she told her mother not to look at her; seems to be distrustful, and does not want to see anyone. She came running in from the street, and said people were looking at her. She sat quietly and alone; her eyes were dim, and she shunned the light. Since this time, the symptoms have returned three times, lasting six weeks each time. This time it has lasted eight weeks, the symptoms just as before, but without the complaints of the eyes. She often cries without cause—imagines people are finding fault with her because she is earning nothing—acts in a childish manner. At the same time heaviness of the head, when the head is in a low position; beating in the temple on which she is lying. After taking cold, diarrhœa. For the past week, coughed when lying down, with stitches in the pit of the stomach; chilly hands and feet; frequent motion in the bowels. *Rhus tox.*—HARTLAUB.

SHOCK OF INJURY.

According to Dr. J. C. Morgan, J. H. M. M., v. V., p. 73 and p. 102, and later communications. It strictly belongs to chapter 45, but is placed here next to mental shocks on account of its great usefulness in this connection. Additions by C. Hg., marked *.

Mind. Injury followed by one fixed and anxious idea of impending death or other dire misfortune: *Acon.*

Anxiety as from conscious danger of death: *Capsic.*

SHOCK OF INJURY. 77

I Acet. ac.*
I Aconit.
I Alcohol.
I Amm. carb.
I Arnica.
II Arsen.
I Calam.
II Camphor.
II Capsic.
II Carb. veg.
I Chamom.
II Cinch. off.
I Chlorof.
II Coffea.
I Cuprum.
I Digit.
II Gelsem.
I Hepar s. c.
I Hydr. ac.
II Ipecac.
I Laches..
II Mercur.
I Natr. mur.
I Nitr. ac.*
II Nux mosch.
I Nux vom.
I Opium.
I Phosphor.
I Pulsat.
I Sec. corn.
II Staphis.*
I Strontian.
I Sulphur.
I Tabac.
II Veratr.

Anguish: *Nux vom.;* with great distress and oppression, despairs of life: *Veratr.;* anxious manner: *Cinch. off.;* after fright: *Opium,* afterwards, *Aconit.;* after sudden, unexpected severe injury: *Camphor.*

Fear of injury: *Gelsem.;* afraid of the surgeon: *Coffea;* of being hurt by persons walking towards him: I *Arnica.**

Overpowering fear, with fatigue: *Gelsem.*

Terror: *Veratr.;* memory of horror: *Gelsem.*

After over-excitement, want of food, exposure: *Alcohol.*

After crushing losses of dearest friends: I *Nitr. ac.**

Following depressing emotions: *Alcohol.*

Intolerance of impressions and of oppositions: *Acon.;* — of all manipulations, they cause great agitation, which interferes with treatment: *Coffea,* — and mental urgency: *Chamom.*

Not to be pacified: *Acon.*

Rather quiet when left alone: *Coffea.*

Great forgetfulness: *Strontian.*

Weeping over his bad luck: *Pulsat.;* preoccupied with lamentations: *Chamom.;* delirium, will dress himself to go home: *Cuprum;* unconscious muttering of anxious sort: *Gelsem.*

Nervous anxiety, mingled with stupefaction of mind: *Camphor.;* increasing stupor: *Laches.;* hardly yielding to any stimuli: *Carb. veg.*

Sensorium. Excessively keen senses: *Acon.;* great sensibility, mental and physical: *Coffea.*

Feels nervous, as if he would fly: *Veratr.*

Vertigo: *Hepar s. c., Nux vom.;* giddiness: *Tabac.;* giddiness and blindness: *Laches.;* with sickness at the stomach, vanishing of sense: *Sulphur.*

Unconsciousness: *Arnica, Chlorof., Opium;* stupefied and cold: *Camphor.;* apoplectic dreaminess: *Nux mosch.*

Faintness: *Sulphur;* from slight causes: *Nux vom.;* from a little pain, is preceded by vertigo: *Hepar s. c.;* on rising: *Acon.*

Syncope immediately after great hemorrhage: II *Calam.;* long lasting syncope: *Hydr. ac.*

Headache after fainting: *Hepar s. c.*

Head. Chronic effects after an injury of the head, such as headache, relieved by sweating: *Natr. mur.*

Paralysis of brain, with symptoms of collapse: *Cuprum.*

Eyes. Bright colors appear before the vision: *Strontian.;* optical illusions: *Digit.*

Loss of vision and hearing: *Carb. veg.*

Pupils dilated: *Hydr. ac., Ipecac.;* inactive: *Digit.*

Eyes fixed unequally: *Opium:* eyelids paralyzed: *Hydr. ac.;* dark areola around: *Laches.;* sunken, with dark margins: *Sulphur.*

Ears. Worse on going to bed, with ringing and roaring in the ears: *Natr. mur.;* want of hearing: *Carb. veg.*

Nose. Nose, ears and forehead very cold: *Laches.*

Face. Distorted features: *Hydr. ac.;* wretched expression: *Sulphur;* motionless features: *Chlorof.;* pallor: *Arnica, Opium, Ipecac.;* pale and sick, pale and languid: *Gelsem.;* pale and weak: *Amm. caust.;* livid: *Opium;* lividly pale: *Camphor.;* bluish paleness: *Digit.*

Bluish face: *Sulphur;* very pale or ghastly: *Cinch. off.;* pale, livid, deathlike: *Veratr.;* hippocratic: *Arsen., Carb. veg.;* cadaverous: *Phosphor.*

Lips. Bluish: *Camphor.;* livid: *Opium.*

Talk. Indisposed to talk: *Pulsat.;* aggravated by it, and by touch: *Chamom.;* speechlessness: *Veratr.*

Mouth. Sticky: *Pulsat.*

Thirst: *Acon., Veratr.;* for little water, and often: **I***Arsen.;* cold water: **II** *Veratr.;* for acids: *Sec. corn.;* with collapse: *Natr. mur.;* no thirst: *Pulsat.*

Appetite. With such as possess a good deal of natural force, and habitually abuse their digestive organs by food or drink: *Nux vom.;* if addicted to the use of liquor: *Alcohol.*

Gastrics. Hiccough: *Hydr. ac., *Nux mosch., Veratr.*

Sickness at stomach: *Cuprum;* nausea: *Ipecac., Pulsat.;* constant deathly nausea: *Tabac.;* loathing of food: *Pulsat.*

Vomiting: *Ipecac., Veratr.;* copious, easy, gushing: *Phosphor.;* especially on moving, better after moving: *Tabac.*

Vomits drink instantly after swallowing: *Arsen.;* as soon as it gets warm in the stomach: *Phosphor.;* vomiting is a good sign after *Arnica.*

Stomach. Deathly feeling behind ensiform cartilage: *Cuprum.*

In gunshot concussion of the stomach after the failure of whiskey: *Amm. caust.*

Abdomen. Colic: *Ipecac.;* colic after cutting a stone out; a fatal symptom, according to George McClellan, was cured in a few minutes by **I***Staphis.**

Struck by a spent ball in the epigastrium: *Amm. caust.*

Abdomen feels cold: *Veratr.;* flatulence: *Nux vom.*

Stool. Tendency to diarrhœa: *Camphor., Gelsem.*

Diarrhœa: *Ipecac., Nux mosch., Veratr.;* very watery, even involuntary: *Sec. corn.;* colliquative, cadaverous odor: *Carb. veg.;* visceral hemorrhage: *Veratr.*

Urine. Shuddering all over with desire to urinate: *Hyper.;* retention: *Hyper.;* suppression: *Sec. corn.*

Sexuals. Emissions next night, very weakening: I *Acet. ac.**

Larynx. Hollow hoarse voice: *Sec. corn.*

Breathing. Rapid breathing, every breath being a loud moan: *Opium.*

Moaning: *Sec. corn.;* groaning: *Chamom.;* sighing: *Cuprum;* incessant sighing: *Laches.*

Respirations few and sighing: *Camphor.;* involuntary deep inspirations: *Hepar s. c.;* heavy anxious breathing: *Sec. corn.*

Rale, the throat emitting the sound of the letter k in inspiration (tubular breathing): *Opium* (one dose high).

SHOCK OF INJURY.

Rattling: *Carb. veg.;* and slow: *Nux mosch.;* and moaning: *Hydr. ac.;* respirations almost stopped, so few and feeble: *Chlorof.;* feeble: *Amm. caust.*

Rolling from one side to the other, at intervals, trying to get a good breath: *Cuprum.;* exhaled air is cool: ‖ *Carb. veg.**

Suffocating feeling in the air passages: *Ipecac.*

Oppression from pit of stomach to chest: *Nux vom.*

"Felt the wind knocked out of him:" *Amm. caust.*

Chest. Anguish, and pressure on it: *Hydr. ac.*

In gun-shot wound of lung: *Amm. caust.*

Heart. Sensation as if the blood flowed warm from it: *Cinch. off.*

Palpitation awaking: *Mercur.;* internal congestion: *Acon.*

Blood feels like cold water in the vessel: *Veratr.;* stagnant circulation: *Carb. veg.*

Sinking feeling at the heart as if dying: *Mercur.*

Pulse. Slow and small: *Digit., Sec. corn.;* — and weak: *Arnica, Mercur.;* — and feeble and irregular: *Tabac.*

Intermitting: *Natr. mur.;* by regular intermission every other beat, apparently slow: ▌*Digit.**

Pulse feeble; *Camphor.;* as if dying: *Chlorof.*

— thready: *Arsen.;* and frequent: *Cuprum;* and tense: *Acon.*

Dying away: *Laches.;* almost imperceptible: *Capsic.;* weak, slow, scarcely perceptible: *Veratr.;* failing: *Cinch. off.*

Frequent and scarcely perceptible: *Carb. veg.;* nearly extinct: *Hydr. ac.*

Back. Aching: *Gelsem.*

— chilly especially externally: *Capsic.*

Injuries of the vertebral region: *Hyper.*

Limbs. Numbness and tingling: *Veratr.*

— feel weak and bruised: *Hepar s. c.;* aching: *Gelsem.*

— cold: *Sulphur;* feet: *Acon.;* — livid: *Chlorof.*

Cold hands and feet, which are dripping with cold sweat: *Ipec.*

Deadness of fingers and toes: *Sec. corn.*

Motion. The least exertion causes great weakness and sleepiness: *Nux mosch.*

Worse by moving or rising: *Arnica.*

Dreads motion or uncovering; uneasy: *Nux vom.*

Position. Wants the head low: *Arnica;* lying with body and limbs doubled up: *Laches.*

Rest. Better by lying still: *Arnica.*

Having led a sedentary life, wants rest and to be covered: *Nux vom.*

Nerves. Nervous agitation: *Cinch. off.;* very irritable: *Hepar s. c.*

Restlessness: *Arsen.;* active and obstinate: *Acon.*

Trembling: *Strontian., Veratr.;* readily excited to it: *Hepar s. c.;* especially on moving: *Sulphur;* from slight exertions: *Mercur.;* on awaking: *Mercur.*

Cramps: *Nux vom.;* convulsions: *Opium.*

Apparently lifeless state, with occasional convulsive movements, followed by greenish vomiting: *Phosphor.*

Weariness: *Sulphur;* feeling of great weakness: *Camphor., Veratr.*

Wants to lie down: *Amm. caust.;* and inertia: *Pulsat.;* debility: *Strontian.*
Faintness, with sweat: *Digit.*
Great relaxation: *Tabac;* with vertigo, fainting: ❙❙*Acet. ac.**
Inertia from over exertion: *Alcohol.*
Sense of great fatigue, with angry despondency: *Nux vom.;* exhaustion: *Gelsem.*
After continued or repeated hemorrhage, prostration: *Cinch. off.*
Prostration: *Ipecac.,* ❙❙*Sec. corn.*
Sometimes a limp prostration, preceded by spasmodic symptoms: *Cuprum.*
Great prostration after a gunshot wound of the lungs: *Amm. caust.*

Collapse. Tendency to collapse, as in cholera: *Arsen.;* threatened collapse, with intermitting pulse and great thirst: *Natr. mur.;* impending death by it: *Opium* (one dose high); from progress of inflammatory lesion: *Opium* (repeated lower doses).

Sleep. Yawning: *Veratr.;* rapid yawning: *Laches.*
Disposed to doze: *Sulphur;* drowsiness: *Gelsem.;* constant sleepiness: ❙❙*Nux mosch., Arnica, Opium.*
Could not get asleep, wide awake: *Coffea.*
Sleepless so long as any noise or light continues at night: *Coffea.*
Jerking of limbs when beginning to sleep: *Sulphur.*
On awaking from a doze, trembling as if frightened, with palpitation: *Mercur.;* dreams of horrible things, as robbers, fire, murder, etc.: *Natr. mur.*
After loss of sleep: *Nux vom.*

Warmth. Wants to be covered up warmly: *Arnica;* and rest: *Nux vom.*
Wants to be uncovered, but the skin is clammy and cold: *Sec. corn.*
Skin cool and sensitive to exposure: *Nux mosch.*
Dreads uncovering: *Nux vom.;* cannot bear a breath of cool air: *Arsen.*
Desires to keep warm: *Strontian.;* wants external heat: *Arsen.*
Pain better from hot application: *Chamom.*
Cannot bear the heat: *Sec. corn.;* cannot bear a warm room: *Pulsat.*
Sluggish manner, as in cold weather, is often seen in persons who have been exposed: *Capsic.*
"Ragged philosophers" who have been much exposed: *Sulphur.*

Chill. Internal shivering from below upwards: *Hepar s. c.*
Chilliness: *Ipecac.;* when uncovered: *Acon.;* increased by drinking: *Veratr.*
General coldness: *Hydr. ac.;* cold and stupefied: *Camphor.;* whole body cold, except the head and face: *Arnica;* most in hands and feet: ❙❙*Veratr.;* especially the legs: *Tabac.*
Whole surface cold and clammy: *Camphor., Capsic., Opium.*
Dry heat after much bruising or sprains: ❙*Acet. ac.**
Can scarcely perspire: *Cinch. off.*
Sweat: *Mercur.;* cold: *Carb. veg., Nux vom., Tabac.;* most in the face: *Veratr.*
Cold, sticky sweat: *Pulsat.*
All over forehead and limbs; sweats when being cold: *Chamom.*
Semi-lateral (r. s.) affections: *Strontian.*

SHOCK OF INJURY.

Pains. "Unstrung" by the pain: *Chamom.*
Extreme pain, with delirium: *Veratr.*
They overcome every thought of civility: *Chamom.*
— especially during aggravation make chilly, but cannot bear a warm room: *Pulsat.;* rheumatic: *Strontian.;* aching, shifting or constant: *Pulsat.;* burning and as if torn: *Chamom.;* burning internally: *Capsic.*

Tissues. Hæmorrhage: *Arnica;* of bright blood: *Ipec., Phosphor.;* of dark blood: *Cinch. off., Nux vom.*
Sequelæ of hemorrhage: *Strontian.;* emaciation: *Strontian.*
When nervous tissues are mainly concerned: *Hyosc.;* tissues of organic life: *Amm. caust.*
Injuries of the tissues of animal life generally, of the feet, the hands, etc.: *Hyper.*
In grave cases, with internal congestions; if in the head, stupor; if in the cheek, stitching pains; if in the abdomen, great tenderness, etc.: *Acon.*
Wherever localized, there is a marked general *uneasiness* and apparent discontent, amounting often to restlessness of a distressing kind; usually thirsty, if conscious; like symptoms to those of Acon., but in *bilious constitutions: Veratr. vir.*

Touch. Fear of: *Arnica;* worse from: *Chamom.;* could not bear to have the broken limb handled: *Coffea.*
Concussion and bruising: *Arnica.*
To prevent bad effects following surgical operations: *Acon.;* cuts by the knife: *Staphis.**
Marked, punctured or torn wounds, lacerations of skin: *Hyper.*
If moved in bed or seat, a very small motion seems to him immensely large: ⅠCoffea.*

Skin. Pale: *Amm. caust.;* moist, cold: *Chamom.;* dry, pinched, cold, livid: *Arsen.;* shrivelled, livid: *Laches.*
Better as soon as an itching begins: ⅠⅠ*Strontian.**
Slovenly people craving spirituous liquors: *Sulphur.*
After allopathic drugging: *Nux vom.*
Liqu. ammon., U. S. Ph., has been useful when taken in drop doses.

Spir. nitr. dulc. might be given according to Hahnemann's direction, how to apply it in typhoid fevers. See Chapt. 40.

According to Dr. J. C. Morgan, the same indications may be used in other forms of collapse, *i. e.:* in the so-called pernicious or malignant intermittent, congestive chills; the symptoms before or after death bear a great likeness. Hence the indications for Lachesis are taken from such a case, and the Cuprum arseniosum, to be relied on in such cases, according to Dr. Eggert of Indianapolis, might also be given in bad cases of "shock."

Acet. ac. is antidote *par excellence* to all anæsthetic vapors; a finger dipped in vinegar rubbed within the lips.—J. C. M.

Ipec. after it if remaining pale and sick, no vomiting but still nauseated and weak.

Model cures, by J. C. M. See end of this Division, page 109.

AILMENTS OWING TO FEAR.

Acon.
Arsen.
Aurum.
! I Bellad.
Calc. ostr.
I Carb. veg.
I Gelsem.
Glonoin.
Hydroph.
Hyosc.
II Lycop.
Natr. mur.
Nux vom.
I Opium.
Platin.
Pulsat.
Rhus tox.
Sulphur.
II Veratr.

"See after a fright."
Continuing fearfulness in the evening: *Acon.* or *Pulsat.*
In the night or the morning: *Bellad.*
Fear of being alone: *Arsen.*
Fear of people: *Pulsat.*
Sees dead bodies: *Arsen.;* imagines thieves to be in the house: *Natr. mur.*
Diarrhœa from fear: *Gelsem.;* cold and trembling: *Veratr.*
Inner heat, outer cold: *Pulsat.*
Body hot, limbs cold: *Pulsat.*
Head hot: *Opium.*
Spasmodic complaints, laughing in sleep, wants to run away: *Hyosc.*

After fear and great anxiety: I *Silic.*

Fear, grief and great sadness in children after punishment; if brought to bed too soon get convulsions in sleep: I*Ignat.;* in case the back is stiff, with twitching and starting and Opium did not help: I*Ignat.*

Suffering from fear of hydrophobia after the bite of a dog, mad or not, or without ever having been bitten: *Hydroph.*

Fear of apoplexy, see Chapter 2.

AFTER ANXIETY.

Anxiety is a frequent concomitant symptom. Causticum has it with all bodily sufferings. Chapter 28, Chest, and 29, Heart, will contain most, next to them Chapter 27, Sleep, and 40, Fevers.

The margin list is analyzed by giving the local observations first, and afterwards the few instances in which other symptoms follow after anxiety.

Anxiety apparently originating in the head: *Apis*, II *Cicuta,* II*Lauroc., Magn. carb., Natr. carb., Phosphor., Psorin., Sarsap.,* II *Thuya.*

In chest, heart and præcordia: II*Acon.,* I*Arsen.,* (also abdominal,) *Calc. ostr., Lycop., Pulsat., Veratr.;* from chest to head: *Acon.*

Pectoral and cardiac: *Nitr. ac., Platin.,* (also abdominal,) *Plumbum, Zincum.*

Pectoral and præcordial: *Arnica, Calc. ac., Colchic., Crot. tigl., Gran. cort.,* (and abdominal,) *Hydr. ac., Ignat., Lauroc., Natr. mur., Nux vom., Phosphor., Sulphur,* (and abdominal.)

Cardiac, præcordial and abdominal: *Cuprum.*

Pectoral and abdominal: *Alum., Ar. mac., Arsen., Platin., Gran. cort.,* and others mentioned above.

Cardiac and abdominal: *Arsen., Cuprum, Platin.*

Præcordial and abdominal: *Gran. cort.*

Pectoral: *Amm. gum., Capsic., Carb. an., Chelid., Cop. bals., Ferrum, Ginseng, Jodium, Kali carb., Mercur., Mezer., Nitrum, Oleand., Opium, Phosph. ac., Pimpin., Pothos., Prun. spin.*

AFTER ANXIETY.

|| Acon.
Alum.
Apis.
| Arnic.
|| Arsen.
|| Aurum.
| Bellad.
|| Bryon.
| Calc. ostr.
|| Caustic.
| Chamom.
Cicuta.
|| Coccul.
Coffea.
|| Cuprum.
| Digit.
Hydroph.
|| Hyosc.
|| Ignat.
|| Laches.
Lauroc.
|| Lycop.
| Mercur.
| Natr. carb.
Natr. mur.
|| Nux vom.
| Opium.
Petrol.
Phosphor.
Phosph. ac.
| Platin.
Psorin.
| Pulsat.
Raphan.
|| Rhus tox.
Sambuc.
Sarsap.
|| Sepia.
Stannum.
|| Stramon.
|| Sulphur.
Thuya.
|| Veratr.

Cardiac: *Ambra., Ant. tart.,* ||*Aurum.,* ||*Bellad., Bromum,* ||*Calc. ostr., Camphor., Canthar., Castor., Caustic., Crocus., Cuprum, Evon., Hæmatox., Magn. mur., Merc. peren., Platin., Spigel., Stramon., Viol. tric.*

Præcordial: *Anac., Bovist., Cannab., Cicut., Cinch. off., Conium, Digit., Droser., Helleb., Hydr. ac., Lactuc., Pulsat., Stannum, Stramon., Thea., Thuya;* left side only: *Phosphor.*

Abdominal: *Amm. mur., Bryon., Calend., Carb. veg.,* |*Chamom.,* |*Cuprum,* |*Euphorb., Moschus, Mur. ac., Rhus tox., Scilla, Sulph. ac.*

Rising up in throat: *Arum mac.;* with heat: *Hyper.;* in chest: *Arum mac.;* from the stomach: *Calc. ac.;* from the hypochondria: *Droser.;* from region of heart: *Arsen., Bellad., Crocus., Cuprum.*

First in head, then in whole body: *Sarsap.*

Originating in upper part of chest: *Arsen., Arum mac.*

As if in the blood: *Mercur., Sepia.*

Mind. Against her will she has to call for somebody: *Thuya.*

Anxiety, with screaming: *Calc. ostr., Chin. sulph., Coccul.,* |*Hyosc.,* |*Lycop., Ran. scel.;* with moaning: |*Acon., Alum., Ant. tart., Arsen.,* |*Chamom., Paris, Phosphor., Rheum.*

Followed by weeping: *Acon., Amm. mur., Carb. veg.*

Fears the dark, desires to look into light: *Calc. ostr.*

Sensorium. A confusedness before the eyes: *Psorin.*

Fainting, interrupts cardiac anxiety: *Arsen.*

Frequently falls into syncope: *Arsen.*

Head. Aches: *Æther, Æthus., Arnic., Zinc.;* hot: *Phosphor.*

Face. Hot: *Carb. veg., Mercur.;* red: *Sepia.*

Sweat: *Arsen., Coccul., Mur. ac., Natr. carb.;* cold sweat: *Arsen., Mur. ac.,* on forehead: *Acon., Nux vom.*

Abdomen. Nausea: *Arnic.;* followed by bellyache: *Æthus., Arnic.;* bursting pain: *Amm. mur.;* has to double up: *Bar. mur.*

Chest. Warmth; blood seems to boil: *Anac.*

Pulsating in different spots: *Alum.;* beating: *Conium, Phosphor.*

Palpitation of heart: ||*Nitr. ac.;* spasmodic quick pulse: *Cuprum.*

Limbs. Hands tremble: *Psorin.;* feet heavy: *Nitr. ac.*

Position. Has to lie down in the afternoon: *Phosph. ac.;* has to sit up: *Crocus.;* it drives him from the seat: *Ant. tart., Silic.*

Nerves. Anguish of conscience causes restlessness: ||*Amm. carb., Arnic.,* ||*Arsen.,* ||*Coffea., Cyclam.,* ||*Graphit., Mercur.,* |*Sulphur.,* ||*Veratr.*

Trembling: |*Arsen., Aurum, Carb. veg.,* |*Chamom., Coffea, Graphit., Laches., Lam. alb., Lycop., Magn. carb., Natr. carb., Phosphor., Platin.,* |*Pulsat., Rhus tox., Sepia;* most in feet: *Sarsap.*

Sleep. Prevents falling asleep: *Kali hydr., Lauroc., Natr. carb., Rhus tox.;* before midnight: *Arsen.;* after midnight turning and tossing about: *Arsen.*

Driving out of bed: **Arsen.**, *Bryon.*, *Carb. veg.*, *Caustic.*, **Chamom.**, *Cinch. off.*, *Chin. sulph.*, **Graphit.**, **Hepar s. c.**, *Natr. mur.*, *Nitr. ac.*
Driving him about: *Acon.*, **Aurum.**, *Conium.*, *Lamium.*, *Silic.*, *Staphis.*, **Tabac.**
Fever. Flushes of heat: *Calc. ostr.;* heat and sweat: *Natr. mur.;* sweat breaking out: *Arsen.*, *Bellad.*, **Caustic.**, *Chamom.*, *Graphit.*, *Magn. carb.*, *Natr. carb.*, *Natr. mur.*, *Nitrum*, ‖*Nux vom.*, *Phosphor.*, *Rhus tox.*, *Staphis.*

MODEL CURE.

Feels the greatest anguish in the head with a whirling before the eyes every day, from 5 A. M. until 5 P. M., *since two years.* He walks up and down the room, wringing his hands, and moaning continually, "Oh, such anguish! Oh, such anguish!" Only when he takes his meals he ceases moaning. His appetite is good: *Psorinum.*—WM. GROSS.

HOMESICKNESS, NOSTALGIA.

Heimweh.

Silent ill humor: *Nitr. ac.*, **Phosph. ac.;** indifference to everything: *Bellad.*
Complains of everything: *Mercur.*
Whimsical and sensitive: *Capsic.*
Longing: *Mercur.;* after his friends: *Ignat.;* sighing and moaning: **Helleb.**
Sorrowful feeling, as if left alone: *Carb. an.;* loneliness: *Magn. mur.;* anxiousness: *Mercur.;* anxious lowness of spirits: *Nitr. ac.*
Inconsolable: ׀*Carb. an.;* cheerful faces increase his woe: *Helleb.*
Whining, sorrowful, as if alone: *Magn. mur.*
Lachrymose: *Phosph. ac.;* frequent weeping: *Capsic.*, *Magn. mur.;* melancholy: *Aurum;* inward grief: *Ignat.;* thoughtless stammering: *Ignat.;* quiet: *Sepia;* reserved: *Helleb.;* depressed: *Nitr. ac.*
Headache, as if bursting when moving: *Capsic.*
Redness of cheeks: **Capsic.**
Long lasting after-taste from that which has been vomited: *Phosph. ac.*
Heat in fauces: **Capsic.**
Hunger, with weak digestion: *Mercur.;* want of appetite: *Phosph. ac.*
Thirst and chilliness: *Capsic.;* insipid, watery taste of all food: *Ignat.*
After eating, burning in stomach: *Capsic.;* with emaciation: *Phosph. ac.;* pain in upper part of belly: *Aurum.*
Diarrhœa: *Phosph. ac.;* with tenesmus: *Capsic.*, *Mercur.*
Disposed to take a deep breath: *Capsic.;* weak chest, unable to talk: *Phosph. ac.*
Short, hacking morning cough, lasting for thirty minutes: *Capsic.*, *Drosera.*
Violent cough in evening and night: *Capsic.*
Frequent palpitation of heart: *Nitr. ac.;* violent palpitation: *Aurum.*

| Aurum.
| Bellad.
|| Capsic.
| Carb. an.
| Caustic.
|| Clemat.
| Eup. purp.
| Helleb.
| Hyosc.
|| Ignat.
| Magn. mur.
|| Mercur.
| Nitr. ac.
| Petrol.
|| Phosph. ac.
| Sach. sach.
| Silic.
| Staphis.

Crawls over the back: *Phosph. ac.*
Pain in limbs at night: *Mercur.*
Wants to run away, inquietude, wants to travel: *Mercur.*
Weak and trembling after slight exertion: *Mercur.;* averse to moving: *Capsic.*
Somnolency, constant inclination to sleep: *Phosph. ac.*
Fear in the night: **|** *Mercur.;* sleepiness: *Capsic., Mercur.*
Warmth of bed aggravating: *Mercur.;* profuse morning sweats: **|** *Phosph. ac.*
Feels as if alone in the morning: *Carb. an.;* evening and night coughs: *Capsic.*

Chilliness, with heat of face, and thirst: *Capsic.;* hectic fever: *Capsic.*
Evening fever, without thirst: *Phosph. ac.*
Night sweats: **|** *Mercur.;* sweats in the morning: *Phosph. ac.*
Phlegmatic constitution: *Capsic.*

Desires to travel, as everything is disagreeable to him; *Spigg. Mart.;* plans about travelling: *Elaps.;* longing to travel early in March: *Laches.;* irresistible propensity to wander from home: *Elater.;* desire to flee: *Hyosc.;* to run away: *Mercur.;* feels homesick when at home with her family: *Eup. purp.;* apprehension, sad, homesick, weeps: *Magn. mur.*

LOVE PANGS.

Liebesnoth.

1. Unhappy love. j. Jealousy. b. Both.

| Apis. j.
| Ant. crud. l.
|| Aurum. l.
| Calc. phos. b
| Camphor. j.
|| Caustic. l.
| Coffea. l.
| Helleb. l.
|| Hyosc. b.
|| Ignat. b.
| Kali carb. l.
|| Laches. b.
|| Nux vom. b.
| Phos. ac. b.
| Sepia. l.
|| Staphis. b.
| Stramon. j.

Unhappy love, disposed to weep, desires to take his life; despair, sudden anger; quarrelsome, or melancholy, with longing for death; alternately joyful and sorrowful; congestion of blood to the head, sparks before the eyes, rushing in the ears; putrid odor from the mouth, excessive hunger and thirst; congestion of blood to the chest, and anxious beating of the heart: *Aurum.*

With jealousy, vehemence and confused talking, quarrelsome: *Hyosc.*

Indignation about undeserved mortification, pushing things away from him: *Staphis.*

With jealous, suspicious despair, weary of life: *Laches.*

With silent grief, one cheek red: *Ignat.*

Not inclined to talk, hectic, red cheeks, sleepiness, morning sweats, emaciation: *Phosph. ac.;* pain in heart, fainting, apparent death: *Laches.*

Complaints of girls for grief about faithless lovers: *Arsen., Calc. phosph. Hyosc., Ignat.*

JEALOUSY.
Eiferſucht.

Apis.
Camphor.
‖ Hyosc.
Ignat.
Laches.
Nux vom.
‖ Phosph. ac.
‖ Pulsat.
Staphis.

Quarrelsome, eager, vehement, with delirious, incoherent speech, rage, mania: *Hyosc.*

With anger, desire to kill; torments others; running about; worse in day-time, mostly women: *Apis.*

With mistrust, suspicion, worse towards evening: *Laches.*

With excessive nervousness, spasmodic attacks, hectic fever, sleeplessness: *Hyosc.*; jealous thoughts rise in his mind: *Camphor.*; during pregnancy: *Laches.*

MODEL CURE.

A very irritable lady, suffering under the most violent and threatening nervous symptoms, even spasms; had hectic fever, sleepless nights, and her mind was nearly deranged; disturbed by unfounded jealousy. After one dose of *Hyosc.*, 30 cent., she soon was well and remained so.—E. STAPF.

GRIEF AND SORROW.
Gram und Kummer.

Alum.
Amm. mur.
Arsen.
‖ Aurum.
‖ Bellad.
Calc. ostr.
Calc. phos.
Capsic.
‖ Carb. an.
Caustic.
Chamom.
Coccul.
Colchic.
Coloc.
Conium.
‖ Cyclam.
Graphit.
Helleb.
Hyosc.
‖ Ignat.
Ipec.
Kad. sulph.
Kali carb.
Laches.
Lact. vir.
‖ Lycop.
Natr. carb.
Natr. mur.
Nitrum.
‖ Nux vom.
Opium.
Phosphor.
Phosph. ac.
Platin.
‖ Pulsat.
‖ Rhus tox.
‖ Sepia.
‖ Staphis.
Stramon.
Veratr.

Mind. Mental derangement: *Arsen., Bellad.*

Sad, indifferent; aversion to everything; full of fears: *Ignat.*

Grief with fear at night, disposition to quarrel, complaining of his relations and surroundings: *Mercur.*

With apprehensions for the future: *Staphis.*

Absorbed in his own thoughts, silent ill-humor; indifference; aversion to speaking; absent minded and dullness of mind: *Ipec.*

Grief and sorrow with shame; suppressed internal vexation, which continues: *Ignat.*

Sensorium. Vertigo: *Ignat.*; in evening: *Phosph. ac.*

Head. Headache: *Ignat.*; mornings: *Phosph. ac.*

Benumbing pain in forehead: *Lact. vir.*; rising up through the neck in the head: *Bellad.*; heat on top of head: *Calc. ostr., Phosphor., Sulphur;* with pressure: *Hyper.*

Nose. Coryza: *Laches.*; running, acrid: *Mercur.*

Throat. Contraction: *Lact. vir.*

Abdomen. Long-lasting after-taste, food often thrown up: *Phosph. ac.*; pressing pain in stomach: *Ignat.*; after every meal: *Phosph. ac.*; emptiness in scrobiculum: *Ignat.*; rolling rumbling in abdomen: *Phosph. ac.*

Stool. Looseness: *Coloc., Gelsem., Phosph. ac.*; involuntary: *Opium;* with tenesmus: *Mercur.*

Sexual Parts. Weakening pollutions: *Phosph. ac.*; amenorrhœa: *Ignat.*

In pregnancy, chorea: *Ignat., Stramon.*; labor pains mostly in back: *Caustic.*

Fainting during parturition: *Ignat.*
Chest. Whooping-cough: *Phosphor.;* weakness of chest causes inability to speak long: *Phosph. ac.*
Palpitation from sadness: *Nux mosch.*
Back. Crawling: *Phosph. ac.*
Spasms. Attacks like epilepsy: *Opium, Phosph. ac.;* fits: I*Ignat.*
Sleep. Prevented by seeing frightful faces: *Mercur.*
Sleepiness in the day-time: *Phosph. ac., Staphis.*
Fever. Without thirst, evenings: *Phosph. ac.*
Tissues. Emaciation: *Phosph. ac.*
After suppressed mental sufferings; seems to be weighed down; broods over imaginary trouble: I*Ignat.*
Chronic complaints after long-lasting grief or sorrow: *Caustic., Laches., Lycop.*
After weeping, nose bleeds: *Nitr. ac.;* throat contracted: *Lact. vir.;* cough, with children: *Arnica, Asar., Chamom.;* moving arms and hands about: *Sambuc.*

BETTER IN COMPANY AND BETTER WHEN ALONE.

According to B. R., each may be reversed, better in company to be the same as worse when alone; better when alone the same as worse in company; the first might be identified with desire to be in company; the second with longing to be alone; the first with dislike to solitude, the second with love of it, and the latter turned into dislike of society. The marks outside of margin list refer to the first, the marks inside to the last. In the text each modality is given separate.

Better in Company. The sad and depressed state: *Bovist.;* sad, solitary feeling: *Kali carb.;* is happy among people, likes company: *Calc. ac., Mezer.*
Better from conversation: *Eupat. perf.*
Desire to be in company: *Arsen., Conium., Caustic., Elaps., Lycop., Mezer., Sepia.*
Dislike to Solitude. Did not want to be alone; great melancholy: *Stramon.;* will not remain alone: *Ran. bulb.;* dare not remain a moment alone: *Sepia;* likes to have one beside him constantly: *Droser.;* dreads being alone: *Conium;* afraid to be left alone: *Lycop.;* frightened to be left alone: *Kali carb.;* cannot bear to be left alone: *Arsen., Bismuth., Calc. ostr.*
Complaints when alone. Has no rest: *Mezer.*
Anxiousness: *Droser, Phosphor., Zincum.*
Fear of ghosts in the evening: *Ran. bulb., Pulsat.*
With fear if people approach: *Conium.*
Fearful: *Arsen., Conium, Droser., Kali carb., Lycop., Ran. bulb.*
Feels forlorn in the morning: *Carb. an.*
Apprehensions: *Bryon.;* hypochondriac: *Arsen.;* irritable: *Phosphor.*
Care and sorrow: *Hepar.;* weeping: *Conium., Natr. mur.*
Sadness: *Kali. carb.*
Room seems gloomy, desolate: *Valer.*
Excited, full of imaginations: *Arsen.*

MIND AND DISPOSITION.

Acon.
Alum.
Ambra. ||
Amm. mur. |
Ant. crud.
Argent. |
Arnica. |
|| Arsen.
Aur. sulph. |
Baryt. **|**
Bellad. ||
| Bismuth.
| Bovist.
| Bryon.
Bufo. sat. ||
|| Calc. ac.
|| Calc. ostr.
Carban. |
|| Caustic.
Cicut. |
Cinch. off. |
Coca. **|**
|| Conium. ||
Cuprum. ||
Cyclam. |
Digit. |
|| Droser.
| Elaps. ||
Eup. perf.
|| Fluor ac. ||
Graphit. |
Gratiol. ||
Helleb. ||
| Hepar s. c. |
Hippom. **|**
Hyosc.
Ignat. |
Jambos.
|| Kali carb. ||
Laches. ||
Ledum. |
|| Lycop. ||
Magn. carb. ||
Magn. mur. |
Menyanth. |
|| Mezer.
Natr. carb. ||
| Natr. mur. |
Niccol. |
Nux vom. ||
Panac. |
Petrol. ||
|| Phosphor. ||
|| Phosph. ac.
| Platin. **|**
Plumbum. **|**
| Pulsat. |
|| Ran. bulb.
Rhus rad. |
Rhus tox. ||
| Sepia. **||**
|| Silic.
Stannum. ||
|| Stramon. ||
| Sulphur. ||
|| Valer.
| Zincum.

Dull mind: *Phosph. ac.*

Always the same idea in his mind: *Arsen., Kali carb., Zincum.*

Cold face, hands and feet: *Calc. ostr.*

Love of Solitude.
Prefers being alone, retired into a corner: ||*Coca.*, ||*Elaps.*, |*Hippom.*; ruminating his thoughts: *Laches.*; rather silent, than to speak: *Menyanth.*; without speaking: *Ant. crud.*

Wishes to pore over his thoughts in solitude: *Magn. mur.*

Wishes to be alone, quiet and at ease: *Nux vom.*; to lie with closed eyes: *Sepia;* everything displeases her: *Hepar s. c.*

Fond of solitude: *Carb. an.*; likes it best: *Cinch. off.*; and great discouragement: *Gratiol.*; and silence from sadness: *Rhus tox.*

Desire for: *Acon., Bellad.,* |*Digit., Panac., Rhus rad.*; to sit alone: *Jambos.*; if interrupted, he gets angry: *Graphit.*; retiring in a corner: ||*Elaps.*; wants quiet: *Bellad.*; with fearfulness and trembling: *Niccol.*; with dislike to people: *Lycop.*

Longing for it: *Alum., Aurum sulph.,* ||*Bellad., Carb. an., Cuprum,* ||*Digit., Gratiol., Jambos., Ledum, Lycop., Magn. mur., Rhus tox., Sulphur.*

Passion for it, and shyness: |*Coca.*

Seeks it: *Aurum;* darkness and silence: *Nux vom.*; full of apprehension: *Natr. carb.*; buried in deep thought, reflects about his future state: *Cyclam.*; plunged in deep meditation: *Conium;* avoids the sight of people: *Cuprum.*

Complaints with the love of Solitude.
Sadness: *Bufo sat., Carb. an., Ignat., Rhus tox.*; and depression: *Alum., Aurum;* unhappiness: *Alum.*; full of fears most every evening in bed: *Kali carb.*; fearful and trembling: *Niccol.*; with apprehension: *Conium, Cyclam., Kali carb., Natr. carb.*

Shyness: ||*Coca;* ill humor: *Gratiol.*; morose: *Cuprum, Ledum;* everything displeases her: *Hepar s. c.*; irritable: *Nux vom.*; gets angry when interrupted: *Graphit.*; thinks her death is near: *Cuprum;* wishes death: *Ledum;* reflects about his future state: *Cyclam.*; full of schemes: *Natr. carb.*; much discouraged: *Gratiol.*; reserved: *Carb. an.*; buried in deep thought: *Cyclam.*; pores over his thoughts: *Magn. mur.*; ruminating: *Laches.*; plunged in deep meditation: *Conium.*

Head as if drunk, with bursting pain in forehead: *Ant. crud.*

In darkness and silence: *Nux vom.*; lies with closed eyes: *Sepia.*

Quiet, every noise disagreeable: *Bellad.*; disturbed by it: *Carb. an.*; by noise of many people: *Petrol.*

Without speaking: *Antim.;* rather silent, does not want to talk: *Magn. mur., Menyanth., Rhus tox.*
Trembling: *Niccol.*
Dislike to Society. Abhorring the foolishness of men: *Cicut.*
With bursts of sarcasm: *Rhus rad.*
Unsocial humor: *Magn. mur.*
Keeps aloof from others: *Bufo sat.*
Dislike to people: *Lycop., Selen., Stannum.*
Avoids people: *Natr. carb.*
Shuns the sight of people: *Cuprum;* the noise of many: *Petrol.;* to hear talking fatigues, hands and feet turn cold: *Aurum.*
Presence of others is disagreeable, visitors loathsome: *Bellad.*
Shuns all conversation: *Carb. an.;* all men: *Cicut.*
Would like to be in a deep cave, seeing no one: *Elaps.*
Aversion to company: *Cinnab., Clemat., Ledum, Natr. carb., Pulsat., Rhus tox.;* dreads society when pregnant: *Laches.*
Worse when other persons are present: *Stramon.*
Fear of approaching people: *Cuprum;* and anxiety when others come near him: *Lycop.;* afraid they might touch him: *Arnica.*
When persons are coming in the room, fear of being hurt: *Arnica;* his cough gets worse: *Phosphor.;* whooping-cough worse among strangers: *Ambra, Baryt.;* when in company anxious: *Bellad., Lycop.,* I*Petrol., Platin.;* unwilling to converse: *Argent.*
In a room with many people, headache; pressure over the whole head: *Magn. carb.*
Worse among strangers: *Ambra., Baryt., Conium, Lycop., Petrol., Sepia, Stramon.*

<small>We may mention a morbid disinclination to leave the bed, lectrophilie (Bettfucht): *Merc. sol., Psorinum,* and shunning of the bed, lectrophobie (Bettſcheu): *Cannab., Caustic., Lycop., Natr. carb.*</small>

Will not be looked at, especially children, they want to be alone, and get out of humor: I*Ant. crud.,* II*Arsen.,* I*Chamom., Cina.*
If any one looks at him he must weep: *Natr. mur.*
Dislike to be spoken to. Ill humor: I*Arsen., Chamom., Gelsem., Natr. mur., Natr. sulph., Nux vom., Rhus tox.;* weeping: *Natr. mur., Staphis.;* coughing: *Arsen.*
Ill humor, worse from friendly persuasion, or soothing words: I*Bellad., Calc. ostr.,* I*Calc. phosph., Cinch. off.,* II*Ignat.,* I*Kali. carb., Mercur.;* I*Natr. mur.,* I*Nitr. ac., Nux vom.,* II*Platin.,* I*Sepia.,* II*Silic.*
Weeping: *Bellad., Calc. ostr., Cinch. off., Ignat., Kali carb. Natr. mur., Nitr. ac., Platin., Staphis.*
Admonitions cause weeping: II*Bellad., Calc., Ignat.,* I*Kali carb., Nitr. ac., Platin.*

THE TALK OF OTHERS INCREASES THE SUFFERINGS.

Alum.
Amm. carb.
|| Arsen.
Colchic.
Conium.
Magn. mur.
Mangan.
Mar. ver.
Mezer.
Nux vom.
Oleand.
Rhus tox.
Silic.
Staphis.
|| Veratr.
Zincum.

Seems unbearable: *Arsen.*
Even the talk of persons dear to him affects his nerves, gets morose and impatient: *Zincum;* cannot bear to be interrupted: *Mezer.;* gets vexed: *Rhus tox.;* and vehement: *Mangan.*
His pains get worse: *Arsen., Magn. mur., Zincum.*
Buried in thought: *Ol. anim.*
Vexed ill humor: *Mangan.;* wrath: *Mangan.;* fatigued: *Amm. carb.*

MODEL CURE.

A child, 3 years old, apparently well, waked often from sleep with a scream, and continued to cry: the more they try by persuasion to quiet it, the worse it gets: Calc. ostr. did not help much; after Calc. phosph., the spells ceased altogether.—LIPPE.

AFTER MORTIFICATION.
Kränkung.

Acon.
Anac.
Arsen.
|| Aurum.
| Bellad.
|| Bryon.
Calc. ostr.
|| Carb. an.
Caustic.
| Chamom.
Crocus.
| Coloc.
Helleb.
|| Ignat.
Ipec.
| Lycop.
|| Mercur.
|| Natr. mur.
| Nux vom.
| Opium.
| Phosph ac.
|| Pallad.
| Platin.
| Pulsat.
| Seneg.
| Sepia.
|| Staphis.
Stramon.
|| Sulphur.
Veratr.

Fearfulness: *Ignat.;* fear and restlessness: *Coloc.;* disposition to cry and weep: *Coloc.;* sad, bursting into tears: *Pulsat.*
Does not like to talk: *Ignat.;* indifference: *Ignat.*
Thinks with pleasure of drowning: *Pulsat.;* anxious; weary of life; sad and gloomy: *Pulsat.*
Melancholy; prefers to be alone: *Ignat.*
Throws things down or pushes them away: *Staphis.;* dissatisfied with everything: *Pulsat.;* aversion to all around him: *Ignat.*
Very easily frightened: *Pulsat.;* bewildered: *Nux vom.;* easily enraged: *Pulsat.*
Derangement of the mind: *Arsen., Bellad.;* continual babbling of stupid phrases: *Anac.;* talking incoherently: *Nux vom.;* everything he attempts he does wrong: *Nux vom.*
Weak memory: *Ignat.*
Heaviness of head: *Ignat., Nux vom.;* headache: *Coloc.*
Losing hair on one side: *Ignat.*
Sees through a fog: *Ignat.;* vacant gaze; sits quietly: *Ignat.*
Hard hearing: *Ignat.*
Frequent profuse nosebleed: *Pulsat.*
Face distorted: *Ignat.;* pale face and sunken eyes: *Coloc.;* earthy pale and sunken: *Ignat.;* pale with pointed nose or red with irritation: *Pulsat., Nux vom.;* earthy, dark ring around the eyes: *Pulsat.*
Bitter sapid taste in mouth: *Pulsat.;* no desire to eat or drink: *Ignat.;* dislikes meat or bread: *Pulsat.;* appetite soon satisfied: *Ignat.*
Nausea with pain in stomach: *Pulsat.*
Bitter, slimy vomiting: *Pulsat.*

Pain in stomach: *Nux vom.;* in left hypochondrium, worse from pressure: *Ignat.*

Cutting in bowels: *Pulsat.;* violent pains in abdomen; squeezing pain, better from outward pressure; cramp in bowels; cramp-colic relieved by extreme pressure; distention of the abdomen: **I** *Coloc.*

Diarrhœa and vomiting every time food is taken: *Coloc.*

Diarrhœa with pain in the bowels: *Coloc.*

Hard scanty stool: *Pulsat.;* increased stool and urine: *Ignat.*

Voice low, trembling: *Ignat.;* labored breathing: *Pulsat.*

Stitches in side when coughing, with frothy bloody expectoration: *Pulsat.*

Pain in small of back: *Nux vom.;* in the hips extending from the region of the kidneys down to the upper part of the thigh: *Coloc.*

Cramp in calves: **I** *Coloc.;* heavy legs: *Pulsat.*

Limbs bruised; swelling on upper part of foot: *Pulsat.*

Staggering walk: *Ignat.;* cannot sit up: *Nux vom.*

General weakness: *Ignat.;* spasms, convulsions: *Opium.*

Later sleep and restlessness: *Ignat.;* sleeplessness: **I** *Coloc.;* starts in sleep: *Ignat.;* anxious dreams: *Pulsat.*

Cold feet, most in evening: *Ignat.;* bilious fever: **I** *Coloc.*

After wounded pride, not getting the praise of others she expected: *Pallad.*

After trying to speak in company, anxious heart beating: *Platin.*

Embarrassment: I *Calc. ostr.*, **I***Sulphur.*

Abashment: I I *Coloc.*, **I***Ignat.*, **I** *Opium*, I I *Phosph. ac.*, I I *Platin.*, *Sepia*, I I *Staphis.*, **I I** *Sulphur.*

From Reproaches: I I *Coloc.*, *Crocus.*, **I** *Ignat.*, **I I** *Opium*, I *Phosph. ac.*, **I** *Staphis.*

MODEL CURES.

Melancholy after deep mortification; heaviness of the head; very great weakness of the memory; forgets everything except dreams; hardness of hearing; sees everything as if through a fog; sits quietly, with a vacant gaze, always thinking of the mortification endured, and knowing nothing of what passes around him; prefers to be alone; thinking of the mortification endured prevents him from going to sleep as early as usual; restless sleep, starts during sleep, much dreaming; pain in the left hypochondria increased by pressure and continuous walk. Loses his hair. Face colorless, hollow; voice low, trembling with distortion of the muscles of the face; does not like to talk; no desire to eat or drink; appetite is very soon satisfied. Always feels cold, especially in the evening. Very weak; staggering walk; walks carefully. Increased stool and urine: *Ignat.*—ATTOMYR.

After mortification sad, gloomy and weary of life. Often pain in the forehead, earthy face, dark rings around the eyes; bitter sapid taste in the mouth; dislikes meat and bread; nausea, with pain in stomach; occasional bitter slimy vomiting; frequent profuse nosebleed; stitches in the side when coughing, with frothy bloody expectoration. Palpitation of the heart; labored breathing, hard scanty stools; frequent cutting pain in the bowels; heaviness of the legs; limbs feel bruised; swelling on the upper part of foot; anxious dreams; thinks of drowning with great pleasure; is sad; bursts into tears; dissatisfied with everything; easily enraged; reticent; very easily frightened; anxious; weary of life: *Pulsat.*—ATTOMYR.

MIND AND DISPOSITION.

VEXATION.
Aerger.

Remedies (margin):
!! Acon.
Aloes.
!! Alum.
Ant. tart.
Apis.
! Arsen.
!! Aurum.
!! Bellad.
!! Bryon.
Calc. ostr.
Calc. phos.
Cannab.
Castor.
Caustic.
!! Chamom.
Cinch. off.
!! Cistus.
!! Coccul.
! Coffea.
Colchic.
!! Coloc.
Crocus.
Cuprum.
Cyclam.
! Hyosc.
!! Ignat.
Ipec.
Kali carb.
Laches.
!! Lycop.
Magn. carb.
Magn. mur.
Mercur.
Mezer.
Natr. carb.
! Natr. mur.
Nux mosch.
!! Nux vom.
Oleander.
! Opium.
!! Petrol.
! Phosphor.
!! Phosph. ac.
!! Platin.
! Pulsat.
Ran. bulb.
Rhus tox.
Sambuc.
Secale.
Selen.
! Sepia.
Silic.
Stannum.
!! Staphis.
Stramon.
Sulphur.
Thuya.
!! Veratr.
!! Zincum.

Ailments after Vexation. Even the slightest brings on ailments or aggravate: *Arsen., Bellad., Cistus., Kali carb., Mezer., Natr. mur., Petrol., Phosph. ac., Rhus tox., Sulphur.*

Easily vexed, and the slightest vexation hurts her very much: *Phosphor.*

She feels slightest vexation through the whole body: *Caustic., Nux vom.*

Long-lasting complaints following vexation: *Alum., Lycop., Petrol.;* great sufferings: *Sepia.*

Serious ailments: !*Natr. mur.;* violent and dangerous: *Chamom., Pulsat.*

After Vexation. Remaining anxiety: *Lycop., Sepia;* about the future: *Staphis.;* full of fear and restlessness: *Chamom.;* in the night: *Arsen.;* with anguish of conscience: *Veratr.*

Disposition to whine: *Bryon.;* wheezing and coughing: *Natr. mur.;* crying about anticipated results: *Staphis.*

Feeling of shame, silent chagrin, sorrowful thoughts: *Ignat.;* fear of being alone, fear of death: *Arsen.*

Cannot forget losses or injuries: *Ignat.*

Ill humor about anything which has happened: *Staphis.*

Stubborn peevishness: *Nux vom.*

Vexation with Indignation: *Coloc., Ipec., Nux vom.,* !!*Platin., Staphis.;* throws away whatever he happens to hold in his hands: *Staphis.*

Disposition to quarrel: *Nux vom.*

With wrath, passion and heat: *Chamom.*

Beside himself: *Nux vom., Phosphor.;* and hot: *Phosphor.*

Very easily frightened: *Nux vom.*

Uses the wrong word: *Laches.*

Is depressed, cannot work: *Calc. phosph.*

Completely absorbed in his own thoughts: *Ignat.*

Derangement of the mind: *Veratr.*

Sanguine sensitiveness: *Chamom.;* over-sensitiveness of senses: *Nux vom.;* very much excited: *Acon.*

Congestion of blood to the head: *Acon., Hyosc.;* fears apoplexy: *Sepia.*

Vertigo: *Ignat., Calc. ostr.;* in attacks: *Nux vom.*

Head. Headache: *Castor., Lycop.,* !!*Magn. carb., Petrol.,* !!*Phosphor., Ran. bulb.;* dull: *Kali carb.;* violent: *Magn. carb., Mezer.;* sudden: *Ran. bulb.;* after a slight vexation: *Ignat., Mezer., Petrol., Ran. bulb.;* the very slightest: *Phosphor.;* in forehead: *Petrol.;* in occiput: *Cannab., Ran. bulb.;* pressing on a small point: *Ignat.;* feels every step: *Natr. mur.;* twinging with heaviness: *Magn. carb.;* increasing from 1 P. M. till evening: *Magn. carb.;* after:

VEXATION.

Mezer.; heat in head: *Bryon.;* attacks of heat and throbbing in the head: *Cyclam.;* with red face, one cheek: *Chamom.;* loss of appetite: *Natr. mur.*

Scalp. Sensitive to slightest touch: *Mezer.;* loss of hair: *Staphis.*

Eyes. Black before them: *Sepia;* pupils contracted: *Coccul.* Full of tears: *Petrol.;* weeping all night: *Natr. mur.*

Nose. Hemorrhage: *Arsen.;* stopped up by cold: *Staphis.*

Face. Hot: *Chamom.;* with cold hands: *Phosphor.;* cold, hippocratic: *Veratr.;* dark blue: *Veratr.;* cold sweat: *Veratr.;* pale: *Arsen.;* yellow: *Kali carb.*

Taste of bile: *Chamom.;* bitter: *Petrol.;* with thirst: *Bryon.*

Throat. Pressure and constriction in pit of throat; worse when swallowing: *Staphis.*

Appetite. Lost: *Petrol., Phosph.;* after whining: *Coccul.;* with headache: *Natr. mur.*

Thirst: *Bryon.;* insatiable: *Chamom.;* little at a time: *Arsen.*

Eating. Worse before dinner: *Phosphor.;* after drinking, cough or vomiting: *Arsen.;* getting sick from eating or drinking soon after the vexation: ‖ *Chamom.*

Belching: *Bryon.;* and sickness: *Petrol.;* bitter: *Bryon.;* and vomiting: *Chamom., Veratr.*

Nausea: *Chamom., Ignat.;* with hot face: *Phosphor.;* gagging: *Kali carb.,* and coughing: *Natr. mur.;* unsuccessful urging: *Natr. mur.;* vomiting: *Acon., Chamom., Ignat., Veratr.;* of bitter water: *Bryon.*

Scrobiculum. Sensitive: *Veratr.;* empty feeling: *Ignat.;* sudden rush to: *Lycop.;* greatest anxiety: ❙*Lycop.;* pain with suffocating spells: ❙*Acon.*

Stomach. Pressing pains: *Chamom., Ignat., Phosphor.;* as from a stone: *Acon.;* pains with fear: *Arsen.*

Hypochondria. Pain in liver: *Bryon.*

Bowels. Cramps: *Ignat.;* belly-ache: *Sulphur;* with diarrhœa: *Chamom.*

Stools. Several thin stools: *Petrol.;* looseness: *Aloes, Calc. phosph., Chamom.,* ❙*Coloc.;* only in the morning or forenoon: *Bryon.;* next morning with agony: *Petrol.;* after a little walk with agitation: *Petrol.;* dysentery: *Sulphur;* costiveness: *Bryon., Nux vom., Staphis.;* burning in anus: *Natr. mur.*

Womb. Cramps: *Ignat.;* catamenia too copious: *Nux vom.;* after it lumps of blood pass off: *Rhus tox.;* catamenia suppressed: *Acon., Coloc., Pulsat., Staphis.*

Amenorrhœa: *Acon.,* etc.

In the fifth month of pregnancy, at night copious hemorrhage from vagina with lumps of coagulated blood, dull headache, yellow face, but no abortion: *Kali carb.;* checked lochia: *Acon., Coloc.*

Chest. Faint speech: *Staphis.;* shortness of breath: *Acon., Chamom.;* want of breath and choking spells: *Arsen.;* suffocating from pain in pit of stomach: *Acon.;* a contracted sensation: *Arsen.;* cramps: *Chamom.;* after midnight with palpitation of the heart: *Veratr.*

Cough: *Acon., Arsen.,* ❙*Chamom., Cinch. off., Ignat.,* ❙*Natr. mur., Nux vom., Sepia, Staphis., Veratr.*

After vexation with fright: *Ignat.;* after fright with vexation: *Acon.*
With grief: *Ignat.;* with indignation: *Staphis.*
If children "get mad:" *Ant. tart., Chamom.*
With gagging and wheezing: *Natr. mur.*
With stitches in chest: *Bryon.;* in left upper part: *Natr. mur.*

Heart. Palpitation: *Chamom., Nux vom., Phosphor., Veratr.*
From the slightest movement: *Staphis.;* with anxiety: *Acon.;* palpitation and trembling; weakness: *Lycop.;* orgasm: *Petrol.*
Pulse altered: *Acon., Chamom., Coloc., Ignat., Natr. mur., Petrol., Sepia, Staphis.*

Back. Pains in small of back: *Nux vom.;* chilliness: *Nux vom.*

Upper Limbs. Burning in arms: *Natr. mur.*
Cold hands and hot face: *Phosphor.*

Legs. Her knees give way, falter: *Caustic.*
Legs get as heavy as lead: *Lycop., Natr. mur., Nux vom.*
Trembling: *Ran. bulb.*

Limbs. Pain when in motion: *Bryon.*
Bruised feeling: *Acon.;* lame and bruised feeling: *Veratr.*

Nerves. Great irritation of the whole nervous system: *Nux vom.;* trembling: *Acon., Ran. bulb., Lycop.;* twitching of limbs: *Ignat.;* all over: *Magn. carb.;* through the whole body: *Petrol.*
Spasms: *Bellad., Cuprum., Ignat.;* violent spasms, wants to run up the wall: *Bellad.;* convulsions: *Bellad., Ignat.;* epilepsy: *Ignat.*
A short, easy walk fatigues much: *Petrol.;* can hardly walk: *Calc. phosph.*
Disposition to lie down: *Nux vom.*
Getting as if lame: *Calc. phosph., Sepia.*
Cannot work: *Calc. phosph.;* gets very weak: *Natr. mur.*
Great weakness: ▮*Arsen., Lycop.;* very infirm all forenoon: *Lycop.;* with fainting and coldness: *Veratr.*

Sleep. At bed time "blood still in motion:" *Petrol.;* sleep improves; heaviness: *Magn. carb.*
Sleepless: *Chamom.,* and restless: *Acon., Arsen.;* restless sleep: *Petrol.;* wakeful all night: *Staphis.;* sleepy during the day: *Nux vom., Staphis.*

Day. Every morning: *Petrol.;* worse morning than evening: *Nux vom.*
Next morning, trembling through the whole body: *Petrol.*
Forenoon: *Ran. bulb.;* infirm, trembling, weak: *Lycop.;* all day: *Carb. veg.*
Sensation of heaviness from 1 P.M., increasing till bed time: *Magn. carb.*
Worse in the evening and morning: *Bryon.*

Warmth. Aversion to fresh air: *Nux vom.;* desire for warmth: *Arsen.*
Chill: *Acon., Arsen., Bryon., Mercur.,* ▮*Nux vom.*
Coldness: *Arsen.;* chilliness in back: *Nux vom.*
Cold or chilly all over: *Bryon.*
Heat: ▮*Acon.,* ▮*Chamom.,* ▮*Nux vom.,* ▮▮*Petrol.,* ▮▮*Sepia,* ▮*Staphis., Phosphor.;* beside himself: *Phosph. ac.*
Attacks of heat and throbbing in head: *Cyclam.*
Febrile motions, with bitter taste and thirst: *Bryon.*

ANGER.

Hot, dry skin, with thirst: *Acon.*

Sweat. |*Acon.*, ||*Bryon.*, |*Chamom.*, |*Lycop.*, |*Petrol.*, ||*Sepia*, |*Staphis.*; constant: *Staphis.*; cold: *Veratr.*

Sensations. Inward suffering, agony; tears always filling her eyes: *Petrol.*; feeling going through the whole body: *Caustic.*; burning pains in different parts: *Arsen.*

Hemorrhages: *Kali carb.*; slightest touch hurts the head: *Mezer.*; after misuse of mercury: *Staphis.*

After ill behavior of others: *Coccul.*, || *Colchic.*, |*Staphis.*

When disturbed at his work: *Pulsat.*

From contradictions: |*Arsen.*, ||*Aurum*, ||*Ignat.*, ||*Lycop.*, ||*Nux vom.*, || *Oleand.*

From the slightest contradiction the blood rushes in his face: *Ignat.*

After offences: *Coloc.*, ||*Mercur.*, *Natr. mur.*, |*Nux vom.*, |*Staphis.*

MODEL CURE.

Especially after mental agitation of a vexatious character, to which she is very subject (in deficiencies of the valves), a trembling and fluttering of the *heart*, distressingly painful in the heart and as far as between the *shoulders;* it extends upwards also into the *head*, where it is felt as an equally painful throbbing; at the same time air, on inspiration, seems so cold that it is felt unpleasantly *cold*, even in the lungs: *Lith. carb.*—N. N.

ANGER.
Born.

Much inclined to anger: *Bryon.*, *Phosphor.*, *Zincum;* long, lasting ailments from it: *Agaric.*, *Zincum;* with mortification: *Staphis.;* vexation: *Chamom.*, *Platin.*, *Staphis.;* indignation: *Coloc.*, *Staphis.;* with wrath and vehemence: *Acon.*, *Arsen.*, *Aurum*, *Bryon.*, |*Chamom.*, *Gratiol.*, *Ignat.*, *Lycop.*, *Nux vom.*, *Veratr.*

Throws things away indignantly, or pushes them away on the table: *Staphis.*

Loss of reason, alternately laughing or crying: *Platin.*

Excessive irritation of mind: *Arnica;* vertigo: *Arnica.*

Head. Congestion: *Arnica;* with unconsciousness or delirium: *Bellad.*, ache: *Mezer.*, *Petrol.*, *Platin.;* headache, heat, red face and thirst: *Bryon.;* hot sweats: *Chamom.*

Face. Burning heat: *Chamom.;* redness: *Bryon.*

Taste. Bitter, as is also the belching: *Arnica.*

Mouth. Putrid breath: *Arnica.*

Thirst: *Bryon.*, *Nux vom.*

Belching bitter: *Arnica;* vomiting: *Coloc.;* bile in the morning: *Nux vom.;* colic: *Chamom.;* looseness: *Acon.*, *Chamom.;* diarrhœa and vomiting: *Coloc.*

|| Acon.
Agaric.
Ambra.
Ant. tart.
Apis.
Arnica.
|| Arsen.
| Aurum.
|| Bellad.
|| Bryon.
|| Chamom.
Coccul.
| Coffea.
| Coloc.
|| Ferrum.
Hepar s. c.
|| Hyosc.
Ignat.
Ipecac.
|| Lycop.
Mezer.
|| Natr. mur.
Nitr ac.
|| Nux vom.
|| Oleander.
Opium.
|| Petrol.
|| Phosph. ac.
|| Platin.
Pulsat.
| Sepia.
| Staphis.
Strontian.
Sulphur.
Thuya.
|| Veratr.
|| Zincum.

Stool. Involuntary passage of it and the urine : *Arnica.*

Womb. Amenorrhœa : *Chamom.;* strangulated prolapsus : *Acon.;* gastric symptoms in pregnancy : *Bryon.;* puerperal convulsions : *Chamom.,* checked lochia : *Coloc.*

Chest. If the motions of the chest are vehement or laborious : |*Rhus tox., Staphis.*

Agony of death; violent, laborious breathing : *Rhus tox.*

Little children lose their breath, or breathe as if the throat was filled with phlegm : |*Ant. tart.*

Cough. Children get angry, and have violent spells of coughing : *Ant. tart., Arnica, Asar., Chamom.*

After screaming or crying, blood spitting : *Arnica.*

Heart. Convulsive beating : *Arnica.*

Circulation disturbed : *Acon.,* ||*Chamom., Coloc., Ignat., Natr. mur.,* |*Petrol.,* ||*Sepia., Staphis.*

Back. Bruised feeling, and in the limbs at every motion : *Arnica.*

Nerves. Trembling after quarrels : *Nitr. ac.;* lameness : *Sepia.*

Cramps : *Chamom.*

Sleep. Drowsy in the evening : *Pulsat.;* by day sleepy, by night sleepless, painfulness of whole body : *Staphis.*

Time of day. Morning : *Nux vom.;* evening : *Bryon., Pulsat.*

Fever. Inner chill, without thirst : *Pulsat.;* with red cheeks and thirst : *Bryon.;* alternating chills and heat, thirst and vomiting : *Nux vom.;* coldness of lower parts, heat of the upper parts of the body : *Arnica.*

MODEL CURE.

Vexation and wrath, followed by fear of being brought before court, because, as she imagines, persons accuse her of having done something wrong. Frightened look on her face. She imagines her neighbors are pursuing her; the devil is lying in wait for her; will come up to her through the floor of the room; sleeps restlessly during the day; hot during the night, with only an hour or two of sleep, disturbed by anxious dreams. She imagines she is falling into a deep abyss. She is pursued, and tries to escape by running as fast as she can. Weakness—the feet feel as if bruised. Lachrymose—she dislikes any one who tries to dissuade her from her idea. Heat in head and face. Cheeks earthy pale, and dark red hollow face. Vertigo. Unable to walk. The body suffers alternately moderate heat and cold. Late, tardy evacuation. Urine with brick-dust like sediment : *Zinc. ox.*—SCHMID.

AFTER EMOTIONS AND EXCITEMENT.

The marks inside of margin-list signify the degree in which heart, pulse and circulation are affected.

❙ Anac. ❙	
Alcohol.	
❙ Alum.	
Al. p. s. ❙	
❙ Amm. mur.	
❙ Ant. tart.	
Apis. ❙❙	
❙ Arnica.	
❙❙ Arsen.	
❙ Asar_t	
❙ Aurum. ❙	
❙ Baryt.	
❙ Bellad. ❙	
Benz. ac.	
❙ Bryon.	
Calc. ars.	
❙ Calc. ostr. ❙❙	
❙❙ Calc. phosph.	
❙ Capsic.	
❙ Carb. an.	
Carb. veg.	
❙ Caustic.	
❙ Chamom. ❙❙	
❙ Cicut.	
❙ Cinch. off.	
❙ Cistus.	
❙ Coccul.	
❙❙ Codein.	
❙ Coffea. ❙❙	
❙ Colchic. ❙	
❙❙ Coloc. ❙	
❙❙ Conium. ❙	
❙ Crocus.	
❙ Cuprum. ❙❙	
❙❙ Cyclam.	
Eryngium.	
❙ Ferrum.	
❙❙ Gelsem.	
❙ Graphit.	
❙ Hep. s. c.	
❙❙ Hyosc.	
❙❙ Ignat. ❙❙	
❙❙ Ipec.	
❙❙ Kali bichr.	
❙❙ Kali carb. ❙	
❙❙ Kreosot.	
❙ Laches. ❙	
❙ Lauroc.	
❙ Ledum.	
Lithium.	
❙ Lycop.	
❙ Magn. carb.	
❙ Magn. mur.	
Mancin.	
❙ Mar. ver. ❙❙	
❙ Mercur.	
❙ Natr. carb.	
❙ Natr. mur. ❙	
❙❙ Nitr. ac. ❙	
❙❙ Nux mosch.	
❙❙ Nux vom. ❙	
❙❙ Oleander.	
❙ Opium. ❙	
❙❙ Pallad.	
❙ Petrol. ❙	
❙ Phosphor. ❙	
❙❙ Phosph. ac.❙	

Mind. Anxiety after hearing of cruelties: *Calc. ostr.;* sad stories: *Cicut.*

Sad and desponding after bad news: *Pulsat.;* much displeased, does not want to say a word, wants to be left alone: *Calc. phosph.*

Vanishing of thought, unconsciousness: *Nux mosch.;* beside himself; sweat breaks out all over him: *Calc. phosph.*

Head. Rush of blood to the head with a spasmodic contraction between the shoulder-blades: *Phosphor.;* from the least little thing so much hurt that it is followed by much pain in forehead, temples and below the chin: *Hura;* after a touching farewell a gradually increasing headache, tension in brain: *Natr. mur.;* nervous headache: *Benz. ac., Eryngium, Gelsem., Kreosot., Natr. mur., Scut. lat.*

Ears. Trembling in them after hearing sad news: *Sabin.*

Nose. The slightest agitation is followed by a red nose: *Vinc. min.*

Face. Red from the slightest emotion or excitement: *Phosphor.* Toothache during pregnancy: *Calc. ostr.*

Stomach. Vomiting and gagging: *Kali carb.;* anxious feeling in scrobiculum: *Phosphor.*

From the least unpleasant emotion a nervous irritation of the digestive organs, expansion of stomach and abdomen: *Nux mosch.;* weak digestion: ❙*Bryon.,* ❙*Chamom.,* ❙❙ *Cinch. off.,* ❙ *Coloc.,* ❙*Nux vom.,* ❙❙*Phosph. ac.,* ❙❙*Staphis.*

Moving to diarrhœa: ❙ *Gelsem.*

Milk scanty with nurses: *Caustic.*

Chest. Asthma: *Cuprum.*

Whooping-cough attack: *Laches., Lob. infl., Spongia;* all kinds of cough increase: *Spongia;* orgasm: *Laches.;* palpitation and short breath: *Sepia;* after the least emotion violent palpitation: *Phosphor.;* after excitement: *Al. p. s.*

Whole Body. Contraction between shoulder-blades: *Phosphor.*

Looking at an offensive object it goes to her limbs, runs through the whole body, and she is nearly beside herself: *Nux vom.;* limbs asleep: *Calc. phosph.*

After every emotion her whole body trembles: *Psorin.;* internal trembling: *Zincum.*

Every event makes a violent impression, with a wave-like trembling in the nerves and sensation of fainting: *Natr. carb.*

Sleep. Sad news makes very sleepy: *Ignat.*

Fever. Exciting news cause flitting chilliness: *Gelsem.;*

MIND AND DISPOSITION.

| Platin.
| Podoph.
|| Psorin.
|| Pulsat.
| Ran. bulb.
|| Rhus tox.
| Sabin.
|| Sambuc.
|| Scut. lat.
| Sec. corn.
| Selen.
| Senega.
| Sepia.
|| Silic.
| Spongia.
| Stannum.
|| Staphis.
|| Stramon.
| Strontian.
|| Sulphur.
|| Thuya.
| Veratr.
| Verbasc.
| Vinc. min.
|| Zincum.

unpleasant news followed by chilliness: *Sulphur;* chill aggravated: || *Calc. ostr.,* | *Cicut.,* | *Ignat.,* | *Mar. ver.;* after unpleasant news beside himself, cannot think, sweat breaks out all over him: *Calc. phosph.*

Affected when thinking about unpleasant things: *Calc. ostr.;* anxiousness: *Phosphor.;* weeps when thinking of old troubles: *Lycop., Natr. mur.;* suffocative oppression of the chest when thinking of adverse things: *Hura.*

Thinking of past troubles accelerates his pulse and takes his breath away: *Sepia.*

Vivid fancy in evening; the mere thought of disagreeable things causes shuddering: *Phosphor.*

Looking at an offensive object affects him: *Nux vom.;* everything that happens causes trembling: *Natr. carb.*

After hearing bad news: ||*Apis.,* ||*Calc. ostr.,* ||*Calc. phosph., Cinnab., Cinch. off.,* ||*Cuprum, Formica,* |*Gelsem.,* |*Ignat.,* ||*Kali carb., Laches., Phosphor.,* ||*Pulsat., Stramon.,* |*Sulphur.*

Affected by sad stories, hearing horrible things, cruelties, etc.: |*Calc. ostr.,* ||*Cicut., Coccul.,* ||*Gelsem.,* |*Ignat.,* |*Laches.,* |*Mar. ver., Natr. carb., Nux vom.,* |*Zincum.*

Much affected by misfortunes, their own or those of others: *Coloc.*

After the slightest annoyance an indifferent, gloomy state of mind: *Kali bichr.*

The slightest depressing emotion hurts much: *Calc. phosph.*

Slight emotion followed by great ailments: *Calc. ars., Cistus, Nitr. ac., Phosphor., Psorin., Zincum.*

Even the slightest thing hurts her affections: *Hura.*

A touching farewell leaves a headache: *Natr. mur.*

Least unpleasant emotion affects stomach: *Nux mosch.*

After the least emotion palpitation: *Phosphor.;* trembling: *Zincum.*

Sentimental people: *Arsen.,* |*Ant. tart., Calc. ostr., Canthar., Cinch. off., Coffea, Conium,* |*Cuprum,* ||*Ignat., Laches., Lycop., Nux vom.,* |*Phosphor., Platin., Sabad.,* ||*Staphis.*

Less sensitive to disagreeable things: *Calc. carb.*

MODEL CURE.

Pressing, stupefying pain in forehead, particularly after mental exertion and emotions. Towards evening restless, anxious and fidgety. Sleep disturbed by dreams; twitching of the whole body; sits up in bed with anxious gestures; weeps, cries out mournfully and wants to run away. Next morning does not remember what occurred: *Bellad.*—BICKING.

SYMPTOMS APPEAR WHEN THINKING OF THEM.

Beim Drandenken.

Agar.
I I Alum.
Argent.
I Arnica.
Arsenic.
Ars. hydr.
Ars. met.
Asarum.
Aurum.
I Baryt.
Bolet. sat.
Bryon.
Calc. ars.
I I Calc. ostr.
I Calc. phos.
I Caustic.
Cinch. off.
I Conium.
Crocus.
I Droser.
Graphit.
I Helleb.
Hura.
I I Hydrast.
I Laches.
Magn. carb.
Mag. sulph.
Moschus.
Natr. mur.
I I Nitr. ac.
I Oleander.
I I Oxal. ac.
I Plumbum.
I Ran. bulb.
I I Sabad.
Sarsap.
I Sepia.
I I Spigel.
I I Spongia.
I Staphis.
I Thuya.

Anxiety, liable to be brought on by thoughts: I *Calc. ostr.*

Comprehends easily when not trying to think, but the harder he tries to comprehend, the more confused he gets: *Oleand.*

Vertigo, as if the bed turned: *Plumbum.*

When thinking of it, rushing in head is increased: *Ox. ac.*

Thinking of his ailments aggravates them; headache, hiccough, bellyache, palpitation of heart: I *Ox. ac.*

Headache: *Ant. crud., Calc. phosph., Camphor.,* I *Conium, Helleb., Hydrast., Ox. ac., Sabad.;* with heat in forehead: *Calc. phosph.;* burning above the left eyebrow, worse in the forenoon: *Ars. met.*

As if something had gotten into the eye: *Calc. phosph.*

Earache as long as he thinks of it: *Crocus.*

Heat in forehead: *Calc. phosph.;* in face: *Staphis.*

Thinking of it increases onesided heat of face: *Spongia.*

Saliva runs together if thinking about the sensation in her throat: *Laches.;* if thinking about eating: *Sepia.*

Distress on seeing any one eat: *Sedinha.*

Desire for food passing off on seeing it: *Crot. casc.*

Cannot smell nor see the food: I *Arsen.*

When thinking of food, nausea: I *Sarsap.*

Aversion to all food if he sees it: *Silic., Squilla.*

Seeing the food, the appetite is gone: *Sulphur.*

Thinking of the meals the appetite comes: *Calc. phosph.*

Disgust and nausea at the mere thought of eating: *Arsen.*

Nausea and disgust when thinking of the taste of the medicine: *Bol. sat.;* when seeing the tincture: *Thuya.*

Greatest disgust and nausea if he only hears them talking about eating: *Cinch. off.;* disgust when thinking of meat: *Graphit.;* or what he has eaten: *Argent., Graphit., Sarsap.*

Nausea: *Argent., Calc. phosph., Droser.,* I I *Graphit., Laches., Mosch., Sarsap.,* I*Sepia.;* of all and everything: *Magn. sulph.;* with good taste: *Graphit., Sepia.;* with emptiness of stomach: *Sepia.;* with drowsiness all day: *Cinch. off.*

Vomituritio when thinking of water: *Ars. hydr.*

Hiccough, bellyache and looseness: *Ox. ac.*

Painful urination renewed or aggravated: *Bellad.*

Prostatic juice: *Natr. mur.* See male parts.

Chest. Thinking of his cough brings it on: *Baryt., Ox. ac.*

Sometimes very strong beats of the heart, it makes him anxious; most at noon; belching relieves it: I I *Baryt.*

Single strong beats after an omission, after thinking of his heart a beat omits: *Ox. ac.* (A strong man who had it for years.)

When thinking about his disease he feels his heart beating: *Al. p. s.*

Limbs. Pain in arms; in the knee: *Ox. ac.*

Cramp in calves: *Staphis., Spongia.*

Sensations. Burning: *Bryon.;* "inch-long" pains, especially in the arms and the hollow of the left knee: ‖ *Ox. ac.*

Oversensitive to pain, when thinking of it, he seems to feel it: ‖ *Aurum.*

The local symptoms which are aggravated by thinking of them, are relieved by the fresh air: *Hydrast.*

BETTER WHILE THINKING OF AILMENTS.

ı Ars. hydr.
ıı Camphor.
ıı Cicuta.
ı Helleb.
Hydroph.
ı Magn. carb.
ı Prun. spin.

When thinking about it, his apprehensions disappear: *Hydroph.;* better from thinking of the pain: *Camphor.*

Feeling of looseness of the brain, early in the morning, disappearing when thinking of the pain intensely: *Cicut.*

Headache, as if the brain were compressed from the top: *Camphor.*

Sensation of constriction in the brain, especially in the cerebellum; the pain ceases when he thinks of it: *Camphor.*

Pressive raw pain in sinciput, goes off immediately on directing his attention to it: *Prun. spin.*

Headache gets better from thinking of it: *Camphor., Cicut.*

Pain in the right shoulder, as if sprained; gets better when thinking of it: *Magn. carb.*

Headache on walking, as if the brain were loose and shaky when walking; disappears when thinking of it: *Cicut.*

Better not thinking about it; every moment he lays the head on another place, violent headache; if he tries to forget it, and forces himself to lie quiet with eyes closed, it ceases: *Helleb.*

BETTER WHEN THINKING ABOUT SOMETHING ELSE.

Attacks of vertigo, with staggering gait and dimness of vision: *Agar.*

Headache and earache: *Thuya;* noises in the ear: *Crocus.*

Pressing headache from outward to inward, with stupefaction and heaviness of the head; worse on moving the head, from exertion; better in the open air and from distraction of the mind: *Helleb.*

Symptoms disappear when busily occupied: *Sepia.*

Digging pain in the left side of the forehead when unoccupied: *Cinch. off.;* pain better for a while when diverted: *Stramon.*

Better from occupying himself.

Turning on a lathe: *Sepia.*

Writing: ‖ *Ferrum,* ı *Natrum.*

Reading: ı *Ferrum,* ı *Natr. carb.*

COMPLAINTS AFTER TALKING, SPEAKING, CONVERSING.

Aconite.
Alumin.
I Ambra.
II Amm. carb.
Arsen.
II Aurum.
Calc. ostr.
II Cannab.
Canthar.
Cinchon.
II Coccul.
Coffea.
Ferrum.
I Fluor. ac.
I Graphit.
II Ignat.
Jodium.
Kali carb.
Magn. mur.
Mangan.
I Mezer..
II Natr. mur.
Nux jugl.
Nux mosch.
Nux vom.
Petiver.
Phosph. ac.
Pulsat.
I Rhus tox.
Sarsap.
Sepia.
I Silic.
I Spigel.
II Sulphur.
I Thuya.

Anxiety and nausea: *Alum.;* vanishing of thought: *Nux mosch.;* omits words: *Chamon.;* confused: *Aurum.*

Vertigo: *Chamom.;* after a long talk: *Thuya;* dullness in occiput, disappearing when shutting the eyes: *Kali carb.;* dullness from the least conversation: *Silic., Staphis.*

Heaviness in head: *Ignat.;* rush of blood: I *Coffea;* trembling in head: *Ambra.;* headache: I I *Acon., Ignat.;* anterior: *Natr. mur., Silic.;* pressing from forehead to vertex: *Thuya;* in temple and both sides of vertex: *Mezer.;* upper part: *Jodium, Mezer., Petiver., Spigel.;* in left side, deep in, pressing and pushing: *Fluor. ac.;* right side: *Ignat., Thuya;* occiput: *Spigel.;* sore headache increases, so that it confuses the mind: *Aurum.*

Shooting: *Natr. mur.;* in left parietal bone: *Canthar.;* cannot talk on account of violent shooting: *Thuya.*

As if bursting: *Ignat.;* beating: *Aurum;* hammering: *Sulphur;* sore: *Cinch. off.*

Hot head and cold hands: *Phosph. ac.*

Face hot: *Sepia;* and disposition to bite teeth together: *Fluor. ac.;* a pressing jar in the face: I I *Silic.*

Teeth aching after their roots had been extracted: *Fluor. ac.;* tearing in left jaw: *Canthar.;* after dinner, irritation: *Cannab.;* and trembling shake in stomach: *Magn. mur.*

Pressing under the ribs: *Natr. mur.*

Inhalations difficult and slow: *Ferrum;* palpitation of heart: *Pulsat.*

Back. Drawing up to head: *Natr. mur.*

Hands. Cold: *Phosph. ac.;* hot: *Graphit.*

Hands and feet cold: *Amm. carb.*

Lower limbs trembling: *Ambra.*

Irritation after much talking, trembling through the whole body, coldness, sleep, headache: *Ambra., Droser.*

Affected: *Calc. ostr.;* irritated: *Ambra., Natr. mur.;* exhausted: *Cannab.;* fatigued: *Amm. carb., Sulphur.*

Lassitude from conversation: *Silic.;* general weakness: *Ferrum.*

Chill, with flushed and red face: *Arsen.*

Heat after interesting conversation: *Sepia.*

Sweat: *Sulphur;* all over: *Graphit.*

All his ailments increase: I I *Coccul.;* all his pains: *Arnica, Sulphur.*

Internal soreness; better after conversing: *Eup. perf.*

If it is the sound of the voice. See hearing, chapter 6.

The exertion of the organs. See tongue, chapter 2; larynx, chapter 25.

HEADACHE FROM EXERTIONS OF MIND OR INTELLECTUAL WORK.

Outside of margin, the marks signify great exertion, overstudy; inside of margin, t, thinking; r, reading; w, writing.

‖ Agar.	׀t.
׀ Agn. cast.	׀r.
׀ Ambra.	
׀ Amm. carb.	‖t, ׀r.
‖ Anac.	‖t.
Angust.	‖t, ׀r.
Apis.	׀r.
׀ Argent.	׀t, ׀r.
‖ Arg. nitr.	׀w.
Arnica.	׀t, ׀r.
‖ Asar.	‖t.
׀ Aurum.	‖t, ‖r, ‖w.
Berber.	
Borax.	׀r, ׀w.
Branca.	׀r.
Bryon.	׀r.
׀ Calc. ac.	׀t, ׀r.
Calc. ars.	׀r.*
‖ Calc. ostr.	‖t, ‖r, ׀w.
׀ Calc. phosph.	׀r.
Cannab.	׀w.
Carb. an.	׀w.
Carb. veg.	׀r.
Carb. sulph.	׀r.
Caustic.	‖r, ׀w.
‖ Chamom.	׀t.
‖ Cina	׀t, ‖r.
׀ Cinch. off.	׀t.
Cinnab.	׀t, ׀r.
‖ Coccul.	׀t, ׀r.
‖ Codeine.	
‖ Coffea.	‖t, ׀r.
‖ Colchic.	‖t.
׀ Conium.	‖r.
‖ Cuprum.	׀r.
׀ Daph. ind.	‖t.
׀ Digit.	‖t.
Droser.	׀w.
Eryng.	׀r, ׀w.
׀ Gent. cruc.	׀t.
׀ Gent. lut.	׀w.
Gran. cort.	׀t, ׀r.
‖ Graphit.	
Gratiol.	׀r.
׀ Helleb.	‖t.
׀ Hippom.	
׀ Hydrast.	
׀ Ignat.	‖t, ׀r, ‖w.
׀ Iris vers.	
Kali carb.	‖w.
׀ Laches.	
Lact. vir.	׀t.
׀ Lycop.	׀r, ‖w.
׀ Magn. carb.	
Mancin.	׀t, ׀w.
Merc. jod.	׀r.
‖ Mezer.	׀t, ׀r.
׀ Morph. ac.	׀r.
׀ Natr. carb.	׀w.
‖ Natr. mur.	‖r, ‖t, ‖w.
Natr. sulph.	׀r.
׀ Nitr. ac.	׀t.
‖ Nux vom.	‖t.

In cases where every exertion of the memory is followed by headache, the temporary touch with a small magnet may overcome the trouble; overtaxed school girls are mostly relieved by *Calc. phosph.*; if reading and writing, and all exertion causes headache: *Calc. ostr., Lycop., Natr. mur., Silic.*

From the least exertions: *Ol. an., Silic., Tereb.;* from the slightest, while lying down: *Nux vom.*

From every acute effort at investigation: *Anac.*

Continual attention: *Psorin., Sabad.;* only with close attention to an orator: *Ignat.;* with excitement and fatigue: *Codeine.*

If the pain does not allow any mental work: *Natr. carb.*

In the brain, as if beaten: *Anac., Aurum, Cinch. off.;* as if sore: *Cinch. off., Daph. ind.*

In the inner head: *Cina;* on a small spot: *Colchic.*

Forehead: *Coffea, ‖Digit., Anac., ‖Arnica, Mancin., Mezer., Ol. an., Pulsat., Rhus rad., ׀Silic., Tereb.;* pressing: *Arnica.*

Pressure like a load: *Digit.;* increasing to stupidity: *Coccul., Petrol.;* want of thinking powers as soon as beginning: *Asar., Mezer.;* after the slightest exertion: *Ol. an.;* heavy pressure: *Arnica.*

Pressure in arcus ciliaris: *Ran. bulb.;* and eyes: *Lactuc.;* tension: *Sulphur;* drawing over eyes: *Calc. ostr.*

From root of nose to forehead: *Natr. mur.;* pressure, worse while walking: *Arnica;* throbbing, better while walking: *Pulsat.*

In forehead and temples, contractive pressure: *Digit.;* as if beaten: *Phosph. ac.*

Forehead, temples and occiput: *Anac.;* right side and occiput: *Calc. ostr.*

Temples: *Anac., Digit., Gent. cruc., Helleb., Mezer., Natr. carb., Natr. mur., Nux vom., ׀Psorin.;* pressure: *Helleb.;* as from a nail: *Anac.;* and tension: *Sulphur;* from one temple to the other: *Mancin.;* tension in brain: *Sulphur;* stitches most in right temple outward: *Lycop.;* one-sided pressure: *Ignat.*

HEADACHE FROM EXERTIONS OF MIND OR INTELLECTUAL WORK. 103

Oleander.	׀t.
׀ Ol. anim.	׀׀t.
׀׀ Ox. ac.	
׀ Paris.	׀t, ׀r.
׀׀ Petrol.	
׀׀ Phosphor.	׀t.
׀ Phosph. ac.	׀׀t, ׀r.
׀ Pimpin.	׀r.
Prun. spin.*	
׀׀ Psorin.	׀t.
׀ Pulsat.	׀t.
Ran bulb.	׀w.
Rhodod.	׀w.
׀ Rhus rad.	׀t, ׀w.
Rhus tox.	׀w.
׀ Sabad.	׀׀t.
׀ Scuttel.	
׀ Selen.	׀t.
׀ Sepia.	
׀ Silic.	׀t, ׀r, ׀׀w.
Spiggur.	׀w.
׀׀ Sulphur.	׀t.
Tabac.	׀r.
Terebinth.	׀t.
Vinca.	׀w.

Vertex : *Carb. veg., Gent. cruc., Natr. mur., Nux vom., Pimpin., Ran bulb.,* ׀׀*Sepia ;* pressing : *Lycop.;* and throbbing : *Nux vom.;* as if beaten : *Phosph. ac.;* as of a foreign body under the skull : *Conium.*

Occiput : *Anac., Calc. ac., Carb. an., Nitr. ac., Rhus rad.;* pressing in the depth of cerebellum : *Colchic.;* drawing, bending backwards : *Cinch. off.*

In forehead, occiput and temples, changing about, better from external pressure : *Calc. ostr.*

Congestion of head by intellectual labor : *Psorin.;* when talking : *Coffea.*

Heat in head, with cold hands : *Phosph. ac.;* heat and sweat : *Kali carb., Phosph. ac., Ran. bulb.*

External pain from writing and reading, increased by pressure of spectacles : *Lycop.*

Pressing : *Anac.,* ׀׀*Arnica, Calc. ac., Chamom.,* ׀׀ *Coccul., Coffea, Colchic., Digit., Helleb., Ignat., Lactuc., Lycop., Magn. carb., Mezer., Nux vom., Ol. an., Paris, Sepia, Silic., Sulphur, Tereb.;* like a heavy load : *Digit.;* urging in whole head : *Arg. nitr.;* as if pressing from in out : *Kali carb.;* asunder : *Nux vom.;* bursting : *Arg. nitr., Nux vom.*

Tension. Forehead : *Sulphur;* as if a bladder was stretched from one temple to the other : *Mancin.;* tension in the brain, with pressure in temples : *Sulphur;* tension pains : *Sabad.;* crampy pressure : ׀׀*Phosph. ac.*

Drawing : *Borax, Calc. ac., Cina, Coffea;* drawing together above the temples : *Agn. cast.;* tearing and pressing : ׀׀*Anac., Ran bulb.;* from glabella to forehead : *Natr. mur.*

Stitches in temples from within outward : *Lycop., Silic., Sulphur.*

Jerks : *Digit.;* throbbing : *Agar., Pulsat.;* throbbing towards the head : *Psorin.;* beating in arteries : *Agar.;* in vertex : *Nux vom.*

Hammering, after an animated conversation : *Sulphur;* congestion : *Agar., Nux vom.,* orgasm : *Cannab.;* heat : *Berber.;* fullness : *Psorin.*

Sore. As if beaten : *Aurum;* as if crusted : *Ignat.;* in the whole brain : *Cinch. off.,* renewed weeks after : *Daph. ind.;* making stupid : *Cinnab.;* sensation in the brain, as if beaten : *Anac.,* ׀*Aurum;* as if the whole head were bruised : *Cinch. off.;* as if mashed : *Ignat.*

Better from mental exertion : aching in head changes places and lessens after exertion of mind : *Calc. ostr.*

Better from thinking; headache undefined : *Amm. carb., Calc. phosph.,* ׀*Ignat., Morph. ac., Natr. mur., Nitr. ac., Paris, Phosphor.,* ׀*Sabad.*

Pressing in one-half of head : *Ignat., Tereb. ol.,* changing place : *Calc. ostr.*

Headache is relieved during mental occupation, but worse after it : *Arsen.*

Head symptoms disappear : *Calc. ac.*

Headache relieved by conversation : *Eup. perf.*

Continued meditation lessens the headache : *Psorin.*

In anterior parts: in temples, tension lessened by intellectual labor; by thinking: *Calc. ac., Sabad.*

Headache, posterior, intellectual labor: *Calc. ac.*

Pressing, tearing headache, which does not interfere with mental labor: *Squilla.*

MODEL CURE.

After *overstudy*, feeling at times of a foreign body under the skull, in vertex: better *during* reading; worse *after* reading; worse on going to sleep, or from excitement, or thinking of the pain; better by touch; the relief during reading seemed to rise from the mind being diverted from the pain. *Conium* 3^m (Jen.). One dose cured.—BERRIDGE.

OTHER COMPLAINTS AFTER MENTAL EXERTION, OVER-STUDY, MEDITATING, ETC.

Nach Geistesanstrengungen.

|| Agar.
Aloes.
| Alum.
|| Ambra.
Amm. carb.
Amm. gum.
| Anac.
| Angust.
Argent.
|| Arsen.
| Asaf.
Aspar.
Aster.
| Aurum.
| Baryt.
| Bellad.
| Branca.
| Bryon.
| Calad.
|| Calc. ostr.
| Cinnab.
| Coccul.
| Colchic.
| Conium.
|| Cuprum.
| Euphorb.
| Evon. eur.
|| Fluor ac.
| Formica.
| Glonoin.
|| Graphit.
Gratiol.
| Hepar.
|| Hyosc.
|| Ignat.
| Jodium.
| Kali carb.
Kali chlor.
|| Laches.
| Lauroc.
|| Lycop.
|| Magn. carb.
| Magn. mur.

Anxiety arising from thoughts: *Calc. ostr.;* after meditating: *Phosphor.;* after over-working the mind, attacks of anxiety which cannot be suppressed or overcome with the best will: *Cuprum.*

After exertion of mind, hasty: *Ignat.*

After over-study talkative mania, speaks in choice phrases, jumping from one subject to another: |*Laches.*^{30}; uses exalted language, corrects herself by substituting another word: *Laches.*^{2m}.

Want of ideas: *Asar.*

Indifference: *Natr. mur.*

After thinking, forgetful: *Amm. carb.*

Forgetfulness when reading: *Viol. od.*

Absent-minded when studying: *Baryt. carb.;* when reading: *Agn. cast., Phosph. ac., Laches., Nux mosch.*

Indisposed to mental labor: *Amm. gum., Cinnab., Colchic., Opium, Ran. scel., Selen.*

Fatigued in head: *Coccul.;* head empty: *Lycop.*

Difficulty of thinking and disinclination to mental exertion: *Spigel.*

Cannot enjoy reading or conversation: *Nux vom.*

Vanishing of ideas: *Canthar., Caustic., Chamom., Evon., Hepar s. c., Mezer., Nitr. ac., Ran. bulb., Staphis.*

When reading thoughts vanish: *Nux mosch.*

While reading sinks into absence of mind: |*Nux mosch.*

Mental work makes weak-minded: *Magn. carb.*

Confused thought: *Oleand.*

Thinking affects the head: *Coccul.*

Inability to think and to perform any mental labor; the head feels stupefied if he tries to exert himself: *Natr. carb.*

OTHER COMPLAINTS AFTER MENTAL EXERTION, ETC. 105

I Mangan. II Menyanth. Morph. ac. II Natr. carb. II Natr. mur. I Nux mosch. II Nux vom. I Oleander. II Opium. II Paris. II Petrol. Phosphor. II Platin. II Plumbum. II Psorin. I Pulsat. II Ran. bulb. I Ran. scel. I Rheum. I Rhodod. Rhus tox. I Sabad. II Selen. II Sepia. II Silic. I Spigel. I Stannum. II Staphis. I Stramon. I Sulphur. I Tarax. Tereb. I Thuya. I Veratr. I Verbasc. II Vinc. min. II Viola od. II Xiphos. I Zincum. Zinc. cyan.	Headache in the forehead; every mental exertion causes him to become quite stupid: *Petrol.* In good humor but cannot work mentally: *Arnica.* Dullness in head makes thinking difficult: *Bryon.* Mental work fatigues: *Aurum;* particularly in morning: *Berber.* Lassitude, thinking and speaking are hard work: *Rhus tox.* When trying to recollect, excitement, convulsions and disturbed feeling in the upper part of the brain: *Aster.;* vanishing of thoughts: *Nitr. ac.* Rushing noise in the head from reading: *Carb. veg.* In the morning happy, clear and decided; after nine o'clock dull and unable to think: *Sulphur.* Dazed feeling, made worse by thinking: *Sulphur;* from writing: *Arg. nitr.;* dazed and sleepy from reading: *Angust.* Mental work makes dull and stupid: *Coccul., Natr. mur., Magn. carb.* Vertigo from thinking: *Agar., Gran. cort.;* from reading: *Branc. urs., Cuprum, Gran. cort., Gratiol., Phosph. ac.;* vertigo and nausea: *Arnica;* from writing: *Kali carb., Rhodod.* Attacks of vertigo and disturbed memory from writing: *Argent.* Vertigo from thinking while walking in the open air: *Agar.;* dizziness towards evening in the open air, aggravated by thinking: *Silic.*

Vertigo after mental occupation, with dull pressure on the temples: *Natr. carb.*

Giddiness and internal soreness of head, senses vanish: *Cuprum.*

Mental work causes congestion to the head: *Nux vom.*

Fulness of the head: *Psorin.*

Dullness and heaviness from mental exertion: *Natr. mur.;* from reading: *Pimpin.;* from writing: *Gent. lut.*

Fainting after thinking or writing: *Calad.*

Crawling in the head: *Thuya.*

Eyes. Darkness before the eyes when reading and thinking: *Menyanth.*

Dull pain in the eyes when reading or from mental occupation: *Cina.*

Pressing pain over the right eyes: *Bromum, Ran. bulb.*

All symptoms appear after reading and writing. See Eyes, Chapter 5.

Ears. Roaring noises in ears from mental exertion: *Conium;* from writing: *Sepia.*

Throbbing when stooping to write: *Rheum, Zincum.*

Nose. Stopped up when reading aloud: *Mar. ver., Verbasc.*

Face. Sudden paleness from reading: *Graphit.*

Heat in the face: *Agar., Amm. carb.*

Thinking causes heat in the face in the evening: *Xiphos.*

Pain in lower jaw when reading: *Hydroph.*

Teeth. Sore, ache: *Nux vom.;* when reading: *Ignat.*

Quiet aching increases to a steady cutting: *Bellad.;* or digging, rooting pain: *Nux vom.;* in hot climate: ııı*Natr. carb.*

Saliva. Tinged with blood: *Nitr. ac.*

Throat. As if torn: *Caustic.;* after dinner, up into the ear and nose: *Conium.*

Nausea: *Asar.;* eructation: *Hepar;* general nausea: *Aurum;* nausea and dizziness from reading: *Arnica.*

After much mental occupation, sitting; costiveness: *Aloes.*

Weak digestion: *Arnica,* ııı*Calc. ostr.,* ııı*Coccul.,* ı*Laches.,* ıı*Nux vom.,* ı*Pulsat.,* ı*Sulphur,* ııı*Veratr.*

After over-taxed mental powers gastric symptoms, nervous irritation of bowels: *Nux mosch.*

Gastric Symptoms. Pressing in the stomach: *Anac.*

Sharp pressing pain in the rectum after meals and after stool; tearing, stinging, constricting pain as from blind hemorrhoids: *Nux vom.;* pressing sore pain as from hemorrhoids: *Ignat.*

Soreness in the hemorrhoids increased by walking and thinking: *Caustic.*

Constricting pain in the forepart of the urethra running back: *Nux vom.*

Urging to urinate, passes a few drops: *Kali carb.*

Emission of prostatic fluid when thinking of lascivious things, without excitement of sexual organs or an erection: *Natr. mur.*

Urging pain in the genitals when sitting bent over and reading: *Bellad.*

Voice. Reading aloud. See Larynx.

Breathing. Anxious breathing when thinking: *Phosphor.*

Deep breathing when writing: *Fluor. ac.*

Dyspnœa from writing: *Aspar.;* dyspnœa relieved by writing or reading: *Ferr. ac.*

Whooping-cough worse from reading: *Cina;* from mental exertion: *Arnica, Ignat., Nux vom.*

Cough worse from thinking and reading: *Nux vom.*

Pressing pain in the chest when writing: *Magn. sulph., Ran. bulb.;* stinging pain when reading: *Euphorb.;* when writing: *Carb. an., Spigel.;* throbbing pain when thinking: *Phosphor.;* when writing: *Magn. sulph.*

Heart. Palpitation from mental exertion: *Ignat., Natr. carb.;* as soon as he turns his attention to one thing his heart palpitates: *Natr. carb.;* when writing: *Natr. carb.*

Pulse feeble, not much more frequent but unequal: *Cupr. ac.*

Coldness at the heart from mental exertion: *Natr. mur.*

Pressing out of the chest when writing: *Asar.*

Drawing pain in the back when reading: *Natr. carb.*

Backache while sitting: *Chamom., Conium.*

When stooping, with throbbing in ears: *Rheum.*

Feet often cold; skin moist, not warmer than usual: *Cupr. ac.*

Excited, crampy, restless sensation in the upper part of the brain similar to that felt in the limbs after severe muscular exertion: *Ast. rub.*

Cannot fix his attention or think, with crawling in the hands and head: *Thuya;* impelled to think, but it makes her body weak, trembling, cold and moist: *Aurum.*

Trembling of the whole body, especially of the hands, with nausea and weakness of the knees: *Borax, Vinc. min.*

Great restlessness in the evening from mental occupation, reading: *Natr. carb.*

Feels tired and weak from reading: *Aurum.*

Easily fatigued from mental work: *Alum., Aurum, Laches., Pulsat., Thuya;* especially from reading and writing: *Colchic.*

Nervous weakness, fatigued from thinking, reading and writing: ||*Arnica,* |*Bellad.,* |*Calc. ac.,* ||*Coccul.,* |*Ignat.,* ||*Laches.,* |*Lycop.,* ||*Natr. carb.,* ||*Natr. mur.,* ||*Psorin.,* ||*Pulsat.,* |*Sabad.,* |*Sepia,* ||*Silic.,* |*Sulphur.*

Mental and bodily exhaustion from long continued activity or night watching: *Cupr. ac.*

Fainting after mental exertion, thinking and writing: *Calad.*

Drowsiness, when thinking: *Natr. sulph.;* when reading: *Natr. mur.;* when writing: *Natr. sulph.*

The least exertion of mind causes somnolency: *Nux mosch.*

Goes to sleep while thinking, after eating: *Natr. sulph.*

Goes to sleep while reading: *Angust., Ignat., Natr. mur., Platin., Prun. spin., Ruta, Sepia.*

Goes to sleep while writing: *Phosph. ac.*

Is worse on going to sleep: *Conium.*

Noises in ear worse when lying in bed, and when waking in the night: *Conium.*

Cannot get to sleep until late: *Chlorum, Kali carb.*

Sleep restless, unrefreshing, confused worrying dreams: *Cupr. ac.*

Coldness: *Aurum;* chill when writing: *Zincum.*

Heat: *Phosphor.;* while reading: *Oleand.*

Heat, as if hot water were poured over her: *Phosphor.*

Sweat in the morning in bed when thinking: *Zinc. cyan.*

Sweat from every mental exertion, reading, writing, etc.: *Kali carb.*

Disagreeable feeling from exerting the mind: *Colchic.*

Jerking pains when writing: *Natr. mur.*

Studying aggravates his pains: *Formica.*

Evening; noises in ear: *Conium, Sepia.*

Thinking and speaking are difficult towards evening: *Ignat.*

During mental prostration (geistige Abspannung), heart and circulation of blood affected: ||*Acon., Asar.,* |*Bellad., Bismuth.,* ||*Cicut.,* |*Cinch. off., Digit., Magn. carb.,* ||*Natr. mur.,* |*Petrol.,* ||*Phosphor.,* ||*Spongia, Stannum,* ||*Stramon.*

Intellectual labor fatigues him: *Pulsat.*

All headwork affects him: *Aurum, Lycop., Pulsat., Silic.*

Head overfatigued from mental labor: ||*Nux vom.,* |*Pulsat.*

Complaints arising when reading or writing: *Aurum, Fluor. ac.;* from writing: *Calc. ostr.*

All mental exertion aggravates or causes ailments: *Calc. ostr., Nux vom.*
Ailments after continual mental labor: *Nux vom.*
Affected by scientific labors: *Graphit.*
Better after exertion of mind, (see Headache) B. R.: ‖ *Crocus,* | *Ferrum,*
| *Natr. carb.*
Longlasting wakefulness: *Laches.*

AILINGS FROM OVEREXERTION OF MIND AND BODY.

In the comparative table, the numbers added indicate the degrees of importance given by B. in his R.   * Signify such as have been altered. The first, after emotions; the second, after exertions of intellect; the third, exertions of the body.

Arnica.	1 1 4
Arsen.	2 2 4
Asar.	1 2 1
Aurum.	3 2 2
Bellad.	3 4 0
Bryon.	3 0 4
Calc. ostr.	3 4 3
Carb. veg.	1 1 4
Cinch. off.	1 2 3
Chamom.	3 1 0
Coccul.	3 3 3
Coffea.	3 1 2
Colchic.	1 3 1
Coloc.	4 0 0
‖ Cuprum.	3 4 3
Hyosc.	4 0 0
Ignat.	4 4 1
	Laches.*	3 4 3
Lycop.	3 4 4
Mercur.	3 0 2
Natr. carb.	1 2 2
Natr. mur.	3 4 3
‖ Nitr. ac.	4 3 2
Nux mosch.	2 1 2
Nux vom.	4 4 2
Oleander.	2 3 2
	*Opium.	4 2 1
Phosphor.	3 1 2
Platin.	3 2 1
Pulsat.	4 2 1
‖ Rhus tox.	2 0 4
Sabad.	0 3 1
Sepia.	2 4 2
Silic.	1 4 3
Stannum.	1 1 1
Staphis.	4 4 1
Stramon.	4 3 0
	Sulphur.	2 3 4
Veratr.	3 1 3
Zincum.	2 1 3

Very sensitive to all moral or physical exertions: *Staphis.*

Mental excitement and perturbations followed by puerperal convulsions: *Act. rac.*

Anxiety, fright or fear: |*Lycop.*

Combined emotions, fright, hearing horrible things, mortification increase all complaints: *Laches.*

Anxious night-watching, care, trouble, scanty milk: *Caustic.*

After longlasting, mental trouble, milk thin: *Laches.*

Watching at the sick bed of a dear friend; losing sleep for a week or longer; cannot sleep at all: *Sulphur.*

After suffering losses or shocks, used up, heart broken. without sleep; in cramps, etc.: | *Opium.*

Great care; loss of sleep: *Hydroph.*

Moral emotions with rapid movements, prolonged walks, overexertion: *Laches.*

Anxiety, overexertion, straining muscles and getting wet when in a sweat, after his house was burnt out: *Rhus tox.*

After most violent emotions of mind, with great mental and bodily exertions and loss of sleep: |*Cuprum.*

MODEL CURES.

After continued loss of sleep, night after night, longlasting anxiety, overexertions of mind and body, from nursing the sick; great anguish of mind from the loss of his dearest friend: ‖*Nitr. ac.*—HAYNEL.

A state of mental and bodily exhaustion after overexertion of the mind, pulse feeble, somewhat frequent, unequal; skin moist, feet generally cold; attacks of unconquerable anxiety; the head giddy and internally painful, feels as if he would lose his senses, sleep full of dreams, restless, unrefreshing: *Cupr. ac.*—SCHMID.

MODEL CURES.

SHOCK OF INJURY.

A soldier, while carrying a wounded comrade, was struck by a spent bullet in the epigastrium—became pale and weak, "felt the wind knocked out of him;" laid down. A drop of *Liquor ammon.* in water relieved at once.

In another case, it helped in shock from gunshot wound of the lung, with great prostration: *Amm. caust.*

Arnica, alternately with *Opium*, both in 1st dec. in water, frequently repeated, relieved shock and concussion in a case of fractured skull in a boy. The fractured edge after some time became indistinguishable (the hat having prevented any scalp wound). The symptoms were, loss of consciousness, sleepiness, pallor; vomiting, after beginning with the medicines.

A young man fell and broke his thigh; was lividly pale, cold, stupefied: *Camphor.*^{6}, speedily followed by relief: *Caustic.*

A boy of five years was run over—thigh broken. Could not bear to have it handled; could not get to sleep; wide awake. Relieved by *Coffea*^{2c}.—J. C. MORGAN.

JEALOUSY.

A farmer's woman who had by jealousy become a raving maniac, and was to be transferred to an insane asylum, got well from one drop of the same remedy, bodily and mentally.—E. STAPF. See Model Cure, page 86.

A young girl was made seriously ill from jealousy and grief about a faithless lover. She suffered with fever most in the hours after midnight; high redness of the face, with constant delirium and desire to run away; she complained all the time of a throbbing toothache. One dose of *Hyosc.* cured the toothache and delirium, and a second week after restored her completely.—BŒNNINGHAUSEN.

AFTER EMOTIONS AND EXCITEMENT.

From disappointed ambition, bewildered, talks incoherently; does everything he attempts to do, wrong; complains of heaviness of the head, pain in the stomach and small of back; feels weak and cannot sit up; face now pale with sharp pointed nose, then red, with irritated pulse: *Nux vom.*—G. HARTLAUB.

OTHER COMPLAINTS AFTER MENTAL EXERTION.

A woman aged 34, nervous temperament after extreme mental exertion, suffered since eighteen months from marked irritation of the intestinal canal; distension of the stomach and abdomen, worse after dinner and from the slightest mental excitement: *Nux mosch.*—HAHNEMANN.

After over-study clicking noise in left *vertex*, on walking and during stool; also in occiput on walking, especially in evening, when tired: *Conium*^{3m} (Jen.). One dose cured.—E. W. BERRIDGE.

A girl, after *excessive study*, uses exalted language; exceedingly particular about the language she uses, often correcting herself after using a word and substituting another of very similar meaning; talks about being under the influence of a superior power. *Laches.*^{2m}.—E. W. BERRIDGE.

BODILY SYMPTOMS CONNECTED WITH THE MIND.
II. Mental Concomitants of Bodily Symptoms.

HEAD.

The stupefying headaches have been placed to Chapter 2. The mental concomitants have not been separated and are given altogether in Chapter 2.
Dreams are placed with Sleep, Chapter 37. Delirium mostly to Fevers, Chapter 40.

ACCORDING TO LOCALITY.

Forehead. Liveliness: *Phosph. ac.*; serenity the first twelve hours: *Caustic.*; contracting, benumbing pain, with ill humor, alternately, with freedom of all complaints, with comfortableness, and excited imagination: *Hyosc.*

Gloomy feeling, and heaviness in occiput: *Ptel. trif.*

Absorbed, sullen mood: *Ol. an.*; hypochondric: *Arg. nitr.*; heat, melancholy: *Stramon.*

Depression of spirits: *Naja tr.*; low spirits: *Ran. bulb., Rhus rad.*; increasing sadness, only in daytime: *Mercur.*; anxiety: *Alum., Caustic., Nitrum*; after precordial anxiety: *Platin.*; anxiety, and heat: *Lauroc.*; fear of going mad: *Ambra*; as if madness would ensue: *Acon.*

Impatience: *Platin., Zincum.*

Morose. Over the right eye: *Rqn. bulb.*; and upper part of head, in the evening: *Mercur.*; as if the bone would burst: *Niccol.*; with vertigo, later in occiput: *Chin. sulph.*; with sneezing, and running of nose: *Clemat.*; heat in upper body: *Platin.*; increasing from 5 P.M.; pressure relieves: *Anac.*

Vexatious ill humor; heaviness: *Aethus.*; heaviness, like a stone; whining about trifles: *Bellad.*; like a weight; incapable of thinking: *Bovist.*; with a painful quivering: *Bovist.*; nausea: *Stannum*; sleepiness: *Calc. ostr.*

Fretful; never gets her work done: *Bryon.*; peevish temper; irritable about others: *Mar. ver.*; moaning and distress; can neither lie nor sit: *Coffea.*

Inclination to work: *Aloes*; desires to hurry his business: *Ptel. trif.*; irresistible inclination to commit suicide: *Mercur.*

Shooting over left eye, extorting cries: *Sepia.*

Sitting alone; would not speak: *Ant. crud.*; disinclined to converse: *Rhus tox.*; to think: *Bromum.*

Aching all day hinders mental exertion: *Amm. gum.*

Diminished intellectual power; difficult comprehension: *Arg. nitr., Calc. ac., Calc. ostr., Ignat., Mezer., Natr. mur.*

ACCORDING TO SENSATIONS.

Inner warmth, stupidity: *Alum.;* on trying to think: *Mezer.;* thinking difficult: *Zincum,* ‖ *Ignat.;* left: *Lauroc.;* impossible: *Mezer., Opium.*

Exalted imagination: *Hyosc.;* delirium: *Chin. sulph.;* delirious, with sneezing: *Mezer.;* as if losing his reason: *Acon., Ambra, Hamam.*

Forgetful: *Calc. ac.;* using wrong words: *Lil. tigr.;* awkwardness: *Bryon.* Loss of consciousness after outward pressure: *Prun. spin.;* after a blow on the crown: *Natr. mur.;* when reading: *Tarax.*

Forehead and Temples. Dull ache, with liveliness: *Phosph. ac.*

Anxiety and sweat: *Nitrum;* after a shock, loud cry: *Stannum.*

Irritable temper: *Lil. tigr.;* depression of spirits: *Naja tr.*

Confuse with obtuse senses: *Crot. tigl.*

Mind exalted: *Anac.;* lively: *Phosph. ac.;* discouraged: *Agar.;* fear: *Agar.;* of return of pain: *Rhus tox.;* anxiety: *Chelid., Nitrum;* anxious, urging to shout: *Mercur.;* ill humor: *Bovist.;* morose: *Coloc.;* singing: *Alum.;* crying: *Kali carb.;* restless: *Ran. bulb.;* forgets the word on the tongue: *Mezer.;* difficult comprehension, weak mind: *Stannum;* difficult to collect thoughts: *Mezer.;* stupor, within inner head: *Lycop.*

Temples and Sides. Sharp shooting, with apprehensions: *Fluor. ac.*

Sides. Uneasiness: *Arg. nitr.;* fearfulness: *Cicut.;* pusillanimity: *Agar.;* ill humor: *Magn. mur.;* morose: *Niccol.;* screams: *Cuprum, Magn. mur.*

Difficult thinking: *Ignat.;* thoughts stand still: *Cannab.;* half-sided, with forgetfulness: *Capsic.*

Vertex. After abatement of pain, exhilarated: *Formica.*

Sadness and apprehension: *Cuprum, Sulphur.*

Anxiety and heat in head: *Hyperic., Strontian.;* precordial anxiety and trembling: *Sepia;* worse from pressing on top: *Benz. ac.;* after talkativeness: *Ambra.*

Fear: *Apis;* despair: *Agar.;* ill humor: *Mercur.;* peevish, whining: *Zincum;* morose: *Mercur., Niccol.;* unwilling to talk: *Phosph. ac.*

Despair, almost amounting to rage: *Agar.*

Loss of memory: *Moschus;* slow thinking: *Cann. sat.*

Occiput. Exaltation: *Anac.;* excitability: *Sabin.;* depression: *Rhus rad.*

Anxiousness: *Bovist., Caustic., Nitrum;* as if danger would approach: *Fluor. ac.;* with vexatiousness: *Kali carb.;* ill humor: *Amm. mur.;* gloomy feeling: *Ptel. trif.;* moroseness: *Chin. sulph.;* bitter complaint: *Phytol.;* has to cry: *Cann. ind.;* screaming: *Petrol.*

Cannot comprehend, weak mind: *Calc. ostr.;* uses wrong names: *Diosc.;* delirium: *Ver. vir.*

ACCORDING TO SENSATIONS.

Sensitive brain and fright: *Laches.*

Heavy head and anxious tossing about: *Mangan.;* and painful confusion: *Calc. ostr.;* and excited talking: *Ambra;* excitement: *Narc. ac.;* ill humor: *Sarsap.;* on top of head, anxiousness: *Sambuc.;* like a stone, fretful and moaning: *Bellad.;* difficult thinking: *Bovist.;* stupidity, worse, stooping: *Lauroc.*

Dullness and difficult comprehension; pressing; morose: *Acon.;* and restlessness: *Ruta.*

As if brain were a lump, with excitement and restlessness: *Cinch. off.*

Constriction, like a tape tightly drawn, with ill humor: *Platin.;* as if too tightly braced, with slowness of ideas: *Carb. veg.;* with stupidity: *Cuprum;* as if a membrane was stretched over the brain, with weak memory: *Helleb.;* internal tension; thoughts stand still: *Lycop.;* as if bound, slow thinking: *Carb. veg.;* as if tied up and cannot get rid of one idea: *Carb. veg.;* as if screwed together and anxious; afternoon; oppression and ill humor: *Magn. carb.*

Pressure and ill humor: *Platin., Silic.,* and obstinacy: *Acon.;* unable to work mentally: *Phosphor.,* unwilling: *Anac.;* anxiety: ||*Arsen.;* whining, moroseness: *Bellad.;* peevish; *Ignat.;* impatient: *Mancin.;* ill humor: *Silic.*

Congestion and difficult comprehension: *Nitr. ac.*

Tension, with stupidity: *Ambra.*

Drawing; and excited mind: *Phosphor.;* and as if senses would leave: *Agar.*

Tearing, shooting and ill humor: *Tongo;* as if losing reason: *Magn. carb.;* difficult comprehension and rage: *Arsen.*

Sensation like lightening, with apprehension: *Fluor. ac.;* shooting, ill humor and vexation: ||*Silic.;* out of humor in the evening: *Magn. carb.;* throbbing, using wrong words: *Chamom.*

Bursting, with loud whining: *Phosphor.*

Pulsating stitches; weak minded: *Stannum.*

Inner heat, excitement: *Arg. nitr.;* gaiety: *Therid.;* anxiety: *Carb. veg., Lauroc., Magn. carb., Phosphor., Ruta., Silic.,* and fear: *Strontian.;* morose: *Lauroc., Platin.;* melancholic: *Stramon.;* ill humor: *Calc. phosph.;* restlessness: *Canthar.;* difficult thinking: *Digit.;* diminished intellect: *Stannum;* laziness: *Calc. phosph., Lauroc.*

Pulsations painless, with fear of dying in sleep: *Nux mosch.;* throbbing and heat after vexation: *Cyclam.;* using wrong words: *Chamom.;* beating, with frightening illusions: *Pulsat.;* pounding, cannot read nor write: *Clemat.*

Boring, forcing to cry: *Sepia.*

Lacerating, with indignant discomfort: *Opium.*

Weak feeling with sadness: *Hyperic.;* lameness of brain, cannot comprehend: *Calc. ostr.;* brain numb as if dead, and unable to work: *Thuya.*

Emptiness, with anxious feeling: *Natr. mur.*

Dullness and depression: *Codein.;* inability to think: *Gelsem.;* with great anxiety: *Chin. sulph.*

WITH HEADACHE IN GENERAL.

Serenity: *Phosphor.;* merriness: *Acon., Crocus;* happiness: *Crocus;* exhileration: *Coca;* foolish laughing: *Sabad.;* better humor: *Amm. carb.*

Discomfort: *Cina, Paris, Ruta;* brain as if contracted: *Gratiol.;* forenoon: *Serpent.*
Unbearable: *Sarsap.;* does not know: *Cuprum.*
Sad, weeping: *Petiv.;* melancholic, after dinner: *Arsen.;* sat on the same place without talking: *Conium, Hippom.*
Sadness: *Arsen., Conium, Crotal.;* low spirited: *Selen.;* fear of death: *Laches.;* depressed, melancholy: ǁ *Crotal.;* ill humored and peevish: *Silic.;* evenings: *Magn. carb.;* lachrymose: *Sepia;* fear of losing reason: *Magn. carb.;* weak memory: *Kreosot.;* dull and confused: *Ailanth.;* vertigo: *Conium;* violent ache: *Conium;* shooting: *Silic.;* when walking in the evening: ǁ *Therid.;* with chilliness: *Helleb.*

HEADACHE WITH ANXIOUSNESS.

Acon.
Aethusa.
Alum.
Ambra.
Ant. crud.
Ant. tart.
ǀ Arnica.
Ars. sulph.
Arsen.
Bellad.
Benz. ac.
Bovist.
Calc. ostr.
Carb. an.
Carb. veg.
Caustic.
ǁ Chin. sulph
ǀ Gelsem.
Glonoin.
Graphit.
ǀ Hyperic.
ǀ Laches.
Lauroc.
Magn. carb.
Natr. carb.
Natr. mur.
Nitr. ac.
Nitrum.
Nux mosch.
ǁ Nux vom.
Ox. ac.
Phosphor.
Platin.
Pulsat.
ǀ Ran. bulb.
Rheum.
ǁ Rhus tox.
Ruta.
Selen.
Senega.
Sepia.
Stannum.
Stramon.
Strontian.
Sulphur.
Vip. red.
Zincum.

Pressing in forehead, with fear of losing his reason: *Ambra;* with mania: *Arsen.;* followed by mania: *Arsen.*
Elastic pressure on top of head: ǁ *Benz. ac.*
Precordial anxiousness with pressing in forehead, heat, red face, and violent thirst till evening: *Platin.;* as if the top of head would burst, with heat and drowsiness: *Strontian.*
Heaviness in occiput: *Ant. tart.*
With the headache, after a few minutes: *Glonoin.*
Pulsating in head on waking from sleep: *Carb. veg.*
Precordial anxiety with red face and bitter mouth: *Bellad.*
Throbbing, shooting with nausea or belching and red face: *Laches.*
With nausea following the headache in afternoon: *Nitr. ac.*
After nausea in the morning or during the afternoon: *Calc. ostr.;* weakness while eating: *Ran. bulb.;* in the chest, better in the evening: *Zincum;* from chest to head: *Acon.;* with restlessness, followed by head and bellyache: *Aethus.;* worse from moving and stooping: *Rheum;* with fear of the slightest touch or motion: *Hyperic.*
Precordial anxiety after the headache with trembling, followed by nosebleed: *Sepia;* weakness: *Ran. bulb.;* driving out of bed, heat in head: *Carb. an.;* when awaking before the fever: *Rhus tox.;* chill, outward or inward: *Arnica.*
With heat in forehead and cold limbs: *Ars. sulph.*
With heat in head and throbbing on vertex: *Hyperic.*
Heat in head after getting angry: *Bryon.;* after vexation: *Cyclam.*
Heat as if sweat would break out: *Platin.*
Sweat, vertigo, staggering: *Nitrum.*
Sweat all over, trembling in every limb, slow pulse: *Chin. sulph.*

8

MIND AND DISPOSITION.

Anxious sweat: *Ant. crud.;* anxious sweat walking in open air: *Ant. crud.;* every day at the same hour: *Platin.*

Afraid to go to sleep, has a painless pulsation in head: *Nux mosch.*

Headache driving to despair: *Agar.*

Inclined to suicide: *Apis, Ant. crud., Cinch. off., Nux vom., Rhus tox.*

HEADACHE WITH ILL HUMOR.

Acon.
Aethus.
II Amm. carb.
Amm. mur.
Anac.
Bellad.
Bovist.
Bryon.
Calc. phos.
Chin.sulph.
Conium.
Cyclam.
Dulcam.
Graphit.
I Hippom.
Ignat.
Kali carb.
Kreosot.
Lachnanth.
Lauroc.
Magn. mur.
Mangan.
Mercur.
Natr. mur.
I Niccol.
Opium.
Panac.
Platin.
II Phosphor.
Silic.
Spongia.
Stannum.
Thuya.
Vip. tor.
Zincum.

Very much vexed with dullness: *Calc. phosph.*

Discouraged: *Agar.;* and peevish, morose, afternoon: *Bovist.;* evening: *Platin.;* forenoon: *Amm. carb.*

Dissatisfied with herself: *Panac.*

With bad humor, she must sing or hum all day: *Natr. mur.*

Whining moroseness: *Bellad.;* sleepy whining mood: *Lachnanth.*

Everything disagreeable, loss of appetite, drowsy: *Spongia.*

Incapable of thinking continuously, with a weight in head: *Bovist.*

As if water in the head, wakes her up morose: *Platin.*

As if lacerated, everything whirling around: *Opium.*

Tearing pain on coming in room: *Tongo.*

Tearing in head and teeth, with heat and sleeplessness and great weakness: *Kreosot.*

Occiput and then the sides of head, screwed in: *Amm. mur.*

Heat in head and face: *Calc. phosph.*

Tearing upwards in left side of the face: *Tongo.*

Stomachache all day: *Amm. carb.*

Every morning with loss of appetite and nausea: *Stannum.*

Nausea and vomiting: *Cyclam.;* and heaviness of all the limbs: *Silic.*

On awaking in the morning and after getting up: *Phosphor.*

Drowsy: *Spongia;* and gaping: *Chin. sulph.*

General sweat in large drops, mostly in face: *Platin.*

Irritable: *Bryon., Mar. ver., Stramon.;* fretful: *Bovist., Calc. ac., Spongia;* trifles bring him into anger: *Hydroph.;* getting angry: *Arsen., Dulcam.;* too harsh with his children: *Hydroph.;* impatient: *Hydroph., Mancin., Pallad., Platin.*

Inclination to sing: *Natr. mur.;* to laugh: *Sabad.;* to weep, with chill: *Bellad., Pulsat.;* weeping bitterly: *Hydroph.*

Shedding tears: *Coloc., Ferr. magn., Kreosot., Phosphor., Platin., Ran. bulb., Sepia.*

Whining: *Bellad.;* groaning: *Laches., Silic.;* sobbing: II*Stramon.;* crying: *Cuprum, Phosphor., Sepia, Stannum, Terb. ol., Tongo;* for help: *Silic.*

Complaining and scolding: *Veratr.;* hasty speech: *Laches.;* hurries when writing: *Ptel. trif.*

Aversion to talk: *Ox. ac.;* dislike: *Agar., Calc. ac., Conium, Thuya;* and to sit alone: *Ant. crud.*

Not inclined to mental occupation and other work: ‖*Alum., Calc. phosph., Cinnab., Dulcam., Lact. vir,, Ox. ac., Phosph. ac.;* head and face hot: *Calc. phosph.*

Excited state: *Ambra, Chin. sulph., Cinch. off., Coffea, Crocus, Narc. ac., Natr. mur.,* ‖*Phosphor., Phosph. ac., Ruta, Viol. od.;* thoughts clearer after the headache: *Aster.;* after sleep in the evening headache, but the mind self-possessed and clear: *Gelsem.*

MODEL CURE.

Irritable, vexed, always quiet, sad, thoughts turned to himself, no ambition to work; heaviness, heat and pain in the head in the morning; backache; spasmodic eructation, thin slimy stool with cutting in the abdomen; pale and emaciated; heavy night and morning sweats: *Petrol.*—KNORRE.

HEADACHE WITH RESTLESSNESS.

‖ Anac.
‖ Arsen.
Bryon.
Calad.
Canthar.
Chamom.
Cinch. off.
‖ Daph. ind.
Gent. cruc.
Kadm. sul.
‖ Kali hydr.
ı Laches.
ı Lycop.
Morph. ac.
Nux mosch.
Ran bulb.
‖ Ruta.
Silic.
Vip. red.

With fear; hurried: *Laches.;* fearfulness: *Kali hydr.;* despair; glistening eyes, red cheeks, yellow face: *Vip. red.*

Restlessness, followed by intolerable headache: *Chamom.;* pressure: *Calad.;* constrictive sensation: *Gent. cruc.;* as if brain were packed together: *Cinch. off.*

Tearing in the whole head, with rigor every third day: *Anac.*

Bursting, tosses about for hours, binding head firmly relieved: *Silic.*

Nervous headache: *Daph. ind.*

Congestive headache: *Ignat.*

Heat of head: *Canthar.*

Followed by headache and vomiting: *Laches.;* and pain in belly: *Morph. ac.;* belly and knees: *Arsen.*

Icy coldness of body, nosebleed, constriction in throat, thirst, nausea and vomiting: *Kadm. sulph.*

Pressing headache: *Petrol.;* heat three successive evenings: ‖*Ruta.*

As if she had to throw hands and feet about, with fainty feeling: *Lycop.*

HEADACHE WITH DIMINISHED INTELLECTUAL POWER.

Almost deprived of thought; pressing asunder: *Prun. spin.*
During the chill: *Cimex.*
Weakness; head pains when he thinks: *Phosphor.*
Difficult performance of intellectual operations: *Calc. caust.*
Difficult comprehension: *Chin. sulph., Silic.,* ı*Phosphor.*

MIND AND DISPOSITION.

Acon.
Agar.
Ambra.
Baptis.
Bellad.
Bovist.
Calc. ars.
Calc. caust.
Carb. veg.
Chin. sulph
Cimex.
Coccul.
Cotyled.
Cuprum.
Hæmat.
Helleb.
Hyosc.
Kreosot.
Laches.
Lauroc.
Lycop.
Magn. carb
Menyanth.
Mezer.
Moschus.
Natr. carb.
Natr. mur.
Nux mosch.
Opium.
Phosphor.
Prun. spin.
Ptelea.
Rhus tox.
Sarsap.
Silic.
Stramon.
Veratr.

Thinking difficult: *Bovist., Hæmat., Lauroc., Mezer.,* ǀǀ*Phosphor.*
Difficult flow of ideas; better in the air: *Menyanth.*
Thinking difficult, pressing pain, spreads from left forehead all over: *Lauroc.*
Complete incapacity for mental work: *Ptel. trif.*
Incapacity to all business: *Calc. ars.*
As if losing their senses: *Agar., Magn. carb., Moschus.*
Unable to speak: *Sarsap.*
As if stupefied, with humming: *Rhus tox.*
Confusion, stupid 4 to 8 P.M., every day: *Helleb.*
Confusion: *Carb. sulph., Cotyl., Ambra, Stramon.*
A "wild" feeling: *Baptis.*
Vanishing of thought: *Lauroc., Prun. spin.*
Dull minded: *Carb. veg., Kali carb., Hyosc., Laches., Lycop., Natr. carb., Nux mosch.*
Loss of intellect: ǀǀ*Acon., Ambra, Coccul., Magn. carb.*
Thoughts and memory left him, could not recollect, with giddy headache of the whole head: *Rhus tox.*
Loss of consciousness: *Sarsap.*
Face red, and sweating: *Glonoin.*
Insensibility: *Carb. veg., Chin. sulph., Crotal., Cyclam., Kreosot.,* ǀǀ*Mangan., Mezer., Nitr. ac., Rhus tox., Sarsap., Silic., Stannum, Sulphur.*

Loss of consciousness followed by drowsiness and headache: *Nux mosch.*

Forgetfulness: *Amm. carb., Capsic.,* ǀ*Caustic.,* ǀǀ*Mezer., Moschus;* weak memory: *Viol. od.*

Loss of reason: ǀ*Kali carb., Rhus tox.*

Weak memory all day, and heat of the forehead: *Kreosot.*

Uses wrong words: ǀ *Caustic.,* ǀǀ*Nux mosch.;* difficult talking: *Thuya.*

MODEL CURE.

A woman otherwise well and strong, had fluent coryza for three weeks. followed by dull pain in the forehead, with forgetfulness, loss of memory, and using the wrong words: *Caustic.* 30 cent. One dose. No return.—GOULLON.

HEADACHE WITH DERANGED MIND.

Distraction of mind: *Helleb.*
Delusions of fancy: *Amphisbœna;* with open eyes: *Crotal.*
Delirious before headache: *Stramon.;* with flow of saliva: *Veratr.*
Low murmuring from 4 P.M., all night on three successive days: *Hepar s. c.*
Mental derangement: *Stramon.;* insane, beside herself: *Zinc. val.;* brings him in a furious rage: *Jodium;* followed by mania: *Arsen.;* furor: *Veratr.;* during the intervals of mania: *Cuprum;* after the mania: *Acon.*

RUSH OF BLOOD TO THE HEAD.

|| Acon.
| Agar.
Argent.
| Arg. nitr.
Aur. mur.
| Carb. veg.
| Cyclam.
Fluor. ac.
|| Glonoin.
Gratiol.
|| Lycop.
Indig.
Kali carb.
|| Lauroc.
| Magn. carb.
Nitr. ac.
Nux mosch.
|| Nux vom.
| Phosphor.
|| Pulsat.
|| Psorin.
Stramon.
|| Sulphur.
Ver. vir.
Vip. torv.

Low-spirited, with throbbing of carotids: *Arg. nitr.*

Anxiousness: |*Acon.*, |*Carb. veg.*, *Lauroc.*, |*Magn. carb.*, |*Phosphor.*, |*Pulsat.*, *Sulphur;* with quick circulation: *Indig.;* anxiety: *Acon.*, *Cyclam.*

Waking from sleep with crawling: *Carb. veg.;* driving out of bed: *Pulsat.*

Disinclined to mental work: *Nux vom.;* shunning it: *Agar.*

Dull mind: *Kali carb.;* obtuseness of senses: *Hyosc.;* difficult comprehension: *Nitr. ac.;* stupefaction: *Lauroc.;* it takes time to think where he was: *Fluor. ac.*

Heavy stupefaction: *Arg. nitr.;* confused stupor with heat: *Psorin.;* unconscious with delirium: *Hyosc.*, *Nux mosch.*, *Aur. mur.*, *Vip. torv.*

Unnatural flow of ideas: *Pulsat.;* and of arguments in conversation: *Argent.*

Wakes from sleep with a crazy-like chaos of ideas: *Psorin.*

Insanity: *Ver. vir.;* mania: *Stramon.;* rage, furor: *Glonoin.*

Did not know where he was and what had happened: *Psorin.*

Cannot recollect herself: *Nitr. ac.*

Sinking unconscious into a chair: *Glonoin.;* incapable to express himself properly and to talk connectedly: *Arg. nitr.*

Inability to find the right words: *Arg. nitr.*

SENSATION OF FULNESS.

Fulness of Head. Not well disposed: *Niccol.;* loss of power of thought: *Arg. nitr.;* deficiency of clearness: *Borax.*

At night with heat and great excitement, during the day a difficulty to attend to mental work: *Arg. nitr.*

Acute mania: *Kali brom.*

Heat in Head. Very joyous, sings: *Therid.*

Anxious: *Magn. carb.*, *Phosphor.*, *Silic.*

Anxious, rising up into head: *Canthar.*

With cold feet: ||*Sulphur;* with cramp in chest, abdominal anxiety, restless, hot hands: *Nitr. ac.*

Pectoral anxiety: *Carb. veg.*

Cardiac anxiety, drives out of bed at night and out of room: *Thuya.*

Anxiousness in the evening; has to rise, which relieves: *Carb. an.*

Could not remain in bed: *Carb. veg.*

Anxiousness and bodily restlessness: *Ruta;* and sweat on forehead: *Phosphor.*

The heat wakens, anxiety follows, fears apoplexy: *Arnica.*

Anxiety, red-hot face and drowsiness: *Strontian.*

Fever heat of body with anxiety: *Stramon.*
Anxiousness and great exhaustion: *Chin. sulph.*
Anguish disappearing in open air, followed by gaping: *Veratr.*
Ill humored and lazy: *Lauroc.*
Unwilling to talk, cold feet: *Laches.*
Uneasiness: *Phosphor.*
Beating of pulse in head, restlessness, cannot fall asleep: *Arsen.*
Restless, changing places: *Canthar.*
Loss of power of thought: *Arg. nitr.*
Difficult thinking: *Digit.*
Increased warmth with dullness: *Phelland.*
Burning in the head with stupidity: *Helleb.*
Only inner sensation of heat with stupidity: *Lauroc.*
The forehead warm and somewhat dull and stupid: *Alum.;* deranged: *Opium.*
Forgetfulness: *Digit., Sulphur.*

In brain-affections children are cross and irritable, or indifferent and dull: *Cuprum.*
With hydrocephalus bellowing in the delirium: *Cuprum.*
Phrenitis with inclination to suicide: *Act. rac.*
Brain affection with moaning, groaning: *Laches.*

OUTER HEAD.

Forehead. As if skin too tight; anxiousness: *Phosphor.;* tension and inability to fix his thoughts: *Colchic.*
Painful crawling, somewhat stupid: *Lauroc.*
Rubbing with the hand, because there is a dullness; sadness: *Plumbum.*
Forehead cold, with anxious heat: *Pulsat.;* warmth and ill humor: *Ant. crud.;* and anxiety; rising from abdomen into the head: *Lauroc.;* outer and inner warmth, with cerebral anxiety: *Lauroc.;* heat and disinclination to think: *Nitrum;* anxious melancholy: *Stramon.;* spreading from forehead over the whole body, with restlessness: *Acon., Opium;* anxious, sweat cold and stupid: *Coccul.;* anxious and fierce: *Acon.;* falling down: *Helleb.;* lying senseless, with groaning: *Bryon.;* warm sweat, with anxiety: *Acon., Arsen., Clemat.. Phosphor., Pulsat., Nux vom.;* covered with sweat; knows no one: *Stramon.;* deranged *Arsen.;* delirium: *Arsen., Bellad.;* mania: *Arsen., Cuprum.*
Wrinkled forehead; morose: *Mangan.*
Furuncle after mania: *Stramon.*

MOVEMENTS.

Convulsions, with illusions of mind: *Hyosc.;* with vanishing of vision: *Stramon.*
Head is thrown involuntarily from side to side after walking, with great anguish: *Caustic.*
Head is turned involuntarily from right to left (repeatedly), with dizziness and anxiety; disappears in open air: *Caustic.*
Spasmodic drawing only sidewise, with cries: *Stramon.*
Turning head left or right, with excessive restlessness: *Colchic.*
Tottering sideways; mania: *Bellad.*
Trembling, and extravagant, as if drunk: *Tabac.;* with mania: *Calc. ostr.*
Sudden jerks backwards, repeatedly, with anxiety: *Alum.*
Frequently lifting up the head; senseless: *Stramon.*

MODEL CURE.

Unwonted restlessness; piercing, fixed look; quick jerking motions of the head; glances now here, now there. Wants to leave the room; sees frightful apparitions, which come to take him away, chickens without feathers on them, a herd of large crabs, which are driven through the gate into the city. Epileptic convulsions: *Hyosc.*—THORER.

POSITIONS.

Has to lay the head forward on the table, with a trembling anxiousness: *Nux vom.;* as if pressed down: *Chamom.*
As if it was pressed down, with loss of recognition: *Cicut.*
Inclination to let it hang down, with sadness and weeping: *Veratr.*
Unwilling to bend backwards, when exerting mind: *Ginseng.*
When bending it forward to the chest, imagines to have a goitre: *Zincum.*
On moving the head, does not know where she is: *Calc. ostr.*
Sudden stupefaction: *Carb. an.;* loss of senses: *Natr. mur., Rhus tox.*

COLD, HEAT, SWEAT.

Icy cold and great anxiousness, fears uncovering: *Mangan.*
Cold chills, weak-minded: *Ambra.*
Chilliness after a merry state: *Hura.*
Hot, confused, joyous: *Therid.;* and anxious: *Carb. veg.,* ‖*Lauroc.,* ‖*Magn. carb.,* ‖*Phosphor.,* ‖*Sulphur;* and ill humored: *Acon., Aethus., Calc. phosph.;* indisposed to think: *Nitrum;* morose: *Lauroc., Platin.;* does not speak: *Aethus., Mephit.;* restless mind: *Canthar., Phosphor.*
Difficult thinking, compression: *Argent., Digit., Natr. carb., Stannum.*
Stupor: *Lycop., Stannum;* deprived of reason: *Stannum;* delirium: *Cuprum, Phosph. ac.*

Raving mad: *Bellad.;* desire to hurry business: *Ptelea;* forgetful: *Digit.*
Loss of memory: *Arg. nitr.*
Anxiety: *Silic.;* and red face: *Strontian.;* flushes and nausea: *Natr. mur.*
Warmth worse on eating warm things: *Magn. carb.;* during catamenia: *Kali hydr.*
Red hot hands; better when standing: *Phosphor.;* laziness: *Calc. phosph., Lauroc.;* 11 P. M.: *Ruta;* while walking, lasts till going to bed: *Strontian.;* at night in bed, better getting up: *Carb. an.*
Sweat of head and anxiousness: *Arsen., Borax, Carb. veg., Mur. ac., Nux vom., Phosphor., Sepia.*
With restlessness of mind: *Phosphor.;* illusions: *Sepia.*
Mania: *Arsen.;* dullness in head, aching in eyes, sore to the touch; sweat of face: *Borax;* fulness in belly as if bursting: *Mur. ac.*
Inclined to take a deep inhalation with stitches in the intercostal muscles: *Borax.*
General fever heat: *Sepia;* when walking in the open air, with hard, quick pulse: *Borax.*
Arms falling down as if lame: *Mur. ac.*

BONES OF THE SKULL.

As if broken when lying down, took away his "mind to live:" *Aurum.*
Aching in left temporal bone over the concha deep in, worse when pressed or on touching the hair: *Agar.*
Pain with stupefaction: *Conium;* with dimness of intellect: *Conium, Nux mosch.;* as if getting mad: *Acon.*

SCALP.

Painful sensitiveness with anxiousness, even his cap hurts: *Nitr. ac.;* with tension on vertex: *Apis.*
Stretched sensation with absence of mind: *Nux mosch.*
Tightness as if from a skin over scalp, unable to think, weak memory: *Helleb.*
As if tied too fast, slow flow of ideas: *Carb. veg.;* anxiety: *Phosphor.*
Shooting on top, as if bruised, and morose: *Niccol.*
Pains with difficult speaking: *Thuya.*
Soreness of single spots with inability to do mental work: *Phosphor.*
As if struck on left side on a small spot, and stupid: *Lauroc.*
Numbness, morose: *Platin.*
As if worms crawled on vertex; sadness: *Cuprum.*
Formication and stupefaction: *Cuprum.*
Itching and excited as from spirituous liquor: *Codein.;* impatience: *Sulphur;* morose: *Clemat.*

Scratching with great impatience: *Natr. mur.*
Erysipelas and delirium: *Stramon.*
As if hair stood on end after fright: *Mur. ac.;* with a chill and anxiousness: *Carb. veg., Pulsat.*

THE WHOLE OUTER HEAD.

As if blown up; crazy feeling: *Spongia.*
As if enlarged, depression: *Mephit.*
As if puffed up, very hot and restless, tossing about: *Amm. carb.*
Swollen; mania: *Opium.*

SIGHT.

Oxyopia. The room and all things appear bright; more friendly, with merriness; happy, as if new born: *Canthar.;* all things in the street are bright: *Carb. an.;* increased power of sight, but cannot think rationally: *Colchic.*

Desire for Light. Wants more light in the room, more candles to be lighted, with melancholy; mania: *Stramon.*

Desire for light with the delirious state: *Calc. ostr.;* light and company: *Stramon.*

Better from daylight shining through the window; anxiety as if shut up in a cellar: *Natr. mur.*

Melancholy, mania with longing to look in the sun and in the fire: *Bellad.*

Fear: *Berber., Calc. ostr., Caustic., Lycop., Pulsat., Rhus tox., Valer.*

Worse in the Dark. Sorrowfulness, sadness: *Stramon.;* depression: *Phosphor.;* melancholy: *Stramon.;* anxiety: *Natr. mur.;* from the slightest darkness; it suffocates her; three or four candles have to be lighted: *Aethus.;* things appear too large: *Berber.;* prevents falling asleep: *Calc. ostr.*

Is afraid: *Calc. ostr., Caustic.;* when a door will not open: *Lycop.;* afraid of pictures: *Lycop.*

Dread: *Lycop., Pulsat.;* in twilight: *Calc. ostr.;* as if he would kill himself: *Rhus tox.;* as if some one would do him injury: *Valer.*

Timid, full of fear: *Graphit.;* full of fright: *Carb. an.;* delirium: *Carb. veg.;* sees horrible figures if the room is dark: *Carb. veg.*

After closing Eyes. Rush of ideas: *Spongia;* exalted imagination: *Ledum;* fear: *Caustic.*

Fear of suffocating, not when closing eyes, all night: *Carb. an.*

Anxiousness: *Calc. ostr.;* in dropsy of chest: *Carb. veg.*

Illusions, things appear too thick or too thin, like the pulse: *Camphor.*

All objects appear as in a fever, with sadness: *Digit.*

Before falling asleep illusions, images, inclination to make verses: *Natr. mur.*

A bright dream after drowsiness: *Stannum.*

Visions: *Bellad.;* sees persons and events; neither fearful nor anxious: **|**Arsen., | *Calc. ostr.*, *Sambuc.;* phantasms: **|***Apis*, *Bellad.*, *Bryon.*, **|** *Calc. ostr.*, *Ledum*, *Opium*, **|***Sambuc.*, **|***Spongia;* disappear: *Kali carb.*

During the night when awake fantastic images appear, which disappear when opening the eyes: *Sepia;* horrible faces: *Aether.*, *Arg. nitr.*, *Calc. ostr.*, *Caustic.*, *Cinch. off.*, *Sulphur;* different images: *Graphit.;* delirium: || *Bellad.*, | *Calc. ostr.*, | *Camphor.*, || *Bryon.*, || *Graphit.*, | *Ledum*, | *Sulphur.*

Horrid visions in typhoid fever: **|** *Calc. ostr.;* when lying awake sleepless and shutting the eyes spirits or animals appear in bright light coming nearer and nearer slowly from a distance; when opening the eyes all disappear: *Thuya;* afraid to shut the eyes that she might never awake: *Aether.*

As if he had lost his mind: *Opium;* senses leave him: *Camphor.;* thoughts vanish: *Therid.*

Unconscious: *Stramon.;* stupefied: *Acon.;* keeps eyes shut, with ill humor: *Thuya.*

Shunning Light. Sensitive to light, fretful, discontented, complains about everything: *Arsen.*

Worse in bright light, fretful: *Arnica;* it puts him quite beside himself: *Colchic.*

Shunning light; quiet, retired state: || *Conium;* with thirst and mania: *Hyosc.*

Melancholy, unwilling to talk, weakness with exaltation now and then; thirst and costiveness: *Hyosc.*

Frightful jumping out of bed, imagining there is too much light in the room: *Ambra.*

On opening Eyes. Visions: *Acon.;* objects appear: *Stramon.;* ill humor: *Ignat.;* sees a sea of fire: *Spigel.*

Better with closed Eyes. In darkness and solitude: *Nux vom.;* wishes to be alone, lying with closed eyes: *Sepia;* inclined to close his eyes, listlessness: *Rhus rad.*

Feels best with eyes closed: *Zincum;* difficult comprehension: *Kali carb.*

Want of recollection: *Kali carb.;* headache lessens when closing eyes: *Acon.*, *Calc. ostr.*

Closing eyes involuntarily, burning pain, anxiety as if he never would be able to open them: *Spigel.*

MODEL CURE.

Fear and mistrust of everyone, great anxiety by day and night, no rest in any place, seeks to fly. Her only pleasure is to look into the sun or the fire. She fled into a forest, built a large fire and remained there four or five days without nourishment. Seeks to be alone, flees society; when alone she cuts up queer antics, screws her mouth in all directions, throws money out of the window. Taciturn; after repeated questioning, she screams her answers loudly and angrily: *Bellad.*—SONNENBURG.

PERVERTED VISION.

Flickering; giddy and anxious; afraid to touch people he meets: *Acon.;* sprightliness and excitement: *Acon.;* after weeping and hiccoughing: *Conium.*

Sparks with anxiety: *Coca;* with restlessness and confusion: *Opium;* with fiery and black spots; rage: *Stramon.*

Different appearance of all things; sadness: *Digit.*

Things appear too large, lifts the legs higher up in walking: *Agar.*

Things around her get more narrow and smaller, with anxiety: *Carb. veg.*

Everything appears smaller; apprehensive, morose humor: *Platin.*

Sees muscæ volantes, frets at not being able to catch them: *Stramon.;* fluids, in mania: *Canthar.;* clouds and rocks: *Magn. mur.;* ciphers, gets stupid: *Phosph. ac.;* animals creeping about; mania-potu: *Arsen.;* imaginary objects, as if stupefied: *Nux vom.;* horrible images at night: *Silic.;* with cardiacal anxiety; despair and suicidal mania: *Calc. ostr.*

Hallucinations, with talkativeness: *Eup. purp.;* with mania: *Stramon.*

Blurred vision, with depression of spirits: *Lil. tigr.;* with fearfulness and apprehensions: *Lil. tigr.;* and great indifference: *Stannum.*

Confusion before eyes, with anxiousness: *Lycop.;* with agony: *Psorin.*

While Reading, feels as if somebody hurried him: *Magn. mur.*

Exaltation: *Coffea, Phosph. ac.;* anxiousness: *Magn. mur.;* distracted attention: *Acon.;* want of attention: *Alum.;* loses himself: *Angust., Coffea.;* distracted: *Laches.;* difficult comprehension: *Fluor. ac.;* vanishing of thoughts: *Nux mosch.;* forgetfulness: *Calc. ac.*

When Writing. Disturbed attention: *Acon.;* dullness of mind: *Nux mosch.;* absence of thought: *Rhus tox.;* confounds right and left sides: *Fluor. ac.* Compare Exertion of Mind.

Exertion. Nausea and anxiousness: *Sepia.*

Looking to one point; absentmindedness: *Bovist.*

Working steadily, one idea remains: *Can. sat.*

Cannot see sharply with all exertion; anxiousness: *Carb. an.*

Can see, but not comprehend what he sees: *Helleb.*

Less shortsightedness and an unusual well feeling: *Plumbum.*

Impaired sight, with diminished intellectual power: *Cyclam., Nitr. ac., Phosphor., Thuya;* vanishing of sight: *Caustic.,* and of hearing: *Stramon.,* and dizzy; with wide open eyes she has to exert herself to know things around her; loud complaints about it: *Arg. nitr.;* weaksighted and fretful, dull brooding: *Carb. an.*

Vanishing of sight from drunkenness: *Nux vom.;* difficult thinking: *Acon.;* absence of mind: *Zincum.*

Dimsightedness and stupidity: *Stramon.,* and indifference: *Stannum;* depression: *Petrol.;* using wrong words: *Lil. tigr.*

Impaired vision, and sadness: *Digit.;* dejected: *Petrol.;* stupefied: *Arsen., Cyclam., Nitr. ac., Phosphor., Thuya;* imperfect sight, with an alternate state of mind, absence and activity: *Alum.*

A veil before the eyes, with loss of thought and weak memory: *Stramon.*

MIND AND DISPOSITION.

Mist before the eyes and loss of consciousness: *Canthar.*

Obscure vision, dark before the eyes, with anxiety: *Bellad., Staphis.;* heat in face and tears in eyes: *Arg. nitr.;* with ill humor: *Sepia;* dull mind: *Arsen., Carb. veg.;* merry madness: *Crocus.*

Black before Eyes, uses wrong words, difficulty of fixing the attention: *Lil. tigr.;* with difficult comprehension: *Mercur.;* unconscious: *Crotal., Gratiol.;* for a moment: *Ol. an.;* senses vanishing: *Crocus;* with confusion of ideas: *Natr. carb.;* fretfulness, anger: *Sepia;* stupid: *Zincum;* excited, fears apoplexy: *Sepia;* anxiety: *Bellad.;* anxious ideas from times past, everything appears as if it was something else, loses all desire to live: *Staphis.;* extremely irritable, his motions are so quick that he finally has to stop and all turns black before his eyes: *Stramon.*

Blindness, loss of sight, suddenly after dinner, with anxious sweat: *Calc. ostr.;* dull minded: *Aethus., Arsen., Stramon.;* mental derangement: *Chamom.;* delirious: *Bellad.;* rage: *Stramon.*

MODEL CURE.

Throbbing pain in the brain, dimness of vision, as if he looked through a sieve; frightful visions appear to him when in the dark, or when closing his eyes; he strikes at them and holds the cross up to them: *Pulsat.*—SZTAROVCSZKY.

EYES.

Pupils. Easily movable; howling or crying for trifles: *Bellad.;* anxiety when in bed: *Chamom.*

Contracted; irritability, fretfulness, ill humor; vexed about trifles, confused, cannot finish anything, lazy, awkward, fribbling: *Coccul.;* mania: *Stramon.;* loss of consciousness: *Morph. ac.*

I Act. rac.	**Dilated Pupils.** Brightness; no sleep: *Secal.;* merry: *Crocus;* tendency to laugh and sing: *Crocus.*
I Bellad.	
Bromum.	
II Crocus.	Stronger memory: *Bellad.*
I Hyosc.	
II Ipecac.	Melancholy, when reminded of having done wrong: *Stramon.*
I Morph. ac.	Inclination to climb: *Stramon.;* crying and moaning: *Bromum.*
II Moschus.	
II Nux vom.	Restlessness: *Nux vom.;* with stammering weakness: *Bellad.:*
I Secale.	feels miserable: *Ipecac.*
II Stramon.	

Whining, ill humor: *Bellad.;* delirium: *Hyosc.;* with nausea: *Act. rac.;* small quick pulse: *Bellad.;* vivid delirium: *Stramon.;* mania, rage: *Bellad., Stramon.;* mental derangement: *Stramon.;* hallucinations: *Hyosc.;* imagines to be three in typhus fever: *Moschus:* stupor: *Morph. ac., Stannum;* unconscious: I*Bellad.*

Pupils Immovable, ill humor: *Chamom.;* unconscious and moving hands and feet: *Stramon.*

Difficult dilation and difficult contraction: *Chamom.*

APPEARANCE.

Lively and bolder talk: *Acon.;* vivid mind: *Opium;* delirium: *Stramon.;* brightness, delirium: *Hyosc.;* fierce: *Acon.;* exalted: *Opium;* glistening, with uneasiness; despair: *Vip. red.;* sparkling, delirious, with walking: *Stramon.;* with raving: *Colchic.;* deranged: *Acon., Bellad., Colchic., Hyosc., Stramon.;* raging; violent mania: *Opium;* takes no notice: *Stramon.;* brilliant, with raging delirium: *Ailanth.;* dazzling in delirium: *Stramon.;* raving mania: *Stramon.;* glaring, with mania: *Crocus, Opium, Stramon.*

Unsteady; anxious with mental restlessness: ||*Aloes.*

Eyes shine; unconsciousness: *Stramon.*

Unsteady and melancholic; hates women: *Pulsat.;* and delirious: *Stramon.;* and wild with laughing; mania: *Veratr.;* wild look and raving: *Bellad.;* mania: *Cuprum, Hyosc., Stramon., Veratr., Vip. torv.*

Eyes rolling, unconscious: *Stramon.;* stupor: *Stramon.*

Eyes wide open; confused talk: *Arsen.;* talking delirious: *Opium,* ||*Stramon.,* |*Veratr.;* talkative mania: *Bellad., Opium, Stramon.*

Fixed. After a fit of scolding: *Moschus;* with insensibility: *Aethus.;* with absence of understanding: *Arsen.;* on the ground, absorbed in contemplation: *Stramon.*

With dilated immovable pupils, senseless: *Stramon.*

On objects with quickly following erroneous ideas: *Cuprum.*

Staring at one point with dull mind, stupidity: *Bellad.*

With anxiety: *Arnica;* with anguish: *Helleb.*

With fretfulness: *Chamom.;* with violent temper: *Moschus.*

With great excitability: *Alum., Cinch. off.*

With uncommon liveliness: *Cinch. off.;* with watery eyes, does not recognize persons: *Opium;* with difficult comprehension: *Cicut.;* with standing still of ideas: *Cannab.;* with maniacal illusions: *Hyosc.;* sparkling, with absorption in his fantasies: *Stramon.;* with delirium: *Chamom., Coffea, Coloc., Veratr.;* with deranged mind: *Bellad., Stramon.;* and a sharp, pungent look with maniacal symptoms: *Hyosc., Stramon.;* with rage and spitting: *Bellad.;* shunning drinks: *Bellad.;* with mania: *Bellad., Stramon.;* with thoughtlessness: *Helleb., Hyosc.;* with unconsciousness: *Stramon.*

Contracted pupils, pulse and skin normal, deranged mind: *Bellad.*

Eyes dim, glassy, broken, full of water; dull mind; anxious breathing: *Opium;* dull brain: *Hyosc.*

Eyes sunken, with entire loss of self-confidence: *Sepia.*

MODEL CURE.

A man æt. 26, a musician, of sanguine temperament, became deranged after the death of his brother, who died in his arms. Scolding, spitting, pushing, tearing clothes, breaking chairs, boring holes into the walls with his fingers. Changes his position from sitting to standing, talks nonsense, imagines at times to be God, at others the devil. Singing. Pupils contracted, eyes listless and sunken, sleepless, no appetite, does not answer when spoken to, avoids people's looks: *Stramon.*—SZTAROVCSZKY.

PAINS.

Aching in eyes and over the forehead, unable to exert mind: *Amm. gum.*, *Pulsat.*; after exerting mind: *Lact. vir.*; as if too large, with a stupid feeling: *Phosph. ac.*

Tearing pains with difficult comprehension: *Natr. carb.*; shooting over left eye extorting cries: *Sepia*; like lightening; apprehension of some evil: *Fluor. ac.*

Drawing backwards with anxiety: *Bovist.*; drawing over right eye with mental exertion: *Calc. ostr.*; hammering over left eye, as if going out of his mind: *Hamam.*

Boring from out in over left eye: *Magn. sulph.*; with stupidity in the whole head, heat and great anxiety: *Nitr. ac.*

Burning pain and weeping mood: *Nux mosch.*; sick headache with fretfulness: *Stannum*; violent pain in the eyeballs and nervous excitement: *Daph. ind.*; delirium: *Plumbum*; pain with confusion: *Carb. veg.*, *Phosph. ac.*; stupefaction: *Stannum*; with forgetfulness: *Guar. trochl.*

TEARS.

Torrents of tears if their personal sufferings are spoken of: *Sepia*; after a running from the eyes her disposition to torment her family is gone: *Fluor. ac.*

Unwilling streams of tears with nightly attacks of agony: *Amm. carb.*; tears force their way between the lashes, with spasmodically closed lids: *Spongia*; pressing weight closes eyes and forces tears out: *Platin.*; tears stand in her eyes but cannot weep, with sadness: *Ars. met.*; with anxiousness, and hot face: *Arg. nitr.*; and involuntary weeping, with sadness: *Veratr.*; burning, with lachrymose mood: *Nux mosch.*

WEEPING.

|| Acon.
|| Ant. tart.
| Arnica.
| Bellad.
| Borax.
| Canthar.
|| Chamom.
| Crocus.
| Cuprum.
|| Hepar s. c.
| Laches.
| Mar. ver.
| Nitr. ac.
| Stannum.
| Veratr.

She laughs over trifles until she has tears in her eyes, which become red: *Natr. mur.*

Shedding of tears following attacks of convulsive laughing: *Formic.*

Weeping even over joyous things: *Platin.*

Nervous unrest, tears start to her eyes: *Apis.*

Weeps when spoken to: *Staphis.*

Much weeping from an idea that she is deserted by all her friends; most intense melancholy with fits of uncontrollable weeping: *Kali brom.*

Homesickness with weeping: *Magn. mur.*

Weeping, inconsolable mood: *Spongia.*

Tears in eyes and sadness: *Veratr.*

Sad and weeping: *Natr. mur.*

Lachrymose, sad: *Natr. sulph.*

When thinking of old forgotten troubles the tears start to her eyes: *Natr. mur.*

Weeping bitterly, as if she could not think nor live any more: *Thuya.*

Tears with anxiety, fear and foreboding: *Arg. nitr.*

Weeping with anxiety: *Cuprum.*

With almost all her sufferings there are sure to be tears and cries: *Pulsat.*

Children fretful: *Graphit.;* with coryza tears rush: *Cepa;* unconsciousness, shedding tears: *Stramon.*

BETTER AFTER WEEPING.

I Anac.
I Digit.
I Graphit.
I Ignat.
I Lycop.
Nitr. ac.
II Phosphor.
Tabac.
Tarax.

Anxiousness: *Digit., Graphit., Tabac.*

Fear: *Digit.;* apprehension: *Graphit., Tabac.*

Sadness: *Digit.;* melancholy: *Phosphor.;* discontentedness: *Nitr. ac.*

Fretfulness: *Platin.;* horrible appearance of the world: *Phosphor.;* hysterical weeping without cause: *Viola od., Rhus tox.*

RED EYES AND OPHTHALMIA WITH DERANGEMENT OF MIND.

I Acon.
Argent.
II Arnica.
II Arsen.
I Bellad.
II Calc. ostr.
I Cinch. off.
Colchic.
II Cuprum.
II Laches.
I Mercur.
I Nux mosch.
II Nux vom.
II Opium.
I Phosphor.
Plumbum.
II Pulsat.
I Sepia.
II Silic.
I Stramon.
II Sulphur.

Eyes injected, pupils enlarged with mania: *Stramon.;* uses wrong words: *Nux mosch.;* blood-vessels of conjunctiva distended with delirium: *Stramon.*

Suffused and sparkling with delirium: *Colchic.,* I*Stramon.;* mania: I*Stramon.*

Red sclerotica, aversion to conversation: *Argent.;* after attempts to study; sparkling eyes; mania: *Opium;* and a wild look; mania: *Cuprum.*

Eyes protruding and inflamed; man : *Opium;* with unconsciousness: *Nux mosch.*

Burning hot or dry, with stupor: *Opium.*

Inflamed with attacks of mania, ending with sweat: *Cuprum;* particularly the left eye, with mania: *Stramon.*

Purulent conjunctivitis with longing for death: *Acon.*

Swelling of eyes with delirium: *Plumbum.*

Swelling, redness or itching of the lower lid with erysipelas under the eye; with frightfulness in the night: *Laches.*

Movements. Eyes in constant motion, anxious restlessness with mania: *Bellad.*

Eyes move upwards and sideways, with silly merriment: *Acon.*

Lids. Heavy; unable to study: *Formic.*

Closed when walking, like a somnambulist, with anxiety: *Alum.;* spasmodically closed with stupor: *Acon.*

Dropping of lids, does not know where he is going: *Nux mosch.*
Lameness, cannot open them; with difficult comprehension: *Nitrum.*
Itching of lids, fright from starting: *Laches.;* and nervous exaltation: *Hura.*
Swollen with delirium: *Plumbum.*
Sunken with anguish: *Vip. torv.*
Dark around eyes, with indifference or ill humor: *Stannum.*
Blue circles; takes no notice: *Stramon.;* with derangements of mind: *Anac.,* ||*Arsen.,* ||*Cinch. off., Coccul., Cuprum, Graphit., Hepar s. c., Ignat.,* ||*Nux vom., Laches., Lycop., Mercur., Phosphor., Phosph. ac., Rhus tox., Secal., Sepia, Staphis.,* ||*Sulphur, Veratr.*

Brows corrugated in delirium with typhus: *Helleb.;* in mania: *Stramon.*

HEARING.

|| Acon.
|| Ambra.
|| Anac.
Ant. crud.
| Bryon.
| Calc. ostr.
| Carb. an.
Caustic.
| Chamom.
|| Coffea.
|| Coca.
| Digit.
|| Graphit.
| Ignat.
|| Kali carb.
|| Kreosot.
| Lycop.
Mangan.
Mercur.
|| Natr. carb.
|| Natr. sulph.
|| Nux vom.
| Phosphor.
|| Phosph. ac.
| Pulsat.
| Sabin.
|| Sepia.
Silic.
|| Stannum.
|| Staphis.
| Thuya.
| Viola od.
|| Zincum.

Music unbearable. Makes sorrowful: *Natr. sulph.*

Oversensitiveness of hearing; the slightest tone rings in his ear; wakes with rush of blood to head; hair standing on end; anxiousness and shuddering; formication from the slightest motion in bed: *Carb. veg.*

When merry: *Crocus.*

The sound of a church bell is doleful: *Ant. crud.*

Doleful when hearing music: *Acon.*

— makes her quite sad: *Acon., Digit.*

— makes her melancholic: *Acon., Natr. sulph.*

Piano-playing causes anxiety in chest: *Natr. carb.*

Cannot bear it in head: *Phosphor.;* much affected by it: *Sepia.*

Timid forebodings: *Digit.;* apprehensions: *Digit.;* bad humor: *Mangan.*

Cannot bear music: *Chamom., Natr. carb., Nux vom., Phosphor., Sabin.*

Everything, even music is unbearable: *Mercur.*

Seeks solitude, darkness and silence: *Nux vom.*

Hates music; peevish, irritable: *Caustic.*

Mind much agitated, even music causes trembling: *Natr. carb.*

Nervousness so great that music becomes quite unbearable, it goes through bone and marrow: *Sabin.*

The sound of church bells moves to tears: *Ant. crud.*

Music makes her weep: *Graphit., Kreosot., Thuya.*

Music, even of a lively kind disposes her to weep: *Natr. sulph.*

Tender and soft mood; music moves him to tears: *Nux vom.*

Makes her sleepy, and shut the eyes; a clairvoyant dream: *Stannum.*

NOISE UNBEARABLE.

!! Acon.
! Alum.
Al. p. s.
! Amm. carb.
!! Anac.
! Angust.
Ant. crud.
! Arnica.
Arsen.
! Aurum.
! Baryt.
! Bellad.
!! Borax.
!! Bryon.
!! Calad.
! Calc. ostr.
! Cannab.
! Capsic.
! Carb. an.
Carb. veg.
Card. mar.
!! Caustic.
! Chamom.
Cicuta.
!! Cinch. off.
Coccul.
!! Coffea.
! Colchic.
! Conium.
Crotal.
Graphit.
Helleb.
Hura.
! Ignat.
!! Ipec.
! Jodium.
!! Kali carb.
Kreosot.
Laches.
! Lycop.
!! Magn. carb.
Mancin.
!! Mangan.
Moschus.
! Mercur.
Narc. mur.
! Natr. carb.
! Nitr. ac.
!! Nux vom.
Petrol.
Phosphor.
! Phosph. ac.
! Platin.
Plumbum.
Ptel. trif.
! Pulsat.
!! Sabad.
!! Sanguin.
! Sepia.
!! Silic.
! Spigel.
! Stannum.
Stramon.
Tabac.
Xanthox.
! Zincum.

With anxiety: *Aurum, Capsic.,* || *Caustic., Natr. carb., Pulsat.,* |*Silic.*; anxiety when among the noise of many people: *Petrol.*

Fear with every noise in the street, full of apprehension: *Caustic.*

Full of care: *Aurum, Baryt.*; irritable and faint-hearted: *Cinch. off.*

Fretful: *Arsen.*; and morose, peevish: *Kali carb.*; ill humored: *Bellad., Phosphor.*

Peevish, irritable: *Ptel. trif.*; cross, all things disagree: *Phosphor.*; displeased with everything, nothing is right: *Arsen.*; angry after contradiction: *Coccul.*

Enraged, angry: *Ipec.*; cannot bear talking of people: *Conium, Mar. ver., Zincum;* vexed: *Rhus tox.*; and angry: *Mangan.*

Cannot bear to hear a person walking in the room, with extreme moroseness and nausea: *Sanguin.*

With every word spoken fright and a shooting in the head: *Cicut.*

Suspicious, as if his life was conspired against: *Al. p. s.*

Unreasonable lamentations, bitter complaints: *Ignat.*; weeping: *Aether., Kreosot.*

Crying and weeping with the slightest noise: *Laches.*

Melancholy, a little noise startles much: *Stramon.*

Reserved mania: *Conium;* men are offensive: *Phosphor.*

Starting. See Hearing, Chapter 6.

With difficult hearing and a dreamy, dull state of mind: *Zincum.*

Difficult comprehension: *Capsic.*; illusions at night: *Carb. veg.*

Stupefaction: *Laches.*

MODEL CURES.

Nervous, sensitive to the least noise, hysterical mood; voice tremulous; fears she is going to die, general chlorotic appearance; amenorrhœa for five months; constipation; scanty, frequent and dark urine; face and legs œdematous: *Xanthox.*

A girl æt. 19. Over-sensitiveness to noise and music, pains in head and ears worse from mental exertion, difficult hearing, sensitiveness of the meatus and tympanum; offensive mucous discharge, buzzing, sensation as if a membrane was stretched before the tympanum; cold feet, tickling cough with dryness in larynx and hoarseness after singing; comedones with itching and burning in the face; desire for sour things: *Calc. ostr.*^{2m}; later other medicine completed this master cure.—RENTSCH.

SUBJECTIVE NOISES.

Hypochondric mood, anxiety: *Pulsat.*
As if some one approached his bed: *Carb. veg.*
Singing: *Chin. sulph.;* humming: || *Coca;* like music: *Pulsat.*
Fretful impatience with a wavering noise (Wuwwern): *Platin.;* wants to be alone: *Conium,* and at rest: *Bellad.;* hates company: *Bellad., Phosphor.;* starting, frightened: *Millefol.,* when falling asleep: *Sulphur;* frightened, starting from claps and cracks (Knallen): *Rhus tox.;* difficult comprehension with buzzing: *Arsen.;* head confused with a rolling noise: *Zinc. cyan.;* dull, stupid with buzzing: *Laches.*
Illusions with buzzing and humming: *Magn. mur.;* imagines he hears some one walking behind him: *Crot. casc., Bromum.*
As if some one were under the bed: *Bellad.;* with a rattling noise: *Canthar.;* over his bed: *Calc. ostr.*
Delirium with singing: *Stramon.;* looking about where the whistling and singing comes from: *Elaps.;* hears voices from the corners of the room: *Arsen.;* hears somebody talk: *Elaps.;* strange voice, follows it and tilts against the door: *Crot. casc.*
Mania, anguish and anxious sweat, with noises as of large church-bells: *Arsen.*
Stupor, with buzzing: *Psorin.*
Distraction of mind and loss of memory: *Camphor.*

DIMINISHED SENSE OF HEARING.

Hears everything, but it makes no impression: *Helleb.*
Does not hear clearly, and makes mistakes in speaking: *Bovist.*
Imperfect hearing and activity, alternating with absence of mind: *Alum.*
Hearing vanishes; stupefaction: *Stramon.*
Difficult hearing, and a dull, dreamy state: *Zincum.*
Deafness, with a dull headache, and with great anxiety, trembling and sweating: *Chin. sulph.;* anxiety in abdomen: *Aloes;* with stupefaction: *Arnica, Carb. an., Crotal., Kreosot., Ol. an., Stramon.*
Pain; ill humor: *Nux vom.*
Ear symptoms. Anxiety: sensitiveness to noise: *Silic., Pulsat.;* musical noise; fear of apoplexy: great noise in the ear, with distraction and loss of memory: *Cannab.;* mental exertion: *Conium;* waking: *Sepia, Zincum.*
Want of memory: *Moschus.*
Insanity; sensitiveness only after loud screaming: half conscious: *Arsen.;* hypochondric humor; confusion of mind: *Agn. cast., Baptis., Carb. an.*
As if drunk: *Magn. carb.*
Does not answer when he is asked: *Magn. carb.*

EARACHE.

Boring, so violent has to scream: *Baryt.*
Stitches, with weeping and weakness: *Silic.;* loud lamenting: *Sepia;* crying out: *Nux vom.*
Large stitches, shooting, fretful and vexed about trifles: *Chamom.*
Stitches with excitement: *Stramon.;* delirium: *Stramon.*
Pains with anxiety in chest: *Kali carb.;* with abdominal anxiety: *Aloes, Glonoin.;* anguish: *Bellad.;* agony all night: *Mercur.;* ill humor: *Chamom.;* confusion: *Hyosc.;* as if it would set him crazy: *Psorin.*
Every time he laughs, a violent drawing, shooting pain from the stomach to the membrana tympani: *Mangan.*
When laughing, cold air out of the left ear: *Millefol.*
After hearing bad news, trembling in ear: *Sabad.*

OUTER EAR.

Heat with anxiety and rigor: *Arsen.*
Hot ear-lobes, peevish and lachrymose: *Alum.*
Tearing and shooting in the right mastoid process, she has to cry out: *Canthar.;* below the right ear shooting, has to cry out: *Baryt.*
With fright, violent tearing, in the left ear, runs into the cheek: *Sulph. ac.*
A pressure over the concha deep in the brain, with complete faint-heartedness: *Agar.*
Tension in the region of ears, with dullness and stupidity: *Asar.*

NOSE.

Smell. Much affected by disagreeable odors: *Acon.;* by odor of flowers: *Graphit., Lycop.;* by light and smell: *Colchic.;* sounds and odors: *Acon.*
Tobacco smoke and soot is unbearable: *Bellad.*
Strong odors put him quite beside himself: *Colchic.*
Illusions when awaking, he smells the burning sponge and sulphur, he dreamt of: *Anac.*
Nosebleed after weeping: *Nitr. ac.;* after aching and dullness in the head: *Carb. an.;* after cardiac anxiousness and trembling: *Sepia;* after mental exertions: *Nux vom.*
Ill humor: *Coffea;* with anxiousness and melancholic mood relieved by nosebleed: *Kali chlor.*
With oversensibility or with anxiety: *Crocus;* preventing sleep: *Bellad.;* restlessness: *Arsen.;* with fear of dying, cannot attempt any business: *Crocus;* ill humor: *Coffea, Kali chlor.;* followed by weeping: *Nitrum;* disinclination to work: *Nux vom.;* vexatiousness: ||*Arsen.*
Excitement, passion: *Arsen.;* restlessness: *Kadm. sulph.*

Answers questions as if frightened: *Bellad.*
Sopor: *Bellad.;* stupid feeling: *Carb. an., Conium.*

Coryza. Sneezing, frequent irritation and fear because it hurts much in the throat: *Phosphor.;* and stupidity: *Graphit.;* dullness, as if coryza would follow: *Stannum;* with violent pain in forehead and delirium: *Mezer.*

As if coryza would come on, ill humor: *Sabin.;* cold, chilliness: *Hepar s. c.*
Ill humor, dull and empty feeling, head like a lantern: *Arsen.*
Running catarrh with lachrymose humor: *Spigel.*
Weeping over his deserted position, nose runs: *Lith. carb.*
Unbearable stoppage: *Psorin.;* obstruction with anxiety: *Zinc. ox.;* can only breathe with open mouth, with anxiousness: *Amm. carb.*
Children are very cross with the sniffles: *Chamom.*
Coryza; is easily agitated: *Arsen.;* disposition to weep: *Spigel.;* melancholy: *Cepa;* with cough, which makes the children cry: *Cina.*

MODEL CURES.

Sad and gloomy for ten days, the following ten days excited. During the first quiet, sad and anxious; picks his fingers; lies in bed most of the time; does not like to answer questions; passes urine often during the night. Confused feeling in the head, often sits lost in thought. He eats and drinks, has only one stool in three days. Weak memory. Timid—cannot be persuaded to work. Sleeps very restlessly.

The ten days following: very much excited, passionate, domineering, quarrelsome, scolds a great deal. Likes to wear his best clothes. Makes useless purchases, cares very little for the things, wastes or ruins them. Does not want to work—goes to play; quarrels with every one—will not bear contradiction; all the time picks his nose, which bleeds easily: *Conium.*—ELWERT.

Hypochondria. Tired of life, inclination to commit suicide, sleeplessness, hysteria, spasmodic twitching, troublesome cough, with stitches in the chest, worse in the evening and at night; coryza with sneezing and watery discharge, also yellow and offensive. Leucorrhœa; retarded and suppressed menses: *Zizia.*—MARCY.

OUTER NOSE.

Illusion, her nose appears to her transparent: *Bellad.*
Dull pain in bones with stupefaction: *Arnica;* over the root of nose, dull gloomy sensation: *Spongia.*
Phlegm in choanæ, torments himself and others with hawking: *Psorin.*
Picks his nose all the time, it bleeds easily: *Conium.*
With itching of nose, stronger memory: *Bellad*
Boring in nose, sitting quiet and silent: *Nitr. ac.*
Itching in the nostrils; water dropping out of them, with cold feet and great impatience: *Sulphur.*
Red nose with the slightest agitation: *Vinca.*

Anxious heat with sweat below the nose: *Nux vom.;* around it: *Ignat.*
Delirium and excoriated nose in scarlet fever: *Phytol.*

FACEACHE.

Faceache. Drawing ache in the forehead; hypochondric mood: *Arg. nitr.*

Pressing pain under the right eye, at night, with anxiety, driving her out of bed: *Arsen.*

Tearing, rending in one side of face, with ill humor: *Tongo.;* tension and stitches in the face and front of neck, with anxiety: *Nitrum.*

Faceache: *Stannum;* with anxiety, driving out of bed: *Magn. mur.;* confusion: *Mur. ac.;* mental exertion: *Carb. veg., Graphit.*

Bones. Pains; frightful anxiety, driving him out of bed; malar bones burning, tearing: *Magn. carb.*

Pain in the jaws after the mania: *Acon.*

Confusion: *Carb. veg., Mur. ac.;* drawing in bones; contractive pressive pain: *Zincum.*

FEATURES, COUNTENANCE.
Gesichtszüge, Miene.

Smiling: in delirium; imagines not to be at home: *Veratr.;* involuntarily when talking: *Aurum;* constantly with a pleasant weakness, as if pining away: *Lauroc.;* in a stupid state: *Bellad.*

Looks disturbed and pale after erysipelas: *Morph. ac.;* in mental derangement, while she is trying to hide it: *Thuya;* with staring, red face and mental derangement: *Hyperic.*

Painful expression, with sighing, indifference, derangement from unlucky love: *Hyosc.*

Sad, and depressed with anxiety: I *Cuprum.*

Anxious and restless: *Acon.;* unsteady look, with great restlessness: *Aloes;* unable to talk: *Laches.;* full of complaints of weakness, apparently well: *Colchic.*

Anxious expression after the opening of an abscess, with an irritable pulse: *Psorin.*

Shows his anger after the most trifling causes, in face and motions: *Fluor. ac.;* very serious, without any depression: *Rumex.*

Morose face; fretful: *Phelland.;* vexed: *Zincum.*

He looks into vacant space with dissatisfaction and vexation: *Mezer.*

Discontent is plainly visible on his face before he is aware of it himself: *Kali carb.*

Dissatisfied with himself; gloomy expressions: *Caustic.*

Discontented and morose expression, people ask him what ails him: *Phosph. ac.*

Wakes up with morose expression: *Ignat.*
Dissatisfied face; in the forenoon: *Magn. carb.*
Dissatisfied and serious expression, does not care to talk during the heat in the head; better towards noon: *Aeth. cyn.*
Sour, disturbed look; morose: *Zincum.;* morose face; out of humor: *Kali carb.*
Sour face; discontented: *Caustic.*
Wildness of countenance, stupid: *Stramon.*
Drunken appearance, sat alone, would not speak: *Ant. crud.*
Drunken look, unconscious: *Stramon.*
Frightful visions take possession of his fancy, and fright and fear are depicted on his countenance: *Stramon.*
Countenance expresses the greatest horror, with dyspnœa: *Gelsem.*
Starting in sleep, whining, painfully sad expression, stamps with her feet, hands and feet white and cold: *Ignat.*
Terrified look: *Pulsat.*
The face expresses fright and stupidity: *Acon.*
Singular countenance, uses wrong words: *Nux mosch.*
Amazed; without consciousness: *Camphor.*
Appearance as if engaged in deep thought and whining: *Nitrum.*
Features confused, weeping and laughing: *Natr. carb.;* delirium: *Secal.*
Consternation with loss of mental faculties: *Laches.;* staring, with absence of mind: *Zincum;* stupor: *Laches.;* apathy, indifference: *Cinchon.*
Unconcern, peevishness, talks in monosyllables, stupid expression, hastiness: *Merc. sulph. nigr.*
Stupid expression, unconcerned: *Calc. phosph.;* staring expression with stupefaction: *Cicut.;* stupid air: *Aster.;* singularly stupid expression: *Opium, Secal.*

MODEL CURE.

An old lady lay in bed free from any inflammatory symptoms, to all appearances in good health. Anxious expression. Complains of lassitude, nausea and great prostration: *Colchic.*—HADEN.

Talking nonsense in her sleep at four o'clock in the morning; disturbed look, stares at people; head hot, carotids throbbing; flushed and bloated face; eyes fixed, pupils dilated; frequent pulse; hair moist, the rest of the body burning hot; great anxiety; singing, followed by weeping and loud screaming, with gasping for breath; beating headache, especially in the vertex; tearing stitches in the brain; crawling in hands and feet, as if they were numb; great thirst, white-coated tongue: *Hyper.*—G. F. MULLER.

FACE MOTIONS.

Inclination to contract and corrugate the eyebrows: **Therid.**
Wrinkled forehead, with vexation: *Mangan.*

After too great merriness feeling as if he must move the muscles of his face; indifference and impatience: *Lycop.*
Muscles of face constantly twitch; mania: *Stramon.*
Twitches in the face and limbs, with derangement: *Bellad.*
Disposition to make grimaces, and push out the tongue: *Bellad.*
Ridiculous grimaces; raving: *Helleb.;* laughable faces; mania: *Hyosc.*
Distorted features, as if discontented: *Arsen.*
Weeping and sobbing, with distorted face: *Alcohol.*
Strange distortion of the face; melancholy: *Stramon.*
Distorted, stretched features, wide open staring eyes, red cheeks, no thirst: *Squilla;* delirium: *Moschus;* with madness: *Opium.*
Foams with anger, and fills the house with cursing and swearing: *Alcohol.*
Face distorted and pale with rage: *Veratr.*
Face distorted with mania: *Veratr.;* stupor: *Acon.*
Loss of all mental functions, with distorted face: *Laches.*

MODEL CURE.

Talks almost continually about fanciful things or such as have really occurred, of faithless love, of her teacher and school days; laughs, sings, dances, weeps, makes grimaces, and gesticulates with her hands. Clings obstinately to her ideas, without, however, growing angry about it. Face distorted, eyes fixed, no desire to eat or drink, things offered her are hastily dispatched: *Platin.*— M. MULLER.

FACE.

Cold face and hands with drops of sweat: *Opium.*
Face, hands and feet cold, with dislike of solitude: *Calc. ostr.*
Face cold and pale, also hands, flying heat, with fear and anxiety: *Pulsat.*
With insensibility: *Aethusa.*
Now cold, now hot; sweat, with ill humor and dislike to talk: *Borax.*
Hot cheeks. Heat in one cheek, inward heat, irritability, talkativeness: Hot cheeks; growing inconsolable: *Nux vom.*
Drawing in the umbilical region from both sides, sometimes ascending to the epigastrium, nausea, with attacks of anxiousness and hot cheeks: *Hepar.*
Flying heat, flushes of heat. With anxiety, anxiousness: *Chamom., Droser., Sepia;* anxiety, dullness of thinking, red face: *Acon.;* cold hands: *Chamom.;* sweating hands: *Calc. ostr.;* cool sweat in palms: *Chamom.*
Flying heat of face, with irresolution, nothing right: *Chamom.;* flushes of heat and ill humor: *Platin.;* lassitude, no ambition to work, irritable, frequent flushes of heat to the face: *Lycop.;* heat rises in face, absorbed in thought: *Bryon.;* flying heat, especially when busily engaged (also when sitting), or when walking fast he gets very hot in the face, with stinging as of needles: *Oleand.;* blood mounts to face with his tendency to hurry: *Ignat.*

Heat in face, with merriness: *Veratr.;* with hypochondric mood: *Hippom., Lycop., Nux mosch.;* with anxiousness: ❙*Acon.,* ❙❙*Arg. nitr., Bellad., Caustic., Copaiv.;* dry heat: *Acon.;* steadily increasing heat: *Carb. veg.;* with apprehension: *Mercur.;* and black before the eyes: *Arg. nitr.;* cold hands and feet: *Graphit.;* sweating hands: *Mercur.;* thirst and bitter taste after anger: *Chamom.*
Anguish: *Carb. veg., Cuprum, Graphit.*
With fearfulness: *Veratr.;* faint-heartedness: *Nux vom.;* morose: *Calc. phosph., Sarsap.;* ill humor: *Asar., Kreosot., Sarsap.;* irritable: *Stannum;* cross: *Sarsap.;* fretful: *Phosphor.;* much vexed after slight causes: *Phosphor.;* with cold hands and palpitation: *Phosphor.;* complaining and weeping: *Nux vom., Sepia;* groaning: *Chamom.;* desire to hurry his business: *Ptelea.*
She does not accomplish anything; heat in the face: *Stannum.*
After suppressed foot-sweat when he sees an open window or a sharp instrument, his face flushes and a sweat breaks out over him, he can scarcely resist the inclination to take his life: *Merc. sol.*
Heat with anxiety, disinclination to work: *Sarsap., Stannum;* to mental work: *Nitrum;* shunning labor: *Agar.*
With excitement, irritation and cold feet, after chill and thirst: *Magn. carb.*
Heat in face without thirst, but a restless mind; restlessness: *Amm. mur.;* before catamenia: *Lycop.*
Indisposition to think; hot forehead: *Nitrum.*
Thinking power leaves him: *Arg. nitr., Bryon.*
Worse from thinking: *Spongia, Xiphos.;* after lively conversation: *Fluor. ac.;* mental work: *Agar.;* mental exertion: *Amm. carb.*
Stupidity in the head, with coryza: *Ruta.*
Mania: *Veratr.;* with a cold body: *Stramon.*
With aggravation of all mental symptoms: *Hippom.*
Cheeks hot and red, with attacks of anxiety: *Pulsat.;* fearful: *Veratr.;* with loud lamentations: *Nux vom.;* inconsolable: *Nux vom.*
Face hot and red, with constant laughing: *Veratr.;* bright mood, excited: *Aloes;* careless humor, indifference: *Veratr.*
Anxiousness: *Strontian;* and dry skin: *Acon.;* and sweat: *Spongia;* and delirium: *Stramon.*
Glowing face from rush of blood, constant unconsciousness with derangement: *Opium.*

SWEAT.

On forehead with heat in head: *Carb. veg.;* and in scrobiculum: *Bellad.*
Warm, with hot and red cheeks, and attacks of anxiety: *Pulsat.*
Cold: *Iberis;* and open fontanels: *Calc. phosph., Mercur.;* anxiousness: *Mur. ac.;* and trembling: *Arsen.*
Anxiety: ❙*Arsen., Calc. phosph., Cicut., Mercur., Mur. ac., Natr. carb., Phosphor.*
Driving out of bed: *Carb. veg.*

I Arsen.	
II Bellad.	
I Borax.	
I Calc. ostr.	
I Calc. phos.	
I Carb. an.	
I Carb. veg.	
I Cicuta.	
II Iberis.	
I Magn. carb.	
I Mercur.	
Mur. ac.	
I Natr. carb.	
Phosphor.	
I Platin.	
II Pulsat.	

Anguish in attacks, several a day: *Natr. carb.*
Colicky tension in the hypochondria: *Arsen.;* followed by a loose stool: *Mercur.*
— — restlessness: *Phosphor.*
— — pulmonary anxiety: *Carb. veg.*
— — it attacks the heart as if he would faint: *Cicut.*
— — frightened feeling: *Iberis;* after a fright in a dream: *Bellad.*
— — trembling: *Arsen.;* of hands: *Cicut.;* and sweat of hands: *Calc. ostr.;* in palms: *Calc. phosph.*
— — and sweat between the feet or on the feet: *Arsen.*
— ill humor: *Borax, Platin.*
— weeping disposition: *Carb. an.*
— inability to think: *Calc. phosph.*
In attacks: *Calc. phosph.;* without pain: *Natr. carb.*
Sweat in large drops: *Platin.*

REDNESS.

Of Cheeks and silly merriness: *Acon.;* serenity: *Argent.*
Like after hearing bad news: *Coccul.;* anxiety: *Hepar s. c.;* anxious heat: *Nux vom.*
Melancholy: *Stramon.;* uneasy to despair: *Vip. red.*
Vexed about every trifle: *Pulsat.;* obstinacy: *Acon.*
As if drunken: *Pulsat.;* talkativeness: *Argent.*
After surprise, such as fright, that she is beside herself, and cannot be quieted: *Mercur.;* stupid when awakening: *Anac.;* distorted, stretched features, open, staring eyes: *Squilla;* delirium: *Stramon.;* talking with open eyes: *Chamom.;* and with circumscribed redness: *Lachnanth.;* one cheek red, the other pale; cold sweat on hands and feet; mind very miserable: *Ipecac.*

Flushed Face, with an anxiety rising up from the abdomen in the head: *Lauroc.;* anxious trembling: *Pulsat.;* a hasty disposition: *Ignat.;* delirium: *Stramon.;* weak minded: *Ignat.;* insensibility, stupid: *Stramon.*
Indifferent: *Veratr.*
Sad and peevish: *Spigel.;* sad and full of fear: *Stramon., Veratr.*
Anxious: *Spongia;* and flying heat: *Acon.;* likes hot water, evenings: *Sepia;* rising up with stitches in heart: *Plumbum;* cardiac anguish: *Bellad.;* uneasy to despair: *Vip. red.*
Fearful: *Veratr.;* from fright: *Opium.*
Shy, embarrassed: *Carb. veg.*
From slight contradiction: *Ignat.*
Inclined to be angry: *Bryon.;* fretful: *Spigel.*
Morose lamenting mood: I I *Acon.;* loud screaming: I I *Opium.*
The infant gets red around the eyes when whining: *Borax.*
From slight emotions: *Nitrate of amyl, Phosphor.;* from animated conversa-

tion: *Sepia;* from excitement in the night: *Aloes;* with restlessness: *Laches.;* beside himself: *Crocus;* dull in head as if drunken: *Caustic.;* delirium and illusions with open eyes: *Crotal.;* with talking: *Opium;* with laughing *Veratr.;* face bloated: *Doryph.;* puffed: *Opium.*

Red in Mania: ‖*Bellad.*, ‖*Cicut.*, ▮*Hyosc.*, ‖*Opium*, ▮▮*Stramon.*,‖ *Veratr.;* sadness, thinking about death: *Stramon.;* anxiety, faint heart, despair: *Veratr.;* violent: *Opium;* strikes at his attendants, tears his clothes, scolding, cursing: *Hyosc.;* lamenting, crying: *Veratr.*

Jumping out of bed, laughing, dancing, jumping, clapping hands, drinking wine all night: *Cicut.*

Great vivacity: *Opium;* restlessness, conversing with spirits all night; fear of bad animals, black dogs: *Stramon.;* raving: *Bellad.;* confused memory: *Stramon.;* unconscious: *Glonoin.*, *Stramon.;* senseless: *Stramon.;* eyes glaring: *Opium*, *Stramon.;* looks wild: *Hyosc.;* staring: *Stramon.;* weeping: *Stramon.*

Face glowing red: *Veratr.;* hot: *Hyosc.;* swollen: *Stramon.*

Stuttering and lisping before a few words come out: *Stramon.*

Thirst very great: *Stramon.;* will neither eat nor drink: *Hyosc.*, *Veratr.;* after frequent drunkenness: *Hyosc.*

Abdomen puffed: *Stramon.;* sexual desire excited: *Stramon.*

Breathing quick and difficult: *Hyosc.*

Cold feet: *Veratr.*

Runs about in his room all night: *Hyosc.;* restless sleep, with strange images: *Stramon.;* no sleep: *Veratr.*

With erysipelas: *Stramon.*

Blue, red, after a slight surprise: *Mercur.;* if she attempts to speak before people: *Carb. veg.;* talkative mania: *Stramon.;* swollen lips, face and head: *Opium.*

Bluish face in madness, with snoring: *Opium;* weeping: *Sambuc.;* bloated: *Sambuc.;* with loss of senses: *Morphin.;* dark blue with screaming: *Veratr.*

Brown and blue after vexation: *Staphis.*

Yellow, and restless to despair: *Vip. red.;* and gloomy humor, forenoon: *Arg. nitr.;* sickly sallow complexion, bloated, with mental alienation, keeping the bed unreasonably: *Aloes.;* complexion livid; disposition sad, irritable: *Kreosot.*

PALENESS.

Easy quiet, mind clear, expecting death, praying for the saving of her soul: *Arnic.*

Happy mind and excessive joy: *Crocus.*

Discomfort: *Magn. carb.*, *Sulphur;* depression: ‖ *Chin. sulph.;* irritable and sad: *Kreosot.*

Infant whining much, crying in sleep: *Borax.*

Child screams, putting fists in its mouth: *Ipecac.*

PALENESS.

Crying and running about: *Veratr.*
Anxious and running about: *Lamium;* with fear of death: *Magn. sulph.;* anxious: *Kali carb., Mangan., Nux vom.,* | | *Pulsat., Spongia.*
— with nausea after pain in stomach passed off: *Kali carb.;* — and restlessness: *Mangan.;* — after dinner, has to lay down: *Nux vom.*
Anguish and cold: *Pulsat.;* or puffed: *Carb. veg.*
Fear: *Veratr.;* of death: *Moschus;* of ghosts: *Pulsat.*
Indifference: *Crotal., Helleb., Stannum.*
Fretful: *Veratr.;* ill humor: *Amm. carb., Stannum;* and drowsiness: *Lycop.;* and fallen away: *Mezer.*
Singing: *Bellad.;* screaming: *Ipecac., Veratr.;* violent scolding: *Moschus.*
Aversion to talk: *Ox. ac.;* to work: *Arsen.*
Overcome from seeing the wounded in the hospital: *Gelsem.*
Starting in sleep: *Lycop.;* mentally and bodily "used up:" *Amm. carb.*
Difficult comprehension: *Cinch. off.;* derangement of onanists: *Hyosc.*
Dull, obtuse mind: *Stannum.*
Illusions: *Hyosc.;* delirium: *Bellad.*
Mania: *Crocus, Mercur., Stannum, Veratr.;* singing, whistling, neither eating nor drinking: *Bellad.;* indifferent; desire to run away and drown herself: *Helleb.;* talks about religious matters, thinks he has been poisoned: *Hyosc.;* vanishing of thought: *Therid.*
Pallor and anxiety: *Spongia.*
Pallid, miserable and indifferent: *Crotal., Mezer.;* discomfort, miserable and sad: *Natr. mur.;* discolored with general discomfort: *Magn. carb.;* emaciated with mania: *Mercur.;* with ill humor: *Mezer.*
Earthy pale and anxious: *Magn. sulph., Pulsat.*
— fear of death: *Magn. sulph.*
— dislikes all kind of exertion: *Arsen.*
— deranged: *Hyosc., Pulsat.*
Hippocratic Face with anxiety: *Arsen.;* with indifference: *Cinch. off.*

MODEL CURE.

After vexation, mental depression; she is in constant dread, with palpitation of the heart, is afraid of every body, considers every one her enemy, despairs of every thing—cries easily—trusts no one. At the same time pale earthy complexion, with dim, desponding look. No appetite, much thirst, limbs feel as if asleep, is weary, weak, cannot sleep at night on account of fear and dread. *Pulsat.*—TH. RUCKERT.

SWELLING.

Sensation of fulness, excited and disinclined to converse: *Ox. ac.*
Puffed up; fear: *Carb. veg.;* and anxious mania: *Bellad.*
Swollen and red from surprise: *Mercur.;* with anxiety in head: *Apis.*
Swollen face and arm, raving about dogs: *Bellad.*
Face and head with madness: *Opium.*
With erysipelas: *Stramon.;* after it struck in: *Cuprum, Stramon.*

SKIN.

Crawling in cheek after fright, shocks: *Sulph. ac.;* as from insects over face: *Crot. tigl.*
An itching pimple above the arcus ciliaris, with coryza and moroseness: *Clemat.*

JAWS.

Tearing, aching, with difficult comprehension: *Natr. carb.*
Spasmodic drawing, wakening about midnight, with anxiety: *Sepia.*
Trismus and stupor: *Acon.;* and rage: *Stramon.*
Lower jaw hangs down, with loss of consciousness: *Stramon.*
Mouth open and looks upwards; gets hot and lachrymose: *Carb. an.*
Distortion and mania: *Opium;* does not want to open it: *Ignat.*
Twitching around: *Glonoin., Opium.*
Moves it backwards and forwards; mania: *Stramon.*
Froth. See Lips.

LIPS.

Tingling sensation and difficult comprehension: *Natr. carb.*
Water touching them enrages him, in delirium: *Stramon.*
Covered with froth in mania: *Stramon.;* froth before the mouth, foaming, with unconsciousness: *Bellad.;* foaming with madness: *Camphor.;* ropy saliva hanging down, with mania: *Bellad.;* corners of mouth covered with foam, in rage: *Stramon.*
Dry with sadness: *Rhus tox.;* with vivid delirium: *Stramon.*
Licks them, with moaning and groaning: *Pulsat.*
Dry and sticky with hypochondric morose mood: *Arg. nitr.*
Red brown streaks in mania: *Opium.*
Blue with passionateness: *Moschus;* in mania: *Hyosc.*
Reddish, blue and swelled; semi-consciousness: *Stramon.;* in madness. *Opium.*
Swollen in mania: *Opium.*
Chin, as if it was growing larger: *Glonoin.*

TEETH.

Toothache. After vexation, following or increasing: ❚*Acon.*, ❙*Chamom.*, ❘*Rhus tox.*, ❙*Staphis.*

After emotions: *Acon.;* if others talk to him: *Arsen., Bryon.;* after getting angry: *Chamom., Nux vom.*

After mental exertion: *Bellad., Ignat.;* meditation: ❘❘*Ignat.*, ❙*Nux vom.;* mental labor: *Bellad.*, ❙*Ignat.*, ❙*Nux vom.;* reading: *Ignat.;* disenabling to all work, especially thinking: *Clemat.*

With Anxiety: ❙*Acon.*, ❘❘*Bellad.*, ❘*Clemat.*, ❙*Coffea*, ❘*Hyosc.*, ❘*Pulsat.*, *Sepia, Sulphur, Veratr.;* and restlessness: *Mangan.;* — as if he would die: *Oleand.;* — and nervous attacks with boring in a tooth: *Natr. mur.;* — and sweat: *Clemat.;* — driving to despair: ❙*Clemat.*, ❘*Nux vom.;* to frenzy: *Arsen.*

Fear it might return prevents sleep: *Rhus tox.*

With mental restlessness: *Mangan.;* with fretfulness and aversions: *Mezer.;* sets to running about: *Nux mosch.;* despairing: *Nux vom.*

With howling and crying: *Ipecac.;* whining: *Magn. carb.;* disposed to weeping: *Chamom., Coffea, Hyperic., Sepia;* weeping: *Acon., Coffea, Hyosc., Sulphur, Therid., Veratr.;* complaining, reproachful: *Nux vom.*

With great irritation: *Alum., Magn. carb.;* as if distracted, screwing the brain together: *Mezer.;* is beside himself: *Acon.*, ❙*Coffea.*

With starting when falling asleep, jerks in the teeth: *Mercur.*

With getting angry: *Arsen.;* in such a rage that she strikes her head with her fists; shortly before catamenia: *Arsen.*

Aversion to everything: *Magn. carb., Mezer.;* reproachful temper: *Nux vom.;* ill humor: *Chamom., Merc. jod. rubr.*, ❙*Mezer.*

With prostration of mental powers: *Hyosc.*

After toothache irritated state of mind: *Chamom.*, ❘❘❘*Lycop.;* cannot sleep: *Sepia;* fainting: *Cinch. off.*, ❙*Pulsat., Veratr.*

Sensations; feel soft and spongy with fear to bite on them, they might fall out: *Nitr. ac.;* — inclines to bite them together: *Phytol.;* — drives to grind them: *Caustic.*

Biting in the tumbler, in the spoon, with brain affection of children: *Cuprum;* attempt to bite things or persons in mania: *Bellad.*, all around: *Cuprum;* biting in delirium or mental derangement: ❙*Bellad.*, ❙❙*Stramon.*, ❘❘*Cuprum, Secal.*, ❘*Veratr.;* tearing with teeth: ❙*Stramon.*

Clapping with lower jaw against the upper in melancholy: *Mercur.;* biting at night in sleep so hard that pain wakens: *Mercur.;* biting firmly together, in melancholy: *Veratr.*

Chattering of Teeth with difficult comprehension: *Capsic.;* with loss of senses: *Camphor.;* with shaking chills and anxiety: *Capsic.*

Grinding Teeth and angry thoughts when awaking: *Kali carb.;* with froth at the mouth in mania: *Bellad.;* raising hands above the head: *Stramon.*

Scrapes her gums while senseless: *Bellad.*

During dentition sleepless with mental irritation: *Chamom., Coca, Coffea.*

Non-appearance of teeth with children and very fretful: *Calc. phosph.*

TASTE.

Sweet, expectoration of blood with anxiety: *Arsen.*
Sour, in the night with restlessness driving out of bed: *Magn. mur.*
Harsh, with heat in precordial region and great anxiety: *Ars. sulph.*
Sweetish bitter, with gloomy humor: *Arg. nitr.*

Bitter, with anxiety: *Amm. mur.;* cardiacal: *Bellad.;* sadness after a slight vexation: *Amm. mur.*

Sad, eyes filled with tears: *Petrol.;* after getting angry, with heat in face and anxiety: *Chamom.;* with moroseness and dullness: *Sulphur.*

Bad taste in the morning and ill humor: *Merc. jod. rubr.;* metallic, herby, slimy, with humor: *Nux vom.*

Flabby, watery, with quiet, silent melancholy: *Ignat.;* insipid, with sadness: *Cuprum.*

Slimy, with confusion of mind: *Cocc. cact.;* ill humor: *Nux vom.*

Loss of taste, smell and feeling, not of sight or hearing, with mind affection: *Opium.*

TALKING.

Excessive loquacity and exaltation of spirits: *Cann. ind.;* continual babbling and unconscious: *Stramon.;* prattling with stupor: *Stramon.;* incessant talking and rage: *Stramon.*

Talks very fast: *Bellad.;* tendency to hurry: *Ignat., Mercur., Phosphor.;* hasty and irritable: *Hepar;* and restless: *Acon.;* bold, and bright eyes: *Acon.;* hurried and hoarse, with a weak voice: *Laches.;* hasty drinking: *Hepar s. c.*

Makes a noise with her tongue in delirium: *Bellad.*

Could not move the tongue right, with anxiety: *Caustic.;* too heavy, fails on some words, while intellect is lessened: *Colchic.;* cannot put it out; in an indifferent state: *Bellad.*

Stammers unconnected words: *Stramon.;* after falling down unconscious: *Helleb.;* with forgetfulness: *Secal.*

Difficult speech with anxiety: *Caustic.;* speaks little, single disconnected words in a higher pitch: *Stramon.*

Inability to speak, knows what he wants to say, but cannot find the right word; if he is told the word, he can say it correctly: *Dulcam.*

Impeded speech and anguish: *Ignat.;* dyspnœa and great lassitude, after anxiety: *Bellad.*

Faint speech from weakness of larynx, otherwise lively: *Staphis.*

When speaking, anxiety: *Alum., Ambra, Platin, Stramon.;* — absent, loses the train of ideas: *Amm. carb.;* forgets the word: *Colchic.;* thoughts leave him: *Mezer.;* talking affects him: *Calc. ostr.;* thinking and speaking are hard work or even repugnant: *Rhus tox.;* does not like to talk; or talks too fast: *Bellad.*

Inability to Speak, words die on her lips when she gets cross about reproaches: *Crocus.;* — in a rage: *Stramon.;* in a stupefied state: *Acon.*

Speechlessness, with anxiety: *Ignat.;* sadness: *Petiv. tetr.;* with throbbing in chest and an indescribable bad feeling: *Mancin.;* unconscious: *Amygd., Mercur.;* absentminded with maniacal gestures: *Arsen.;* cannot even write his thoughts: *Arsen.*

MODEL CURE.

Great restlessness, confused memory. Red face and staring eyes. Sadness, weeping, thoughts of dying. Stammering, gets the words out with great difficulty. Cold feet, restless sleep with wrong visions. Fear of wild animals and black dogs: *Stramon.*—BETHMANN.

TONGUE.

Sticks it out a long way in delirium: *Bellad.*
Numbness of it, with thoughtlessness: *Sepia.*
Crawling, ascending from throat to the tongue and lips, stiffening the tongue, with an attack of great anxiety: *Natr. mur.*
Dryness of tip of tongue and lips without thirst, with anxious sweat: *Nux vom.*
Apparently livelier, but the tongue drier and increased thirst: *Clemat.*
Tongue dry and very red, vivid delirium: *Stramon.;* with raving: *Bellad.*
Sensation of dryness of the moist tongue, with anxiousness: *Mangan.;* with fevers: *Natr. mur.*
Tongue moist, no thirst, indifference; typhoid fever: *Arsen.*
— — and white, red borders with uneasiness to despair: *Vip. torv.*
Whitish furred tongue; morose: *Uran. nitr.;* idiotic state: *Opium.*
Coated tongue, with anxiety and forgetfulness:. *Guar. trichl.;* with confusion: *Cocc. cact.;* delirium: *Stramon.*

MOUTH.

Cramp-like pain and fear wakens: *Sepia.*
Child sticks fists into its mouth and screams violently: *Ipecac.*
Sensation of dryness, but tongue moist; irritable mood: *Bellad.*
Dry; after violent scolding: *Moschus.;* with rage: *Stramon.*
— with costiveness and difficult comprehension: *Chin. sulph.*
— and thirsty, with anxiety and restlessness: *Canthar.*
He imagines in his derangement that his breath is offensive: *Hyosc.*
Froth about the mouth, with semi-consciousness: *Stramon.;* unconscious: *Bellad.;* with maniacal rage: *Camphor.*
Saliva runs, when thinking about her throat: *Laches.*

Sticky and slimy, with very bad humor: *Platin.*
Full of rattling phlegm, when intending to scream in mania: *Stramon.*
Full of Saliva; mouth dry, anxious heat, drink repugnant: *Nux vom.*
Flow of saliva; sweating all night, in delirium: *Veratr.;* unconsciousness: *Morphin.,* and stupor: *Veratr.*
Has to spit all day long, with prickling stitches under the tongue, and fear of hydrophobia: *Hydroph.*
Much spitting, with vexation: *Calc. ostr., Kali carb.*
Spitting and biting in delirium: *Hyosc.;* with madness: I*Bellad.*
Spitting at others in mania: I*Bellad., Cannab., Cuprum;* with insanity: *Mercur., Veratr.*
Spits continually without ejecting any saliva: *Stramon.*
Ejects copious, frothy saliva in attacks of rage: *Canthar.*
Saliva discolored with blood, after mental labor: *Nitr. ac.*
Spitting blood, with screaming and weeping from the slightest noise: *Laches.*

ROOF OF MOUTH AND PALATE.

Stinging until he drinks, after fever heat, with anxiety: *Stramon.*
Dryness in roof of mouth without thirst, with anxious heat: *Nux vom.*
Heat, with homesickness: *Capsic.*
A sensation in the fauces and upper throat forces to hawk, is almost intolerable; obstinately refuses to gargle, insisting it did not relieve; annoy their families exceedingly; some emaciate from the constant efforts, get hectic fever and die: I I*Lycop.,* I*Mar. ver.,* I*Psorin., Sabad.;* if bending the head back relieves: *Lycop.;* if imagining horrible inner diseases: *Sabad.*
Mucus in throat; fears he will suffocate if closing his eyes; lessens when opening eyes and sitting up; keeps him awake all night: *Carb. an.*

THROAT.

Dryness, with uneasiness and horrible anxiety: *Rhus tox.;* with flashes of heat and anxiety: *Sepia.;* with disagreeable, anxious heat: *Sulphur;* with scraping and ill humor: *Platin.*
— sore and painful, with thirst, stupid slumber, dull after waking: *Anac.*
— of fauces and pharynx with difficult comprehension: *Chin. sulph.*
Tensive pain, with anxiousness: *Pulsat.*
Sensations; stitches producing a cough; after mental excitement: *Cistus.*
Severe pain with sneezing, fears something will tear out: *Phosphor.*
A tearing sensation, not when swallowing, but from exertion of mind: *Caustic.*
Burning with stupor: *Stramon.,* and a tickling in larynx and anxious constriction: *Mezer.*
Sore sensation with anxiety, most at night: *Zincum;* pain with anxiety:

Kali carb.; in attacks: *Spongia;* pain with anxious expression: *Arsen.;* with hopelessness and despair: *Apis;* pain when swallowing, with very ill humor and sour sweat at night: *Thuya.*

Sensations upwards; oppressed breathing from stomach up; anxious, restless, like from a bad conscience, or as if something was going to happen: *Ignat.*

Great distension of abdomen, felt in the throat, with dyspnœa and anxiety: *Magn. mur.*

Crampy sensation rising from chest into throat; wakes with anxiety: *Veratr.*

Rush of blood from throat to head, with difficult comprehension: *Fluor. ac.*

Burning and soreness rising from pit of stomach up, behind the sternum to roof of mouth, with great restlessness: *Mangan.*

Easily startled, and each time a hot sensation rises up in her throat, with apprehensions and anxiety: I I *Hyper.*

Throbbing in chest is felt in throat, with heat in face and restlessness: *Amm. mur.;* jerks from stomach up into the throat, with anxiety: *Pulsat.*

Sensation as if a semi-liquid fluid would rise from the throat to the palate, with fear of fainting: *Spigel.*

Sensations downward; pain from occiput down in the throat, with difficult comprehension: *Arg. nitr.*

Unbearable, painful pressure and throbbing in right temple, going down into throat, with very ill humor: *Bovist.*

A burning down the swallow, with mental alienation, keeping the bed unreasonably (lectrophilie): *Alum. p. s.*

Burning from throat down into stomach, with trembling anxiety: *Evphorb.*

Constriction in throat and chest, as when about to weep, and moody and sensitive after the meal as long as digesting: *Iodum.*

— violent, caused by inclination to weep from grief: *Lact. vir.*

— with great anxiety: *Sarsap.;* in chest, and anxious feeling in throat, has to take a deep breath: *Cannab.*

Spasmodic — of muscles, with a tormenting anxiety: *Tereb.*

— with headache, nausea and restlessness: *Kadm. sulph.*

— cannot swallow a drop without great anxiety: *Canthar.*

— hydrophobia with furor uterinus: *Gratiol.*

— visible outside with overhasty speech: *Laches.*

Dysphagia. Clawing with the hands at the throat, anxiety, relieved after something hot: *Arsen.*

Impediment in swallowing, stitches in throat, anxiety: *Nitrum.*

After eating cannot swallow, with anxiety: *Merc. subl.*

Swallowing difficult and painful, particularly fluids, with stupor, unconsciousness: *Stramon.;* pain in throat when swallowing or inability to swallow, in rage: *Stramon.*

As if swollen in throat, chest constricted and great anxiety: *Glonoin.;* oppressive feeling and out of humor: *Iodium.;* swelling of throat and windpipe, pressure causes anxiety: *Natr. sulph.;* sensation as of a plug in the throat, also felt when not swallowing; as if raw, with burning pain and anxiety, as if the throat would close: *Natr. mur.;* like a plug and sore, wakes at night, same fear: ‖*Natr. mur.;* in diphtheria remarkable nervous phenomena: *Phytol.*

After bursting of abscess in quincy, there remains anxiety in the face: *Psorin.*

THIRST.

<small>The marks on the margin signify the degree of intensity.</small>

Acon.
‖ Ailanth.
‖ Anathem.
‖ Arsen.
Bellad.
Capsic.
ǀ Chin. sulph
ǀ Clemat.
Crotal.
Cuprum.
ǀ Hepar s. c.
Nux vom.
ǀ Opium.
‖ Platin.
‖ Podoph.
Ruta.
‖ Stramon.
Sulphur.
Thuya.
Ver. vir.
ǀ Vip. red.

Great serenity, with a flushed, red face: *Clemat.;* bright mind, fever heat and sweat: *Opium.;* exalted state: *Opium.;* waking with sorrowful ideas about midnight: *Platin.;* uneasiness, to despair: *Vip. red.;* sadness: *Cuprum, Sulphur;* and restless tossing about: *Arsen.*

Anxiousness: *Chin. sulph.;* anxiety: *Bellad., Cuprum,* increasing with heat: *Platin.,* and difficult breathing: *Thuya;* anxious heat: *Nux vom.,* with the dying: *Crotal.;* and moroseness: *Capsic.;* irritability: *Acon.*

Suffocating, has to scream: *Arsen.;* lamentation and moaning, wringing of hands day and night, much thirst, with but little appetite, although she swallows food hastily: *Sulphur.*

Hastiness, speaks hastily: *Hepar s. c.;* with great agitation, spasms: *Anath. mur.*

As if drunken: *Stramon.;* difficult comprehension, coldness: *Capsic.;* during delirium: *Ailanth., Stramon.;* with burning heat, talking from 4 P.M. all night: *Hepar s. c.;* loquacity during the fever: *Podoph.;* mania: *Stramon.;* after erysipelas: *Stramon.*

Semi-conscious, unconscious, stupor: *Stramon.,* a.m.m.; comes when getting conscious: *Acon., Ver. vir.;* with a stupid feeling in the head, is intense, but after drinking once, it is gone: *Ruta.*

Thirstless and peevish: *Pulsat.;* anxious heat without thirst: *Cinchon.;* frightened in sleep, burning heat, very little thirst: *Lycop.*

HUNGER.

Appetite comes with the thought of food: *Calc. phosph.*

Wants to eat all the time, when thinking of food his mouth waters: *Sepia.*

Good appetite, but eating distresses, with moroseness: *Uran. nitr.*

Hungry after eating: *Aloes.*

Desire greater than the demand; eats and drinks too much: *Arsen.*

Increased appetite, with great depression: *Chin. sulph.;* with weariness of life: *Nitr. ac.;* with imbecility: *Secal.;* with sensitiveness and vexation: *Calc. phosph.*

Hungry for want of something to do: *Aloes.*

Hunger with contemptuous, haughty humor, greedy, hurried eating: *Platin.*

Anxiety if he does not eat every three or four hours; cannot eat much at a time: *Iodum.*

Sharp appetite, but the least thing disagrees and upsets his spirits, cannot endure it: *Mercur.*

A hungry and empty feeling wakes him in the morning, with restlessness: *Natr. mur.*

Swallows food and drink hastily, mania: *Bellad.*

Unnatural hunger, flares up easily: *Crot. tigl.;* with apathy and idiocy: *Veratr.;* with emptiness and anxiety: *Nitr. ac.;* and thirst with fever, restlessness, moaning and groaning: *Podoph.*

DIMINISHED APPETITE.

I Indisposed for food, little appetite, diminished appetite. II No appetite, want of it, no desire, loss of it. I Complete want, total loss. II Refuses food and drink.

|| Arg. nitr.
I Arsen.
I Bellad.
|| Borax.
|| Carb. veg.
I Clemat.
|| Coccul.
I Coca.
II Crocus.
|| Drosera.
II Hyosc.
|| Ignat.
I Kali bichr.
II Kali chlor.
|| Lepid.
|| Lil. tigr.
Lycop.
I Mercur.
I Opium.
I Platin.
|| Phosphor.
II Phosph. ac.
II Pulsat.
|| Spongia.
I Stramon.
|| Sulphur.
|| Valer.
II Veratr.
|| Viola od.

Very much elated: *Coca;* when eating taste good, with indifference of mind: *Mercur.;* with discomfort and ill humor: *Valer.;* with great sadness: *Clemat., Cuprum, Sulphur;* in the evening: *Platin.;* with melancholy: *Ignat.;* discomfort, low spirits: *Valer.;* mental depression: *Droser., Ignat., Kali bichr., Lil. tigr., Platin., Valer.;* with anxiety: *Arsen., Veratr.;* anxiousness: *Carb. veg.;* with fearful apprehension: *Lil. tigr.;* out of humor: *Spongia;* with fretfulness: *Coccul., Phosphor., Pulsat., Spongia;* morose: *Pulsat.;* after weeping about the least thing vexing her: *Coccul.;* with a weeping mood: *Platin.;* everything is disagreeable: *Spongia;* nursing children refuse the breast, weep, start from sleep, and grow pale and wilted: *Baryt.;* with lamentations and thirst: II*Sulphur;* is anxious and concerned: *Droser.;* anxiety and nausea: *Veratr.;* swallows hastily, moaning: *Sulphur;* thinks he ought to die by hunger: *Kali chlor.;* silent: *Ignat.;* with relaxed mind: *Lepid.;* confusion: *Carb. veg.;* with idiocy: *Opium;* childish derangement: *Viol. od., Phosph. ac.;* with delirium: *Bellad.;* when persuaded to take something she becomes furious: *Arsen.;* drinks, with attacks of mania: *Crocus, Hyosc.;* with mania: *Stramon., Veratr.*

DESIRES AND AVERSIONS.

Desire for acidulated drinks; delirium: *Stramon.;* longing for acids; mania: *Ignat.*

Thirst for beer, with anxious heat: *Nux vom.*

Aversion to bread, with depression of spirits: ||*Lil. tigr.*

Aversion to coffee, nausea when thinking of it, with fearfulness and apprehension: *Lil. tigr.*

Aversion to food, with weeping mood: *Platin.*
Want of appetite, vexed, everything is disgusting: *Spongia.*
Aversion to food and drink; stupor: *Coccul.*
Disgust for all nourishment except beer, with hypochondria: *Mercur.*
Aversion to food, with depression of spirits, disposed to weep: *Lil. tigr.*
By being made to eat, becomes furiously angry: *Arsen.*
Aversion to fluids, they pass down with difficulty: *Bellad.;* semi-conscious or spasmodic symptoms: *Stramon.*
When drink is forced upon her, she becomes furious: *Bellad.*

BEFORE, WHILE, AND AFTER EATING AND DRINKING.

Better while Eating or while Drinking. While eating the anxiety of mind disappears: *Aurum;* and tearfulness: *Sulphur.*

Anxiety relieved by drinking cold water: *Acon.;* only when he takes his meals he ceases to moan about his anguish: *Psorin.*

Better after Eating. Sensation of fulness and tension is followed by brightness and mental and bodily activity after eating: *Ant. crud.*

After dinner anxiousness better: *Sulphur.*

After supper headache and stomachache are relieved, with better humor: *Amm. carb.*

After meals better humor: *Amm. carb., Amm. mur., Kali bichr.*

Nausea better, but hot face and despair: *Acon.*

Better after eating in the evening; inability to think: *Silic.*

Delirium better after eating: *Bellad.*

Worse before Eating. Before eating, anguish: *Mezer.*

Before breakfast, out of humor: *Natr. phosph.*

Before breakfast, dull headache: *Conium.*

Before dinner, vexed, fretful: *Phosphor.*

While Eating. When beginning to eat, toothache and headache, is overcome: *Euphorb.*

Anxiousness while eating: ||*Sepia*, and after: *Carb. veg., Sepia.*

While eating supper, anxiousness: *Magn. carb.*

Anxious mood after a meal in the morning: *Conium.*

Hastily swallowing her meals under lamentations: *Sulphur.*

During dinner fretful: *Mar. ver.*

During breakfast weak mind; absent-minded: *Guaiac.;* after it ill humor: *Conium.*

Cold feet; itching in nostrils makes him very impatient; everything molests him: *Sulphur.*

Drunken feeling during and after a meal: *Gratiol.*

While eating warm food anxious: *Magn. carb.*

During breakfast mental relaxation: *Guaiac.*

MENTAL STATES AFTER EATING. 149

After Eating a little too much. Anxiety and restlessness: *Phosphor.*
Vexation, headache and gastric symptoms: *Cinch. off.*
Such ill humor that he can hardly stand it: *Mercur.*
It is difficult to persuade her to eat something; after it she gets conscientious scruples: *Ignat.*
Peculiar kind of hypochondria kept up by slight errors of diet: ‖*Natr. carb.*

After Breakfast. Anxiety rising upward from the abdomen: *Ignat.*
Ebullition from abdomen up the back, with heat and anxiety: *Lauroc.*
Anxious heat over the whole body: *Phosphor.*
Trembling, want of confidence: *Arg. nitr.*
Ill humor and drowsiness: *Calad.*
Ill disposed: *Conium;* with pressure in stomach: *Natr. carb.*
Inclination to write is gone: *Spiggur.*
Suddenly after lunch, 1.30 P.M., loses memory and power of thought: *Calc. sulph.*

After Supper. Unusual vivacity: *Colchic.;* followed by drowsiness: *Bellad.*
Excessive gaiety: *Bellad.*
Indisposition: *Petrol.;* trembling anxiety: *Caustic.*
Burning pain in the epigastrium, with anxiety: *Nux vom.*
Pressing pain in the loins towards the spine, causing anxiety: *Nux vom.;* after drinking, great ill humor, with pressure in epigastrium, liver and spleen: *Natr. carb.*
Weeping and vexation, will not listen to anything: *Arnic.*
Unconquerable drowsiness, with stretching and impatience: *Nitr. ac.*
Shocks of vertigo, as if senses would leave: *Sepia.*
Very irritable humor, disgusted with everything, would like to run away: *Mezer.*

MENTAL STATES AFTER EATING.

b. after breakfast; d. after dinner; s. after supper. If only after one of the three meals, an * is added. In all others the meal has not been specially mentioned.

Acon.
Agar.   d.*
‖ Aloes.
Ambra.
Amm. carb.
Amm. mur.
Anac.
Ant. crud.   d.
Arg. nitr.   b.d.
Arnic.   s.
Arsen.   d.
Asaf.
Bellad.   s.*
Borax.
‖ Bovist.   d.
Bryon.
Calad.   b.*
Calc. ostr.   d.*

Cheerfulness: *Carb. veg.*
Not sleepy, but indifferent and repelling: *Aloes.*
Very cheerful, inclined to singing and dancing, talking and laughing: *Mezer.*
After dinner drowsy, with gaping, which disappears as soon as he begins work: *Natr. carb.*
Trembling of the head and hands; very merry as if drunken: *Tabac.*
Hysterical laughter after meals: *Pulsat.*
After dinner thirsty, chilly; in evening burning face, with cold feet and mental excitement: *Magn. carb.*
Sadness: *Anac., Arsen.,* ‖ *Cinnab., Hyosc., Nux vom.,*

MIND AND DISPOSITION.

Cannab.
Canthar. d.
Capsic.
Carb. an. d.*
Carb. veg. d.
Caustic. s.*
Chamom. d.
Chelid.
Cinch. off.
Cinnab.
Colchic. s.*
Conium. b.
Cyclam. d.*
Digit.
Ferrum. d.*
Graphit.
Gratiol.
Hyosc. d.
Ignat. b. d.
Iodum.
Kali carb.
Kali hydr. d.*
Laches.
Lauroc. b.*
‖ Magn. carb. d.*
‖ Magn. mur. d.
‖ Mar. ver. d.*
Mercur.
Merc. subl.
Mezer. s.
Millef. d.*
‖ Natr. carb. b. d. s.
Natr. mur. d.
Nitr. ac. s.
‖ Nux vom. d. s.
Ol. anim. d.*
Petrol. s.
Phelland. d.*
‖ Phosphor. b. d.
Phosph. ac. d.
‖ Plumbum. d.*
Pulsat.
Ratanh. d.*
‖ Rhus tox. d.
Sepia. s.*
Silic. d.*
Spiggur. b.*
Tabac. d.
Thuya.
Tilia. d.*
Turpethum. d.
Uran. nitr.
Veratr. d.
Ver. vir.
Viol. tric.
‖ Zincum. d.*

Ol. anim., ‖ *Pulsat.*; soon disappearing: *Caustic.*; with headache: *Arsen.*

Melancholic: *Arsen.*, *Pulsat.*; low spirits: *Canthar.*; dispirited: *Nux vom.*, *Ol. anim.*

Hypochondriacal humor: ▮ *Anac.*, ‖ *Canthar.*, ▮ *Cinch. off.*, *Moschus*, ▮ *Natr. carb.*, ▮ *Nux vom.*; three hours after dinner: *Zincum.*

Indifference. Mental relaxation, sits by himself without speaking, no inclination for mental or physical occupation: *Aloes.*

Anxiety. In region of scrobiculum: *Cinch. off.*

After dinner precordial anxiety: *Arg. nitr.*

Anxious sensation in abdomen, with distension: *Rhus tox.*

Anxious pressing in abdomen, with distension: *Phosphor.*

Fulness and anxiety in chest; sour eructations; thin stools: *Capsic.*

Anxiety with constriction in chest after dinner: *Phelland.*, *Phosphor.*

Anxiety in chest: *Carb. an.*; rapid pulse with anxiety and dyspnœa: *Natr. mur.*; anxiety with painless uneasiness in back: *Carb. an.*; after dinner anxiety as if he was threatened by a sad event: *Hyosc.*

Fear and apprehension: *Canthar.*, *Laches.*, *Magn. mur.*

After dinner sudden blindness with anxious sweat and nausea: *Calc. ostr.*; sudden attack of paleness, nausea, anxiety, trembling and weakness: *Nux vom.*

Fulness and discomfort with anxiety: *Phosph. ac.*

Fulness, anxiety, tearing pain in back, going into abdomen: *Chamom.*

After dinner palpitation with anxiety: *Silic.*

Sensation of dysphagia after eating, great fear of suffocating with it: *Merc. subl.*

After dinner increased warmth with anxiousness, as if sweat would break out: *Phosphor.*

After eating, hot face, sadness and despair: *Acon.*

Anxiety: *Ambra*, *Asaf.*, *Carb. veg.*, *Hyosc.*, *Kali carb.*, *Laches.*, *Magn. mur.*, *Natr. carb.*, *Nitr. ac.*, *Nux vom.*, *Phelland.*, *Thuya*, *Veratr.*, *Viol. tric.*

Indifference in the evening: *Aloes.*

Fainthearted, anxious with palpitation: *Thuya.*

After dinner discouraged: *Tabac.*

Dissatisfied with his position, despairs of success; after dinner: *Turpeth.*

Ill humor: *Ambra*, *Bovist.*, *Carb. veg.*, *Chamom.*, *Iodum*, *Kali carb.*, *Natr. carb.*, *Pulsat.*, *Turpeth.*

Very bad humor, and sticky and slimy in the mouth: *Platin.*

MENTAL STATES AFTER EATING.

Burning in stomach with heaviness and ill humor soon after eating: *Graphit.*

After dinner a great feeling of roughness on the chest, with a pressure in pit of stomach which makes him ill humored: *Natr. carb.*

Morose, ill humor: *Carb. veg., Kali carb., Natr. carb., Pulsat., Thuya, Turpeth.*

Distress after eating, with good appetite; dispirited; morose: *Uran. nitr.*

After eating dinner morose: *Chamom.*

After breakfast morose thoughts: *Conium.*

After dinner out of humor: *Carb. veg., Phosphor.*

All the time during digestion out of humor: *Iodum.*

After eating anxiety and apprehension; *Laches.;* irritable: *Mar. ver.*

Hypochondria, the least thing affects him: *Nux vom.*

During and after dinner ill humor; cannot bear to hear others talk: *Mar. ver.*

In the morning fretful: *Conium.*

Ill humored after dinner: *Cyclam.;* and supper: *Natr. carb.;* with good appetite, distension and fulness; better in open air: *Borax.*

Pressing in stomach, as from a stone; ill humor: *Bryon.*

Fulness in head, ill humor after it: *Kali hydr.*

Anything that crosses him after dinner makes him violent and irascible: *Millef.*

Anxious and tearful after dinner: *Magn. mur.*

Lachrymose: *Arnic., Iodum, Magn. mur., Pulsat.*

After dinner whining: *Magn. carb.*

Red-hot spots on cheeks, throat, and front part of neck, with lamentations and despair: *Nux vom.*

After dinner and supper drawing toothache, changing from upper to lower molar, and from there to the front, with lamentations, self-reproach and despair: *Nux vom.*

Violent stitch under left ribs at dinner, screams: *Ratanh.*

Taciturn and indifferent, as if hurt: *Aloes.*

No desire to work, inactivity; after dinner: *Agar.;* drowsiness and inactivity: *Anac.*

Disgust of everything: *Bovist*

Distension, heaviness, no desire to work: *Digit.;* lassitude, goes to sleep over his work: *Ignat.;* drowsy and monosyllabic: *Amm. mur.*

Disinclined to talk, quiet manner: *Plumbum.*

Aversion to move: *Zincum;* sluggishness: *Chelid.;* and inclination to lie down: *Ant. crud.;* drowsiness: *Zincum;* yawning and stretching: *Magn. carb.*

Disagreeable taste and restlessness: *Petrol.;* after dinner and in the evening great anxiety and heat in the face: *Amm. mur.;* and mental inquietude: *Veratr.;* hypochondric depression, weakness: *Anac.*

Repulsive, sluggish humor: *Alum.*

After dinner difficult comprehension: *Phosphor.;* weak and languid, even reading and writing affect him: *Cannab.*

Incapacity for intellectual operation: *Graphit.*

After dinner drowsiness and disinclination to mental work: *Ferrum;* inclination to lie down, unable to think: *Natr. mur.;* languid and drowsy, falls asleep while standing and talking: *Magn. carb.*

After mental work tearing, stinging pain in rectum as of hemorrhoids: *Nux vom.;* mental dullness, absence of thought: *Rhus tox.*

While walking after dinner absent-minded: *Rhus tox.*

After dinner dull and drowsy: *Cannab.*

Vertigo and dullness, better in open air: *Magn. mur.*

Dullness, vertigo, dark before the eyes, better in open air: *Mercur.*

After dinner stupefaction: *Tilia;* congestion in head with stupor: *Acon., Ver. vir.*

Many unpleasent ideas: *Conium;* could not hold fast one idea: *Jalap.*

Stomach puffed up after the meals; mania: *Veratr.*

Moral and more nervous disturbance in attacks, particularly after dinner: *Arg. nitr.;* weak mind: *Tabac.*

During Digestion. Constricting sensation in throat and chest as when about to weep, moody and sensitive: *Iodum.*

Eating particular Food. Ill humor, fulness in head after eating apples with mutton: *Borax.*

After eating salad in the evening she awoke after midnight with nausea, rising up, diarrhœa and soreness in anus: *Phelland.*

Ill humor, disagreeable feeling in abdomen after salt herring: *Fluor. ac.*

After soup heat in abdomen with anxiety and sweat on stomach and chest: *Ol. anim.*

Beer soup caused heat and anxiety: *Ferrum.*

After Drinking. One swallow of cold water lessened spasmodic attack of anxiety with lameness of tongue: *Caustic.*

Believes to be double and that other men were in bed with him; he does not believe that the drink gets into the stomach, that the stomach has gone on a journey, or that some one else was in there who drinks it for him: *Anac.*

Dullness in head after drinking: *Conium;* does not recognize his relations: *Hyosc.*

Violent headache, which almost deprives him of the power of thinking during the chill, worse when he drinks: *Cimex.*

Drink is swallowed hastily; unconsciousness: *Stramon.*

After milk, irritated: *Sulph. ac.*

After Stimulants. Anxiety, from acids: *Sulphur.*

Melancholy from the long use of wine: *Cuscuta Epithymun.*

After wine or coffee very forgetful, confused: *Millef.*

After drinking beer, stupefied: *Coloc.*

After spiritual drinks, loquacious: *Therid.*

Delirium tremens of drunkards: I*Laches.*

From coffee anxiety: *Chamom., Ignat.,* I*Nux vom.;* out of humor: *Calc. phosph.*

Better humor after coffee: *Kreosot.*

After smoking anxiety: *Sepia.*

GASTRIC SYMPTOMS.

Hiccough from anger, if contradicted: *Stramon.;* with dullness and drowsiness: *Graphit.*

When thinking of it: *Ox. ac.;* — before catamenia, mania: *Sepia;* — after catamenia: *Alum.;* — uninterrupted, threatening to suffocate; melancholy, worse in rest: *Stramon.;* desperate, furious grimaces: *Sepia.*

With vomiting of bile, palpitation, anxiety, quick, weak pulse, lassitude and failing of vital powers: *Colub.*

Eructations. Spasmodic, irritable and vexed: *Petrol.*

Relieve confused mind: *Sanguin.*

Relieve anxiousness with violent cramp in stomach, constriction and anxiety caused by lying on the right side: *Kali carb.*

Timorousness ceases after frequent belching: *Veratr.*

After the wind has passed up or down, cheerful disposition: *Carb. sulph.*

After futile attempts empty eructation without relief: *Mangan.*

Would like to belch with anxious pressure on chest, but cannot: *Spigel.*

Empty eructations with apprehension: *Crot. tigl.;* with anxious sweat and burning: *Mezer.;* with distension after mental exertion: *Hepar s. c.*

Eructations with ill humor: *Agn. cast.;* with anxiety: *Acon., Thuya;* and drowsiness: *Bovist.*

— bitter. With anxiety and fear: *Amm. mur.;* and palpitation: *Phosphor.;* with sadness: *Amm. mur., Cuprum;* with fear: *Veratr.*

— sour. With hilarious good humor: *Calc. sulph.;* with nausea and anxiety: *Carb. an.;* gulping up of food, after a great uneasiness in the pit of stomach: *Kali carb.*

Great constriction and anxiety in the chest with warm rising from the epigastrium to the throatpit: *Platin.*

Waterbrash with cough, anxiety and fear of fainting: *Spigel.*

ANXIOUSNESS, ANXIETY, ANGUISH, WITH NAUSEA AND VOMITURITIO.

As if she would faint: *Nitr. ac.;* dark before the eyes: *Carb. veg.*

When straining the eyes: *Sepia.*

With fever and chilliness; hot ear: *Arsen.*

Heat in left cheek and toothache: *Oleand.*

During conversation: *Alum.;* as if water was running together in the mouth; as if she had to belch; alternately ravenous hunger in attacks: *Nitr. ac.*

Loss of appetite, white tongue: *Carb. veg.*

With desire to vomit: *Cyclam., Laches., Veratr.*

Vomituritio: *Bar. mur., Crotal., Pulsat., Tabac.*

Nausea in scrobiculum with anxiety: *Cannab.; Pulsat.;* with fearfulness: *Gratiol.*

Diarrhœa twice after midnight, with pressure and tenesmus in anus, afterwards soreness: *Phelland.*

MIND AND DISPOSITION.

Acon.
Aethus.
| Alum.
Amm. mur.
Arnic.
|| Arsen.
Baryt.
Bar. mur.
|| Bellad.
|| Calc. ostr.
Cannab.
Carb. veg.
Caustic.
| Crotal.
|| Cyclam.
| Digit.
|| Graphit.
Gratiol.
Helleb.
Kali carb.
Laches.
Ledum.
| Mangan.
Mercur.
|| Nitr. ac.
| Nux vom.
| Oleander.
Phelland.
Platin.
Plumbum.
| Pulsat.
| Rhus tox.
Sabad.
| Sepia.
Spongia.
Squilla.
| Tabac.
| Tarax.
Veratr.

With urging to stool: *Mercur.*
Frequent urination and toothache: *Oleand.*
Before menses, thick black blood: *Mangan.*
Takes a deep breath at intervals: *Squilla;* followed by dry cough: *Nux vom.*
Anxiety across the chest: *Arnic.;* on the whole chest: *Laches.;* in the heart: *Plumbum;* with palpitation: *Baryt.*
She cannot sit still, with sweat: *Graphit.*
Better when walking about: *Tarax.*
With darkness before the eyes; has to lie down toward evening: *Carb. veg.*
With great lassitude and trembling feeling in the whole body: *Platin.*
Nausea with anxiety and trembling: *Nitr. ac.*
With yawning, eructation and heat: *Kali carb.;* with drowsiness: *Ledum.*
Attacks coming at night: *Cyclam.;* awaking about midnight with sweat: *Bellad.;* followed by diarrhœa and tenesmus: *Phelland.;* with deep breathing: *Squilla;* vomiting, fainting and diarrhœa: *Nitr. ac.*
In the morning before breakfast: *Calc. ostr.;* with palpitation: *Baryt.;* better in the open air: *Rhus tox.*
In the afternoon with headache: *Calc. ostr., Nitr. ac.*
When coming into the house after a walk; while speaking: *Alum.*

Preceded by heat coming from below and rising up; the nausea goes downward: *Bellad.*

Sweat: *Bellad., Calc. ostr., Graphit.*

In attacks with great depression of mind: *Digit.;* with faintiness, bulimia and waterbrash: *Nitr. ac.*

The anxiety follows the nausea: *Nux vom.*

Nausea and other Mental Symptoms, with uneasiness and sleeplessness: *Secal.*

Squeamishness, with mental excitement: *Ambra;* with uneasiness: *Asar.*

Sad thoughts: *Acon.;* sick feeling with sadness: *Amm. mur., Arsen., Digit., Petrol., Veratr.*

Depression of spirits: *Lil. tigr.;* in attacks with melancholy: *Sepia;* nausea with melancholy: *Veratr.;* disagreeable dejection: *Codein.;* low spirits: *Mephit.*

Apprehension of some impending evil, nausea when thinking of it: *Lil. tigr.;* as if going to die: *Digit., Laches., Oleand.*

Nausea; apprehensiveness: *Tabac.*

Anxiety. See separate margin list above.

Despairing thoughts: *Acon.;* after vexation, with weeping all night: *Natr. mur.;* and lassitude: *Strontian;* with vexation: *Canthar., Phosphor.*

Tired of life: *Pulsat.;* fear of death: *Tabac.;* fearfulness: *Lil. tigr.*
Dullness and ill humor: *Magn. carb.;* and headache: *Stannum.*
Extreme moroseness, with *nausea*, cannot bear to hear a *person walk in the room: Sanguin.;* with irritability: *Kali bichr.;* nausea, with hot face and fretfulness: *Phosphor.*
Depression of spirits and disposition to weep, with *nausea* and pain in the *back*, aversion to *food: Lil. tigr.;* after nausea, weeping: *Tabac.*
With thoughts of suicide: *Clemat.;* nausea in scrobiculum and inclined to self-destruction: *Pulsat.;* — getting awake in the morning; could drive her to suicide: *Lil. tigr.;* afterward: *Sepia.*
With dullness and indifference: *Asar.*
With mental restlessness: *Calc. ostr., Helleb., Mangan.;* sweat, restlessness: *Graphit.*
Aversion to food, with mental and physical depression: *Lepid.*
With a pale face and mental and physical depression: *Amm. carb.*
With derangement: *Arg. nitr., Opium;* incapability after heavy labor: *Coca.*
With delirium: *Stramon.;* vertigo and raving: *Chelid.*
In afternoon with thoughtlessness: *Calc. ostr.*
Stupid and *sleepy* feeling: *Corn. circ.;* loss of senses: *Pœonia;* after nausea loss of consciousness: *Sarsap.*
Vanishing of thoughts, with *paleness* and sickness at the stomach on closing the eyes: *Therid.;* with stupidity: *Thuya, Veratr.*
Nausea in abdomen and using wrong words: *Chamom.*
Nausea with every mental emotion: *Kali carb.*
Brought on by thinking of it: *Droser., Lil. tigr.*
Aggravated when thinking of it: *Laches.*
The mere thought of food causes nausea: *Argent., Arsen., China, Graphit., Magn. sulph., Moschus.*
Loathing or nausea when thinking of the food eaten: *Sarsap.*
Aversion of meat when thinking of it: *Graphit.*
Nausea worse from reading: *Arnic.;* brought on by mental exertion: *Aurum;* and trembling: *Borax.*

MODEL CURE.

Anxiety, burning in stomach and contraction in abdomen; fear drives out of bed; walks about moaning; anxiousness in evening twilight, with palpitation and heat; dullness in head; puffed face, red and flushed; pulse 80 and rather weak; gnawing in the epigastrium, with waterbrash; urging to urinate, scanty urine: *Arsen.*—NEUMANN.

VOMITING AND ANXIETY.

Acon.
|| Ant. crud.
|| Arg. nitr.
Arnica.
Arsen.
Ars. hydr.
Asar. can.
Bar. mur.
Bismuth.
Calc. ostr.
|| Cuprum.
Cupr. sulph.
| Dulcam.
Guar. off.
| Helleb.
Laches.
Lycop.
Nitrac.
Nux vom.
Sanguin.
Secale.
|| Senega.
Silic.
Sulphur.
Tabac.
Turpeth.
Thuya.
Vip. torv.

After vomiting, anxiety worse: *Arnic.*
After anxiety vomiting: *Sanguin., Thuya.*
Fear of death: *Arsen.;* and despair: *Ars. hydr.;* fearfulness: *Cupr. sulph.*
Has to leave the bed: *Silic.;* restlessness: *Calc. ostr., Thuya.*
Delirium: *Secal.;* rage: *Cuprum.*
Forgetfulness during the fever: *Laches.*
Vertigo: *Nux vom.;* with the headache: *Laches.;* heaviness in head: *Sulphur;* screwing the head together: *Arg. nitr.*
Pain in eyes and coated tongue: *Guar. trich.*
Vomiting of food and bile at night: *Lycop.*
Irritation of stomach: *Arg. nitr.;* in scrobiculum: *Digit.*
Lump in pit of stomach: *Arg. nitr.*
Bellyache, cramps in the bowels: *Turpeth.*
Urging to stool: *Sulphur;* diarrhœa: *Ant. crud., Turpeth.*
Oppression of chest: *Guar. trich.*
Has to cough and drink: *Nitr. ac.;* dry cough: *Silic.*
Glassy phlegm, drawing out in threads: *Arg. nitr.*

Chest painful: *Guar. trich.*
Anxiety in the heart: *Lycop.*
Weakness in arms: *Sulphur.*
Trembling: *Sulphur,* and weakness: *Arg. nitr.*
At midnight awaking: *Arg. nitr.,* at night: *Nitr. ac.*
Chill and sweat: *Digit.;* external heat, with crawls of chilliness: *Digit.*
Heat: *Dulcam.;* sweat: *Silic., Sulphur.*
At 5 and 6 P. M. for several days: *Digit.*
In the evening: *Sulphur.*

Vomiting and other Mental Symptoms; after it unable to work: *Zincum;* ill humor and headache: *Cyclam.;* neuralgia, with boring pain, causing him to cry out: *Sepia.*

— day and night with fearful screams: *Arsen.*

— with whining about shooting in ear: *Silic.*

Before — hasty and restless with headache: *Laches.;* derangement of mind and delirium: *Secal.;* want of mind: *Asar.*

With — she chokes herself; in madness: *Bellad.;* delirium: *Vip. red.;* and stupor: *Aethus., Doryph.;* and collapse: *Podoph.;* loss of consciousness: *Laches., Natr. mur.*

After — stupid and dull in occiput: *Cannab.*

Vomiting blood with desire for death: *Phytol.;* depressed and stupid: *Ox. ac.*
From anger vomiting and diarrhœa: *Coloc.*

Inclination to Vomit, Gagging, Retching. Anxiety at three in the morning, heat with nausea: *Arsen.;* retching, nausea and anxiety: *Bar. mur.*

Worse after supper, hypochondria: *Nux vom.*

Inclination to vomit, with melancholy: *Veratr.*

Gagging, ineffectual efforts, delirium, semi-consciousness: *Stramon.*
Inclination to vomit, with stupor: *Stramon.*
Retching aggravates all symptoms except dullness in head, which is relieved: *Asar.*

As soon as he commences to think, nausea follows; he is obliged to give it up, as he finds he is very stupid: *Asar.*
Nausea with vomiting from every mental exertion: *Natr. mur.*
Anxiety and other Mental Symptoms, relieved after Vomiting.
After vomiting of bile mental quietude: *Hyosc.*; hopeful: *Acon.*; less apprehensive and less anxious: *Tabac.*; less anguish: *Helleb.*
Before the vomiting spell less mental strength; after it, better: *Asar.*
Improved after vomiting; rush of ideas; want of mind; loss of senses: *Tabac.*

STOMACH SYMPTOMS WITH ANXIETY.

Ant. crud.
Arg. nitr.
Arsen.
Aurip.
Baryt.
Bar. mur.
Calc. ostr.
I Canthar.
Carb. veg.
Chamom.
Cinch. off.
Ginseng.
Glonoin.
II Graphit.
Guaiac.
Helleb.
Jatroph.
II Kali carb.
Kobalt.
Mercur.
Nux vom.
Opium.
Osmium.
Petrol.
Phytol.
I Phosphor.
Ran. bulb.
Rhodod.
I Sulphur.
Sulph. ac.
Thuya.
Zincum.

Driving to despair, to suicide by drowning: *Ant. crud.*; restlessness with pain: *Kobalt.*; and uneasiness, fidgety: *Osmium*; disagreeable sensation: *Graphit., Helleb.*; anxiousness, as if from the stomach: *Calc. ostr.*; restlessness: *Glonoin.*; as if having committed a murder: II *Canthar.*; around the region of stomach: *Pulsat.*; disagreeable sensation: *Graphit.*; oppression: *Bar. mur.*; pressure: *Phytol., Sulphur*; violent, with retching, has to double up: *Bar. mur.*; dull pressure in morning after an anxious night: *Aurip.*; as if filled up to bursting: *Arg. nitr.*; as if overloaded: *Cinch. off.*; great fulness: *Canthar.*; and heat: *Thuya*; drawing together from both sides with increased warmth: *Zincum*; violent heat, then sweat: *Kali carb.*; cramp at night: *Kali carb.*; with the stool: *Kali carb.*; screwing together, with difficult breathing: *Guaiac.*; with agony of death: *Opium*; grasping, snatching: *Petrol.*

Burning in pylorus and cardiacal anxiety: *Ran. bulb.*; burning in stomach; driving out of bed: *Arsen.*; with coldness of body: *Jatroph.*; hot rising into chest, and sweat on forehead: *Phosphor*; burning, with convulsions, crawls, cold limbs: *Phosphor.*

Pains: *Baryt., Calc. ostr., Carb. veg., Chamom., Graphit., Mercur.*

Stomach and other Mental Symptoms. Stinging and cramps, with mental agitation: *Ananth. mur.*; faint sensation in stomach, with fear of losing her reason: *Kali sulph.*

Distress, wakes up moaning, screaming, crazy, crying: *Arsen.*

Weak digestion, with mania, alternately with melancholy: *Digit.*; affection of stomach, with despair, depression and faintheartedness: *Laches.*; uneasiness, with ill humor: *Mangan.*

Stomachache and ill humor: *Amm. carb.;* after eating a little too much: *Mercur.;* pressure with fretfulness: *Phosphor.;* ill humor: *Bryon., Conium;* gloomy: *Coloc.;* and unconscious: *Calc. ostr.;* pain with crying: *Phytol.;* whining: *Ox. ac.;* gnawing, with frequent sighing: *Eupat. purp.;* burning; sudden frightening: *Sulph. ac.;* with dullness in head: *Sulph. ac.;* with lectrophilie: *Al. p. s.;* stupor: *Stramon.*

Sensitive to touch; delirium: *Stramon.*

Distension; delirium: *Veratr.*

Distension after the least mental emotion: *Nux mosch.;* pains aggravated: *Ananth.;* pressure after mental exertion: *Anac.*

Feels as if the soul was in the stomach; unable to think: *Acon.*

ANXIETY IN SCROBICULUM.

| Acon.
| Argent.
|| Arg. nitr.
| Arsen.
|| Calc. ostr.
|| Calc. phos.
| Cann. sat.
| Carb. an.
| Carb. veg.
| Chamom.
| Chelid.
| Cicut.
| Cinch. off.
| Colchic.
| Conium.
| Crotal.
|| Cuprum.
|| Ferrum.
| Ferr. mur.
| Glonoin.
| Graphit.
| Guaiac.
| Hydr. ac.
| Ignat.
| Lactuc.
| Lycop.
|| Mercur.
| Mezer.
|| Natr. mur.
| Nitrum.
| Nux vom.
| Phosphor.
| Pulsat.
| Rhodod.
| Rhus tox.
| Sepia.
|| Silic.
| Stannum.
| Stramon.
|| Sulphur.
| Sulph. ac.
|| Sambuc.
| Thuya.

Unbearable: *Arsen.;* with children: *Calc. phosph.;* anguish: *Hydr. ac.;* suicidal inclination to drown herself: *Silic.;* anxiety if people come near her: *Lycop.;* apprehensions: *Mezer., Rhus tox.;* when thinking of unpleasant things: *Phosphor.;* from vexation: ||*Lycop.;* unpleasant sensations: *Graphit.;* empty feeling: *Ignat.;* feels very ill: *Arg. nitr.*

Pains: *Calc. ostr., Carb veg., Chamom., Cicut., Crotal., Ferr. mur., Mercur.;* scraping: *Rhus tox.*

Whining and lamenting: *Arsen.;* screaming, with sweat: *Chamom.;* sighing and sadness: *Ignat.*

Pressure: *Argent., Carb. veg., Natr. mur., Sambuc.;* deep in: *Sambuc.;* with palpitation: *Sulphur.*

Jerks: *Calc. ostr.;* throbbing: *Acon.;* palpitation: *Calc. phosph., Ferrum, Thuya;* spasmodic: *Chelid.*

Appearing suddenly: *Mercur.;* rising upwards: *Arsen.;* into the head: *Thuya;* as from swinging: *Lycop.* (*Borax*); sudden drawing together, interfering with breathing: *Sulph. ac.*

Sensation as if too narrow: *Cicut.;* deep in: *Rhodod.;* impeded breathing, with inhalation like asthma: *Ferrum;* stopping breath: *Carb. an.;* difficult breathing: *Guaiac.,* ||*Stramon.;* anxious breathing: *Chelid.;* as if screwed together: *Arsen.;* anxious pressure, wishes he could belch: *Spigel.*

After the meals: *Cinch. off.;* with a drawing pain from kidneys down to the glands in the groin: *Cannab.;* scraping in region of heart: *Rhus tox.*

When lying down, better after pressure: *Stannum.*

With trembling followed by nosebleed: *Sepia.*

Desire to go out doors to cool himself: *Cicut.;* after attack of fever, painful swelling: *Arg. nitr.;* dry heat of body: *Stramon.*

Sweat in scrobiculum: *Nitrum;* hands sweat; face gets hot: *Mercur.;* cold sweat: *Stramon.*

Scrobiculum, with other Mental Symptoms. Beating in scrobiculum, with concern about the future: *Ant. tart.*

Throbbing in pit of stomach, morose: *Acon.;* and stupid in head: *Magn. mur.*

Pressing, with irritability: *Natr. carb.*

Tickling sensation causes him to laugh at serious subjects: *Anac.*

Burning, cramp-like pain, driving to despair; would like to commit suicide by drowning: *Ant. crud.*

Tenderness to touch, with lectrophilie: *Al. p. s.*

Pains excite much: *Millef.;* drive to madness: *Canthar.*

Sweat after waking from a frightful dream: *Bellad.*

Cannot think; seat of mental functions seems to be in the scrobiculum: *Acon.*

After a fright pain with distress: *Acon.*

Vexation is felt in pit of stomach, followed by heaviness in the legs: *Lycop.*

HYPOCHONDRIAC REGIONS.

Region of Liver. Disorder, with hypochondriac mood: *Podoph.*

Pressure under the short ribs on right side and disinclined to work, sad: *Zincum;* from same region proceeds an inclination to laugh: *Conium.*

Stitches from the least motion, has to scream aloud: *Nitr. ac.;* the same with burning or biting: *Zincum;* liver diseases, with mania: *Mercur.*

Region of Spleen. Anxiety, with pressing and drawing: *Rhus tox.;* with accumulation of wind: *Sulphur.* Compare *Lycop.*

A fixed idea of having something alive in her abdomen; she hears a deep voice in the region of the spleen, and a fine one on the right side between the ovary and the liver; feels a creeping sensation as of something moving: *Thuya.*

MODEL CURES.

Moaning, groaning and restlessness during the fever; ravenous hunger with thirst during the fever, white tongue, heat in the abdomen, especially in the region of the liver, liver indurated; asthmatic cough: *Podoph.*—W. WILLIAMSON.

Great depression of spirits; unhappy state of mind, always associated with "pain about and under (not below) the short ribs in the back, on the left side, and extending outward nearly to the left side; this embraces the posterior aspect of region of spleen:" *Lob. coerul.*—J. JEANES.

PRÆCORDIAL ANXIETY.

Acon.
Arg. nitr.
! Arsen.
Bellad.
Canthar.
Cina.
Cinch. off.
Coccul.
Coffea.
Conium.
Cuprum.
Digit.
Droser.
Kali carb.
Laches.
Lauroc.
Lycop.
Naja trip.
Nitr. ac.
Opium.
Phosphor.
Phosph. ac.
Platin.
Pulsat.
Rhus tox.
Staphis.
Stramon.
Sulphur.
! Thuya.
Zincum.

As if death were near: *Rhus tox.;* as if he ought not to live: *Phosph. ac.;* dragging, with great grief: *Naja trip.;* after dinner: *Arg. nitr.;* with nausea: *Nitr. ac.;* collection of wind: *Coffea, Cinch. off.;* rising upwards: *Droser., Rhus tox.;* tension and drawing together: *Digit.;* tension across, oppression: *Staphis.;* tension, like colic: *Arsen.;* and beating: *Conium;* around the heart: *Acon.;* alternately with a throbbing pain: *Hydr. ac.;* pressure while standing: *Phosph. ac.;* several attacks during the day: *Nitr. ac.;* painful: *Kali carb.;* sleeplessness after midnight (from 2 to 7 A. M.), with colicky distension under the ribs, causing anxiety and sensation of heat over the whole body without sweat, except above the nose; no thirst; desire to uncover: *Coffea;* with heat and headache with heat: *Aurip.;* if people come too near her she feels an anxiety in the præcordia: *Lycop.*

Constriction in the hypochondriac regions, very much excited, as if an accident would happen: *Hura.*

Spasm of the diaphragm after vexation: *Staphis.*

Anxiety and pains, with feeling as if the diaphragm cut off the chest from the abdomen: *Arsen.;* diaphragmitis, with nymphomania: *Stramon.*

ABDOMINAL COMPLAINTS WITH ANXIETY AND OTHER CONCOMITANTS.

Head. Headache: *Arnic.;* following: *Aeth. cyn.;* in head and in hands: *Nitr. ac.,* worse in head: *Magn. carb.*

Earache: *Aloes, Glonoin.*

Nose. Stopped up: *Bellad.*

Face. Hot: *Bellad.;* when eating warm dishes: *Magn. carb.*

Abdomen. Hollow: *Chamom.;* heat: *Bellad.;* unpleasant warmth: *Bovist.;* here and there pressing wind: *Nux vom.;* accumulation of wind: *Cicut.;* dull pressure deep in, with fever: *Caustic.;* painful pressure waking at night: *Mezer.;* does not know what to do with himself: *Mezer.;* a heavy load in region of navel: *Opium;* on going out of doors after eating, agony, better after belching: *Mezer.;* tension and pressure, several hours after dinner: *Sulphur;* violent tearing: **!** *Arsen.;* as if the chest was cut off from the abdomen: *Arsen.;* as if contracted, cannot work, stay anywhere, has to run about: *Moschus;* cramp-like contraction in abdomen and great anxiety, thoughts of self-destruction: *Aurum;* gurgling with anxiety: *Nux vom.;* pulsation in different places of abdomen with anxiety: *Alum.;* pulsation with anxiety, feeling as of cramp: *Lycop.;* soreness with anxiety: *Euphorb.;* painful to the touch: *Caustic., Plumbum;* anxious feeling, causing him to bend double and change his position: **!** *Arsen.;*

ABDOMINAL COMPLAINTS WITH ANXIETY AND CONCOMITANTS. 161

|| Aloes.
|| Alumin.
|| Amm. mur.
| Agn. cast.
| Apis.
| Arsen.
| Asaf.
|| Aurum.
| Bellad.
| Borax.
| Bovist.
| Bryon.
|| Calend.
  Calc. ostr.
|| Carb. veg.
| Caustic.
|| Chamom.
| Cicut.
  Colchic.
  Coloc.
| Crocus.
|| Cuprum.
| Digit.
| Euphorb.
| Glonoin.
| Gran. cort.
| Ignat.
|| Lycop.
| Mezer.
| Moschus.
|| Mur. ac.
| Natr. mur.
| Nitr. ac.
| Nux vom.
| Opium.
|| Platin.
| Plumbum.
| Rhus tox.
|| Squilla.
|| Sulphur.
| Sulph. ac.
  Terebinth.

disagreable warmth and weight in abdomen with anxiety: *Bovist.;* sensation of flying inner heat: *Opium;* hot burning in abdomen: *Calc. ostr.*

Belly. Colic, see separate margin list.

Heaviness with anxiety: *Mezer.*

Constant moving in the bowels: *Chamom.;* with restlessness, disagreeable warmth and heaviness alternating with cold feeling: *Bovist.;* with heaviness, as if the abdomen would burst, better from sleep: *Amm. mur.;* with pain in whole abdomen to os pubis, and tension: *Carb. veg.;* painful pressure and tension, wakes from sleep, borborygmus: *Mezer.*

Stool. With pains after a fright, urging to stool: *Platin.* Better after wind and stool passes: *Mur. ac.*

Urine. From continual ineffective urging to urinate: *Natr. mur.*

Breathing. With short breathing: *Bryon.;* bellyache with dyspnœa, better from walking: *Bryon.;* takes his breath and drives him from place to place: *Arsen.;* difficult breathing and moaning: *Arsen.;* or pain in abdomen with it: *Arsen.*

Chest. Rumbling from chest down, when expiring, followed by palpitation: *Aurum;* spasmodic constriction: *Nitrum;* pain in chest and ear with deafness: *Aloes.*

Heat. Heat in hands and head: *Nitr. ac.*

Limbs. Weakness in feet: *Sulphur;* cutting pain, has to walk bent: *Coloc.;* violent pain, restlessness and despair of recovery: *Arsen.*

Motion. Trembling with tearing in abdomen: *Arsen.* Inward trembling with weak feeling in feet: *Sulphur.*

Time. In the morning in bed: *Sulph. ac.;* sensation of hollowness in evening, attacks with anxiousness: *Chamom.*

Fever. With fever and thirst: *Arsen.;* stupefaction with inner heat: *Opium.*

Directions. Pressing from in out: *Angust.;* wind in stomach, seems to urge upwards, causing anxiety: *Nux vom.;* anxiety rising upward: *Ignat., Stramon.;* falling sensation from the heart to the feet: *Crocus;* tearing sensation rising from right of umbilicus upward: *Calc. phosph.*

MODEL CURE.

During the latter portion of pregnancy: face pale, earthy, distorted, anxious; voice weak; burning, pinching, contracting pain in stomach and both sides of abdomen, with dyspnœa; drawing under the umbilicus; in attacks every half hour. Vomiting of mucus and bile with violent retching, burning in throat and œsophagus like fire, thirst without desire to drink. After the attack empty eructation, retching, dyspnœa, great restlessness and sensitiveness of the abdomen, lively motion of the child: *Arsen.*—SCHELLING.

COLIC WITH ANXIETY.

Aethusa.
Al. p. s.
Amm. carb.
Ant. crud.
Ant. tart.
|| Arnica.
|| Arsen.
|| Aurum.
| Bellad.
| Borax.
| Bovist.
Bryon.
|| Calc. phosph.
Capsic.
| Carb. veg.
Caustic.
| Cepa.
|| Chamom.
Chin. sulph.
Cinch. off.
Coccul.
| Colchic.
|| Coloc.
Cuprum.
Hepar s. c.
Kali bichr.
Kali chlor.
Lycop.
Mezer.
Morphine.
Moschus.
| Natr. mur.
| Natr. sulph.
Nux vom.
|| Opium.
Pæonia.
Phosph. ac.
Plumbum.
Rhus tox.
Sepia.
|| Spigel.
|| Sulphur.
Terebinth.
|| Veratr.

Anguish: *Arsen.;* moaning: *Sepia;* despair: *Arsen., Carb. veg., Cepa, Cuprum, Phosphor.;* as if he had to die: *Arsen., Rhus tox.;* agonizing tossing about: *Chamom.;* rolling on the ground in despair: *Arsen., Cepa.*

Unbearable, tormenting anxiety and restlessness, compelling him constantly to seek another position: *Morph. ac.*

Loud cries that some one should kill her, the pain is so intense: *Arsen.;* oversensitiveness: *Coccul.*

Body. Dullness: *Sulphur;* afterwards stupid: *Chamom.;* gagging: *Sulphur.*

Intolerable headache, following the anxiety: *Chamon.;* and bellyache: *Aethus.*

Pain causes intense anxiety, the face is distorted, the eyes sunken, and he screams out loud: *Platin.*

Tensive feeling under the short ribs, worse at night: *Cinch. off.*

Distension, causing anxiety: *Lycop.*

Does not know what to do on account of pain and anxiety, squirms like a worm, presses the abdomen furiously against a bed post: *Coloc.*

Cutting: *Natr. mur., Sepia;* as if screwed together: *Spigel.*

Contracting sensation in stomach: *Natr. mur.*

Tearing in abdomen: *Chamom.*

As if intestines were held by strings which might tear: *Coloc.*

Sensitiveness of abdomen with terrible anxiety mostly in the evening: *Sepia.*

Pain commences in right groin, with great tenderness of abdomen, restlessness and misery: *Natr. sulph.*

As the pains increase the abdomen becomes more distended and painfully sensitive to pressure: *Veratr.*

Cold skin; burning in abdomen, especially during stool: *Carb. veg.;* fear that fæces will pass off involuntarily: *Sepia;* no stool: *Coccul.*

A small spot over the right ovary is very sensitive: *Arsen.*

Very lively motion of the child in the womb: *Arsen.*

Breathing difficult: *Al. p. s., Plumbum, Spigel.;* takes breath away: *Arsen.*

Slow, small, intermitting pulse: *Carb. veg.*

Extreme weakness: *Arsen.;* great lassitude: *Carb. veg.*

Sleeplessness: *Arsen., Carb. veg.;* starting in sleep, lies with one arm under the head: *Coccul.;* before midnight: *Natr. mur.;* at night: *Sulphur.*

In attacks: *Bellad., Coccul., Coloc.;* icy coldness of the whole body, with indescribable anxiety, in half an hour followed by heat: *Arsen.*

With children: *Aurum, Calc. phosph., Chamom.*

COLIC WITH OTHER MENTAL CONCOMITANTS.

Uneasiness, pain also in head and knees: *Arsen.*
Homesickness: *Bellad.;* low spirits: *Kreosot., Magn. mur., Sulphur;* hypochondric mood: *Millef., Rhus tox.;* tension and pressure: *Sulphur;* desponding mood: *Rhus tox.;* tired of life: *Aurum.;* weary of life, during catamenia: *Berber.;* melancholy and tired of life: *Nux vom.*

Dry humor: *Ant. crud.*

Apprehensive feelings rise from the abdomen to the heart, with restlessness, inward trembling and confusion: *Thuya;* and faint-heartedness: *Chamom.*

Discontent and tearfulness about inanimate things, with cutting in umbilical region: *Capsic.*

Disagreeable sensation, with discontented humor: *Fluor. ac.*

Ill humor: *Aloes, Capsic., Ferrum, Magn. mur., Tarax., Thuya.*

Obstinacy, with red, flushed cheeks; burning in umbilical region and pressing headache: *Acon.;* sudden anger: *Seneg.;* irritability: *Sulphur.*

Irritable and vexed, with cutting pain: *Aloes, Petrol.*

Distressing sensation causing dyspnœa; complaining: *Arsen.*

Restlessness, weeping and despair, with tension and pressing pain in abdomen: *Carb veg.*

Anguish and lamentation: *Arsen., Plumbum, Sepia.*

As if she had to weep: *Sulphur.*

Screaming, with violent, cutting bellyache and boring pain in knees: *Canthar.*

Loud screams about dull, shooting shocks: *Clemat.*

Piercing screams, with pain in limbs: *Cuprum.*

At night cramps in the abdominal muscles, which get very hard; pain causes to scream out aloud: *Lycop.*

Loud screams, with bellyache: *Ox. ac.;* and weeping: *Pedic.*

Screaming about bellyache, before the cough: *Phosph. ac.*

Pain in stomach, crying out: *Phytol.*

Cramp-like contraction, with longing for death: *Aurum;* violent pain, weary of life: *Berber.;* prepares for suicide: *Plumbum.*

Cutting all day; indisposed: *Ant. crud.;* indisposed to walk in the open air, but it improves the cutting in belly: *Aloes.*

Ill humor, vexation and shunning people, with bellyache: *Aloes.*

Agitation: *Veratr.;* restlessness: *Ant. tart., Bovist., Chamom., Kobalt., Sarsap.;* with pain in the knees: *Arsen.*

In umbilical region, with restlessness: *Morph. ac.;* — feeling of surprise: *Alum.;* — and as after a fright: *Pæonia.*

In the morning, after coming into the cold, cramp in left side, with inconsolable mind: *Rhus tox.*

Obtuseness of head: *Calc. ostr.;* dullness and vertigo in the beginning: *Coloc.;* confusion: *Kali bichr.;* pain in belly, cutting and stupefaction: *Vip. torv.*

Unbearable pain, restlessness, mental confusion and fainting; swelling of abdomen, painful to touch, with delirium: *Plumbum.*

Lead-colic combined with delirium tremens: *Sulphur.*

With madness: *Mercur.;* pressure on abdomen in mania: *Canthar.;* bellyache in mania: *Cuprum.*

Intellect and memory weakened: *Plumbum;* memory lost: *Bellad.;* incoherent answers: *Plumbum.*

Vexation, mental activity not diminished: *Asaf.*

After a fright stitches from abdomen into chest: *Chamom.*

After vexation violent colic: **ǁ** *Coloc.*

Colic and dysentery after vexation: *Sulphur.*

Throbbing and buzzing in the abdominal tumor worse after mental excitement: *Laches.;* abdominal pains made worse by reading: *Carb. an., Sulphur;* when thinking of it: *Ox. ac.*

Bodily Symptoms. Dullness: *Sulphur;* headache following the anxiety: *Stramon.;* contraction in stomach: *Natr. mur.;* tenesmus in rectum: *Magn. mur.;* fearing involuntary stool: *Sepia;* diarrhœa, with insanity: *Hyosc.;* costive: *Vip. red.;* diuresis: *Vip. red.;* bearing down of sexual parts: *Magn. mur.;* breathing difficult: *Spigel.;* heat in chest: *Bellad.;* can hardly walk: *Sulphur;* trembling: *Arsen.*

Morning early in bed: *Acon.;* after coming in the room colic: *Sulphur;* after taking cold, spasmodic pain in abdomen: *Rhus tox.;* anxiety and warmth particularly in head, while eating warm food: *Magn. carb.;* pressing bellyache, with anxiety after eating and walking in open air: *Mezer.;* in the right side of abdomen spasms: *Rhus tox.;* neither touch nor pressure painful to abdomen; senseless: *Stramon.;* children, with fearfulness: *Aurum.*

Dropsy, with fulness: *Apis.*

Extract of a case published by S. HAHNEMANN, 1797. *See Lesser Writings, translated by* R. E. DUDGEON.

A compositor, æt. 24, lean, of pale, earthy complexion, suffered for years after eating carrots, all sorts of cabbage, especially the white and sourcrout, every species of fruit, pears in particular: violent attacks of neuralgia; a certain movement was felt about the navel, then suddenly, always at the same place a pinching as if by pincers followed, with the most intolerable pain lasting half or a whole minute; each time it went away with borborygmus, extending to the coecal region. There occurred also a sensation of constriction above and below, preventing flatus from passing. Attacks of anxiety and pain increase from half to a whole hour, abdomen swelled and became painful to the touch. Along with all this: inclination to vomit, chest constricted, breathing shorter, more and more difficult, cold sweat, stupefaction and total exhaustion. Could not swallow a drop of liquid, much less any solid food. He lay many hours stupified, unconscious, with a swollen face and protruded eyes, without sleep. After wind passed up or down it went off. *Ver. alb.*, four powders, each containing four grains of the powdered root, caused a dreadful aggravation, followed by a perfect cure.

OTHER ABDOMINAL SENSATIONS, WITH MENTAL CONCOMITANTS.

Startling stitch in left side of abdomen: *Millef.*
Painful and penetrating stitch in right side of abdomen, darting like lightning towards the right side and startling her: *Ol. an.*
Abdomen tense; senseless: *Stramon.*
Chest and right side of abdomen yellow; nervousness, twitches when approached by strangers: *Thuya.*
In abdomen living animal, fixed idea: *Thuya.*
Discontented, with unpleasant feeling in abdomen: *Fluor. ac.*
Restlessness, with shuddering and heaviness in abdomen: *Turpeth.*
Disagreeable warmth in abdomen alternately with coldness in whole body: restless mind: *Bovist.*

FLATULENCY.

Noises and Motions. Rumbling with uneasiness: *Crocus;* with anxious restlessness: *Alum.;* rumbling and anxiety: *Borax.;* and weeping, with lachrymose mood: *Rhodod., Rhus tox.*
Stupor with muttering and *loud rumbling* in the *bowels*: *Doryph.*
Anxiety with rumbling: *Borax.;* lachrymose humor and weeping: *Rhus tox.*
As if something alive moved in abdomen, startled: *Kali hydr.*
Rumbling in bowels with stupefaction: *Morph. ac.*
Wind colic about midnight, with anxiety: *Aurum;* intestines feel as if tied in a knot, pressing pain: *Cinch. off.*
With anxiety and vexation: *Cicut.;* with bodily heat and anxiety in pit of stomach: *Stramon.*
Flatulent distension with despondency: *Aloes.*
Uneasiness: *Calad.;* with pressing pain and aversion to mental labor: *Kali carb.;* with dullness and heaviness in head: *Graphit.;* in delirium: *Stramon.;* with burning and stupor: *Stramon.;* with raving: *Bellad.*
Flatulency with hypochondria: *Nux mosch.*
Flatulent complaints with hypochondria, hysteria: *Staphis.*
Restless, anxious, despondent: *Mephit.*
With mental symptoms: *Bellad., Carb. veg., Cinch. off., Coccul., Graphit., Lycop., Natr. carb.,* ǀǀ*Nux vom., Phosphor.,* ǀǀ*Pulsat.,* ǀǀ*Sulphur, Veratr.*

ABDOMINAL DISEASED STATES.

Abdominal complaints with maniacs: ǀ*Arsen.,* ǀǀ*Bellad., Calc. ostr., Canthar.,* ǀ*Caustic.,* ǀ*Cinch. off.,* ǀ*Coccul.,* ǀ*Coloc., Cuprum,* ǀ*Hyosc.,* ǀ*Ignat., Laches.,* ǀ*Lycop.,* ǀ*Mercur.,* ǀǀ*Nux vom.,* ǀ*Phosphor.,* ǀǀ*Pulsat.,* ǀ*Stramon.,* ǀ*Sulphur.*
Abdominal complaints; shunning labor: *Ant. crud., Laches.*

Chronic gastric illness with ill humor: *Psorin.*
Ill humor from relaxed intestines: *Ferrum.*
Melancholia abdominalis: *Bellad., Nux vom.*
Plethora abdominalis: *Stramon.*
Abdominal sufferings with hypochondriacs: *Nux vom.*
Gastric complaints after overtaxing the mind: *Nux mosch.*
Irritable, vexatious humor with lassitude and abdominal complaints: *Terebinth.*
Asthenia of abdominal functions with insanity: *Aloes.*
Dropsy, with fulness and anxiety: *Apis;* — stupor and dullness of mind; *Eup. purp.*
Emaciation and dropsy with abdominal complaints: *Chin. sulph.*
Inflammation of bowels shortly before death, anxiety and twitching: *Plumbum.*
Chronic abdominal diseases with ill humor in high degree, during climacteric years: *Psorin.*

LOINS.

Pressing pain worse in rest and from cough; has to scream: *Nitrum.*
Digging, pressing, shooting pain in left loin, from in out, towards the ribs, with anxiety: *Asaf.*
Pinching in hypogastrium towards the loins, causing anxious sweat: *Sulph. ac.*
Burning pain in right loin (region of liver?) on a place as large as a hand, which makes him very ill humored, sad and unable to think and to work: *Nitr. ac.*
With pain in loins; uneasy, to despair: *Vip. red.*
Swelling with delirium: *Plumbum;* uneasiness, like urging to stool: *Baryt.*

EMISSION OF WIND.

Anxiety as a concomitant to flatus: *Crot. tigl.,* according to the Cypher Repertory.
Fear that the stool might pass with the wind: *Aloes.*
Difficult emission of loud flatus with short anxious breathing: *Mezer.*
Anxious pressure in the chest relieved by passage of wind: *Spigel.*

LOOSENESS FOLLOWING EMOTION AND EXERTION.

After sudden joy: ❙*Coffea,* ❘*Opium;* exalted imagination: *Arg. nitr.;* after fright: *Gelsem.;* with internal heat and external coldness: *Pulsat.;* particularly if better in the open air and throbbing of heart in connection with it: *Pulsat.*
After suddenly hearing bad news, or from fear even in a dream: ❙*Gelsem.*
Slight vexation proves very hurtful; bitter taste, loss of appetite, lassitude,

eructations, restless sleep, trembling in the morning, diarrhœa, sadness, eyes fill with tears: *Petrol.*

After being much vexed, with indignation: ❚ *Coloc.;* with grief: *Calc. phosph.;* after chagrin: *Aloes, Chamom.;* getting angry: *Acon., Chamom., Sacch. off.;* worse when alone: *Stramon.*

After depressing emotions: *Coloc., Gelsem., Phosph. ac.;* mental or moral excitement of soldiers: ❚ *Gelsem.*

After all mental emotions: *Thuya;* mental exertions: *Nux vom.;* thinking of it: *Ox. ac.*

MODEL CURE.

Miss ———, æt. 48, nervous temperament. Troubled for six years with diarrhœa, which occurred only in the morning and *hurried her out of bed.* She had a severe attack when I saw her, aggravated by a *suppressed perspiration.* Gave *Sulphur*^{9c}. No apparent relief in several weeks. From the fact that, if she composed *three lines even, in the afternoon, she would wake up the next morning with diarrhœa,* showing the preponderating influence of *mental labor,* I gave *Nux vom.*^{1m}. The diarrhœa disappeared and *congestive headaches, to which she was formerly subject,* reappeared. They in their turn went away without any other medicine. The patient remained unusually well for three months, when an undue amount of mental work brought it on again, but it as readily yielded to the remedy.—E. A. FARRINGTON.

LOOSENESS OF BOWELS, WITH MENTAL CONCOMITANTS.

Pleasurable Feelings. After loose stools cheerful and happy: *Natr. sulph.;* exhilaration: *Ox. ac.;* tendency to laugh: *Nux. mosch.;* diarrhœa and cholera, with ecstacy: ❚ *Jatroph.;* looseness with sentimental mood: *Ant. crud.*

Painful Feelings. Looseness, with homesickness: *Capsic.;* with over-sensitiveness: ❚❚ *Coffea, Colchic.,* ❚ *Nux vom., Phosphor.;* with sadness: *Crotal.;* despondency, melancholy: *Chelid., Gamboy., Hepar s. c., Kali bichr., Natr. carb., Nitr. ac., Pulsat., Sulphur, Veratr.;* with diarrhœa, much depressed: *Apis;* indifferent, melancholy, avoids society: *Crotal.;* with a thin, slimy stool, cutting pain, irritable and vexed: *Petrol.*

Unpleasant Feelings. Diarrhœa in the morning after rising and after breakfast some bellyache; the greatest care and apprehension about his business: ❚ *Ambra;* bloody stools, followed by anxiety and dyspnœa: *Kali carb.;* with anxiety in the pit of stomach: *Mezer.;* with anxiety: *Acon., Canthar., Carb. veg., Magn. carb., Secal., Thuya,* concerning the illness: *Nitr. ac.;* fear of death: *Acon., Arsen., Raphan., Secal.;* in cholera: *Cuprum;* with nausea and thirst: *Crotal.;* cold, anxious sweat in the face: *Mercur.;* feeling like diarrhœa with anguish: *Agn. cast.;* anguish: *Arsen., Camphor., Raphan., Veratr.*

Neutral Feelings. Looseness, with seriousness: *Alum.;* apathy: *Opium, Phosph. ac.;* indifference: *Phosph. ac., Rhodod.;* in cholera: *Cuprum;* fretfulness with debility: *Kali phosph.;* changeable mood: *Alum.*

MIND AND DISPOSITION.

ı Aethus.
Aloes.
Amm. mur.
ıı Ant. crud.
ı Bellad.
ı Bryon.
ıı Calc. ostr.
Canthar.
ı Chamom.
Cina.
ıı Colchic.
Coloc.
Dulcam.
Hepar.
Hydroph.
Ipec.
Kali bichr.
Kali carb.
Mur. ac.
Natr. carb.
Nitr. ac.
ıı Nux mosch.
Nux vom.
Petrol.
Phosphor.
Pulsat.
Rheum.
ıı Silic.
ıı Staphis.
Sulphur.
ı Sulph. ac.

Irritability, ill humor, with white bloodstreaked stool: *Calc. ostr.;* screams, will be carried: *Carb. veg.*
— fitful mood: *Nux vom.;* nothing pleases her: *Coccul.*
— obstinacy: *Silic.;* — willfulness: *Calc. ostr.;* with a child: *Pulsat.*
Rejects things when offered: *Chamom., Cina;* with anger: *Aloes.*
Indignation: *Coloc.,* ı*Staphis.*
Distrustful mood: *Ant. crud.*
After excitement and over-work: *Coffea.*

MODEL CURE.

A little girl, æt. 4, had diarrhœa for a week. Stools greenish-yellow, thin, with mucus, tenesmus after stool; passages more in the morning and forenoon.

Continual thirst, but no appetite. Very fretful, calling for things and refusing them when offered. Fever at night. Had taken *Acon., Bellad., Chamom.* and *Pulsat.* with no benefit. *Aethus.*^{10m}, (F.), two doses, twenty-four hours apart, cured in two days.—C. R. NORTON.

Conations. Loquacity: *Laches., Stramon.;* cholera with groans and moans: *Cuprum.*

Crying: *Bellad., Borax, Chamom., Cina, Gambog., Jalap., Ipec., Rheum, Valer.;* sudden cries in cholera: *Cuprum.*

Easily startled: *Bellad., Borax, Kali carb.;* desire to be quiet: *Gelsem.;* desire to be carried: *Chamom.;* desire to be naked: *Hyosc.*

Aversions. To being alone: *Arsen.;* to being looked at: *Ant. crud.;* to being disturbed: *Gelsem.;* to mental and bodily exertion: *Corn. circ., Hepar, Rhodod.;* to light: *Camphor.;* to sound of scratching on cloth: *Asar.;* to noise: *Kali carb., Nitr. ac., Nux vom.;* to downward motion: *Borax;* to open air: *Nux vom.;* to washing: *Sulphur;* to being in bed after cholera: *Cuprum.*

Exaltations. Excitability: *Agar., Coffea, Phosphor.;* things seem too large: *Hyosc.;* drunkenness: *Gelsem.*

With cholera and after it restlessness: *Cuprum.*

Diarrhœa; sluggish flow of ideas: *Nux mosch.;* derangement: *Hyosc.*

Productions. Takes a long time to answer: *Nux mosch.;* imagines that another person is sick: *Petrol.;* carphologia: *Hyosc., Opium;* wandering of thought: *Apis;* delirium: *Bellad., Bryon., Hyosc., Mur. ac., Opium, Phosph. ac., Stramon.;* delirium in *typhoid fever*, with black *diarrhœa: Ver. vir.;* mental derangement with looseness: *Hyosc.;* vanishing of thought: *Nitr. ac.;* purging, vomiting and unconsciousness: *Laches.*

COSTIVENESS AND CONSTIPATION, WITH MENTAL SYMPTOMS.

!! Aloes.
! Ambra.
! Apis.
! Bellad.
!! Borax.
!! Bryon.
Calc. phosph.
Chamom.
!! Chin. sulph.
!! Clemat.
Cuprum.
Gnaphal.
! Hyosc.
Laches.
Lil. tigr.
!! Lycop.
!! Mercur.
! Nux vom.
! Oleander.
! Opium.
!! Platin.
!! Psorin.
Rhus. rad.
! Spigel.
!! Stramon.
!! Sulphur.
Vip. red.
Zinc. ox.

Sadness: *Cuprum, Platin.;* cardial anxiety: *Opium.*
Depression of spirits: *Rhus rad.;* after: *Calc. phosph.;* with copious, clear urine: *Vip. red.;* with chill and headache: *Chin. sulph.;* eats nothing: *Lycop.*
Melancholy: **!** *Oleand.;* frequent weeping, backache; after *Pulsat.:* **!!** *Ambra;* with dislike to talk, shunning light, thirst and intercurrent states of exaltation: *Hyosc.*
Hypochondria: *Chamom., Mercur.,* **!** *Nux vom., Zinc. ox.*
Hysteria; mind symptoms improve as soon as she gets costive: *Psorin.*
Fear: *Laches.;* anxious and ill humored: *Sulphur.*
Anxiety, thinks she will not get well, afternoon: *Nux vom.*
Mental uneasiness to despair: *Aloes, Vip. red.*
Ill humor: *Clemat.;* about trifles: *Chamom.*
Irritable temper: *Gnaphal.;* and nervousness: *Apis, Opium;* nervous and irritable: *Sulphur;* angry about himself: *Aloes;* lies in bed, indifferent to everything: *Bryon.*
Intolerable condition of mind: *Aloes.*

Difficult comprehension: *Chin. sulph.;* inactive: *Rhus rad.;* absorbed in himself: *Platin.;* weakness of imaginative faculty: *Chin. sulph.*

Dreads insanity, fears an internal disease from which she will not recover: *Lil. tigr.;* congestion to the head, red face, maniacal state: *Bellad.;* the same, with meteoristic abdomen: *Opium;* with dilated pupils, hallucinations and convulsions: *Hyosc.;* obstinate constipation in mania: *Stramon.*

Forgetfulness: *Platin.;* slow recollection: *Chin. sulph.*

Absent-minded, distracted: *Platin.;* stupor: *Stramon.*

MODEL CURES.

She has a fixed idea that there is a strange odor in the room, and asks to have it removed. Feels very unhappy, fearful and anxious; despairs of her salvation. Easily frightened, hides when persons come into the room. Does not recognize her son or her physician. Constipation, with congestion to the head and flushed face: *Bellad.*—ENGELHARDT.

Griping in the umbilical region towards evening. Pressing and urging in the rectum, hard stool coming out in pieces; forgetful, absent-minded, sad and melancholy; fear of death; thinks he is better than his wife: *Platin.*

He thinks he lives away from home, and invites people into his house. Will not brook opposition. Face flushed and hot, stupor which makes him forgetful, does not recognize his friends; anxiety; wildness, sleepy but cannot sleep. Constipation, with tympanitis; retention of urine, as if caused by the abdominal distension. When smoking forgets to draw. Very cheerful manner in spite of his drowsiness: *Opium.*—SCHUELER.

MENTAL COMPLAINTS BEFORE, DURING AND AFTER STOOL.

bef. before; dur. during; aft. after.

Agar.
I Aloes.
II Alum.
II Ant. crud.
Apis.
I Arsen.
Bellad.
I Borax.
I Calc. ostr.
I Camphor.
Canthar.
I Capsic.
II Carb. veg.
I Caustic.
I Chamom.
Chelid.
Chin. sulph
Cinch. off.
I Coffea.
Colchic.
II Coloc.
Conium.
Corn. circ.
II Crot. tigl.
Cuprum.
I Ferr. magn.
Gambog.
Guaiac.
II Gelsem.
Hæmat.
Hepar s. c.
I Hyosc.
Jatroph.
Kali bichr.
II Kali carb.
Laches.
Magn. carb.
Magn. mur.
I Mercur.
Natr. carb.
I Natr. sulph.
I Nitr. ac.
Nux mosch.
Nux vom.
Ox. ac.
Petrol.
Phosphor.
Phosph. ac.
II Platin.
I Pulsat.
I Raphan.
Rhodod.
I Rhus tox.
Sabin.
Sanguin.
II Secale.
Sepia.
Silic.
I Stramon.
II Sulphur.
I Tabac.
I Veratr.

Contented with himself and the world, serene and happy contemplation of the future, aft.: *Borax;* cheerful, aft.: *Natr. sulph.;* better humor, aft.: *Aloes.*

Looseness relieves: *Sanguin.;* exhilaration: *Ox. ac.*

Sentimental mood: *Ant. crud.;* gloomy: *Coloc.;* homesick: *Capsic.*

Depression, sadness, despondency, melancholy: *Chelid., Chin. sulph., Gambog., Hepar s. c., Kali bichr., Natr. carb., Nitr. ac.,* I*Pulsat., Sulphur, Veratr.*

Anxiety, bef.: *Ant. crud., Magn. mur., Sabin.;* with heat: *Kali carb.;* bef. and dur.: *Arsen., Chamom.,* II*Mercur.;* bef., with trembling of whole body: *Mercur.;* dur.: *Acon., Camphor., Canthar., Magn. carb., Platin., Raphan., Secal., Sepia, Stramon., Sulphur, Tabac., Veratr.,* etc.; bef. and aft.: *Borax, Calc. ostr., Ferr. magn., Hæmat., Jatroph., Kali carb., Rhus tox.;* dur. and aft.: *Carb. veg., Nitr. ac.;* bef., dur. and aft.: *Crot. tigl., Mercur.;* aft.: II*Caustic., Coloc., Nux vom.;* with irritability: *Nitr. ac.*

Anguish: *Arsen., Camphor., Raphan., Veratr.;* bef., dur. and aft.: *Mercur.;* with oppression: *Crot. tigl.;* fear of death: *Acon., Arsen., Raphan., Secal.*

With apprehension of apoplexy: *Veratr.*

Anxiousness and general uneasiness: *Nitr. ac.;* about his health: *Nitr. ac.*

— aft., with heat in face: *Caustic.;* as if diarrhœa would follow: *Platin., Sabin., Sepia;* aft., with puffed up abdomen: *Caustic.;* aft., with trembling sensation and involuntary motion: *Carb. veg.;* — aft. with trembling, bef. with tenesmus: *Mercur.*

Pectoral anxiety: *Calc. ostr., Caustic.*

Heat, bef.: *Kali carb.;* inclination to sweat, aft.: *Caustic.;* general malaise and over-irritability: *Nitr. ac.*

Seriousness: *Alum.;* indifference: *Phosph. ac., Rhodod.;* apathy: *Opium, Phosph. ac.*

Ill humor, bef.: *Aloes,* I*Calc. ostr.;* aft.: *Nitr. ac.*

Fitful mood: *Nux mosch.;* changeable mood: *Alum.*

Great despondency: *Calc. ostr.*

Wilfulness: *Calc. ostr.;* obstinacy: *Silic.;* irascibility; *Guaiac.;* anger: *Aloes.*

Peevish, low-spirited, lazy and dissatisfied, bef.: *Borax;* fretful, bef.: *Calc. ostr.*

Distrust: *Ant. crud.*

Loquacity: *Laches., Stramon.;* tendency to laugh: *Nux mosch.*

On going to stool groans and grunts: *Pulsat.;* moaning, bef.: *Pulsat.;* and groaning: *Sepia;* crying: *Bellad.*, I*Borax*, I*Chamom.*, *Cina*, *Rhus tox.*
Child cries bef. and is quiet aft.: *Rhus tox.*
Obstinate weeping: *Sulphur.*
Fear of being alone: *Arsen.*
Desire to be quiet: *Gelsem.;* desire for things, which are rejected: *Chamom., Cinch. off.;* desire to be naked: I*Hyosc.;* desire to be carried: I *Chamom.*
Aversion to being disturbed: *Gelsem.*
— and taciturnity: *Ferr. magn.*
Aversion to mental exertion: *Corn. circ.*, *Hepar s. c.*, *Rhodod.;* to being looked at or touched: *Ant. crud.*
Easily startled: *Bellad.*, I*Borax.*, *Kali carb.*
Over-sensitiveness: *Coffea*, *Colchic.*, *Nux vom.*, *Phosphor.;* agitation: *Arsen.*
Excessive irritability: *Ferr. magn.;* irritability, aft.: *Nitr. ac.*
Excitability: *Agar.*, I*Coffea*, *Phosphor.*
Wandering of thoughts: *Apis.*
Imagines that another person is sick: *Petrol.*
Vanishing of thoughts: *Nitr. ac.*
Stupefaction: *Stramon.*, *Tabac.*
Complaints after over-exertion of mind: *Arsen.*

MODEL CURE.

After over-study clicking noise in left vertex, on walking, and during stool; also in occiput on walking, especially in evening, when tired: *Conium*^{sm} (Jen.). —E. W. BERRIDGE.

TENESMUS AND INVOLUNTARY STOOL.

Ineffectual urging, as if it would tear the abdomen asunder; hot hands with anxiety: *Phosphor.*
With anxiety, cannot bear company: *Ambra.*
An ineffectual urging, with pain, anxiety and flushed face: *Caustic.*
Uneasiness, anxiety, with apprehension of evil: *Caustic.*
Urging to stool with anxiety: *Chamom.*
Ill humor: *Magn. mur.;* and disposition to scold: *Kreosot.*
As if diarrhœa would set in: *Crot. tigl.*
Feeling as if he must go to stool, loses consciousness: *Spigel.*
Involuntary Stool. Pinching and cutting in the intestines, with groaning and anxiety that stool might pass involuntarily: *Sepia.*
After fright, with icy coldness of the body: *Veratr.;* after nervous excitement: *Gelsem.;* with weak-mindedness: *Ant. crud.*
Involuntary stool: *Opium;* with mania: *Ant. crud.*, *Cuprum;* — and urine; in mania: *Hepar s. c.*

RECTUM.

Pressing, with depression of spirits: *Lil. tigr.*
Cramp, with great anxiety; has to walk about: *Calc. ostr.*
Cutting and shooting, with loss of energy: *Graphit., Mercur., Natr. carb., Phosphor., Sepia.*
Hæmorrhoids. Tenesmus, pains cause screaming: *Ratanh.;* irritability: *Apis.*
The lumps or knots sore after thinking: *Caustic.*
After mental exertion sore pressure: *Ignat.*
Painful, with apprehension: *Lil. tigr.*
Derangement of Mind. Mental ailments in connection with hæmorrhoidal discharges: *Anac., Ant. crud., Arnic., Arsen., Bellad., Caustic., Cuprum, Hyosc., Ignat., Laches., Lycop., Nux vom., Phosphor., Sepia, Sulphur, Veratr.*
Coagulated blood with the fæces; mania: *Mercur.*
Bleeding from rectum, with hypochondric mood: ❙*Psorin.*
Sphincter paralyzed after nervous excitement: *Gelsem.*

ANUS.

Pressure and shooting after mental exertion: *Nux vom.*
Violent pain, with anxiousness; warm flannel relieves: *Phosphor.*
Burning, with piles: *Ratanh.;* after vexation: *Natr. mur.*
Creeping and restlessness: *Mar. ver.*
Itching in anus from worms, causing furor: *Stramon.*
Moisture exsuding from — causes great vexation and ill humor: *Zinc. cyan.*
Sensation of excoriation, after mental exertion: *Ignat.*
Condylomata, great depression: *Caustic.*

UROPOETIC ORGANS.

Drawing pain from region of kidneys to inguinal glands, with anxiety in scrobiculum: *Cannab.*
Anxiety with unsuccessful urging to urinate, without there being much urine in the bladder: *Chamom.*
Apprehensive of danger without fear, with pain in bladder: *Fluor. ac.*
Afraid of wetting the bed, with weak feeling in bladder and sexual organs: *Alum.*
Retention of urine with a boy of eleven months, screams awfully, throws things away from him: *Staphis.*
Weeping, groaning and wringing of hands with renal colic; vomiting: *Ocimum.*
Talkative delirium, with violent pains in bladder: *Bellad.*
Albuminuria with insanity: *Phytol.*

Urine passed off unconsciously in mania : *Cuprum.*
When busily occupied she has to stop and pass quickly a few drops of water : *Kali carb.*
Urinary symptoms worse when thinking of them ; painful urination : *Helleb.*
When thinking of it a contracting pain running backward from the fore-part of the urethra : *Nux vom.*
Urine Copious. Cheerfulness after copious urination : *Hyosc.*
Much thirst, much urine and great exhaustion : *Chin. sulph.*
Great flow of clear urine ; uneasy to despair : *Vip. red.*
Frequent urination, always crying before ; with sucklings : *Borax.*
Profuse flow of burning urine, drunken feeling : *Stramon.*
A large quantity of urine, passed all at once ; clear like spring water, confused all night : *Stramon.*
Water-like urine in quantities, vivid delirium : *Stramon.*
Urine Scanty. Frequent desire to pass urine, but in small quantities, with apprehension of some impending evil : *Lil. tigr.*
Urine pale and scanty with attacks of mental derangement : *Crocus.*
Scanty and much reddened, with hallucinations : *Bellad.*
Scanty and red colored, with idiocy : *Opium.*
Very little, but frequent discharges of milky urine, with unconsciousness and delirium in hydrocephalus : *Apis.*

COMPLAINTS BEFORE, DURING AND AFTER URINATION.

Everything looks brighter after urination : *Jambos.*
Burning after urinating, causing ill humor and despondency : *Alum.*
Anxiety and restlessness before urinating : *Phosph. ac.*
Anxiety during urination : *Chamom.;* and pressure in the bladder, with scanty urine : *Sepia.*
Great depression and anxiety before and after urination : *Digit.*
Impatience before urinating : *Sulphur.*
Before, during and after urination violent cutting pains in the urethra, has to bend double and scream : *Canthar.*
Is kind of frightened when going to urinate : *Alum.*

SEXUAL DESIRE.

Increased. With sadness : *Bellad.;* hypochondric melancholy : *Veratr.*
Hypochondria from denial of sexual intercourse, with single men : *Conium.*
Sexual desire when suppressed is followed by great mental activity : *Laches.*
With restlessness felt in the whole body, cannot sit still : *Ant. crud.*
Thoughts run on sexual subjects, which torment him so that he fears insanity : *Graphit.*

Continued erection without desire; no inclination for mental or physical work: *Bufo*.

Mind dwells on sexual subjects: *Conium, Staphis*.

Lascivious imagination without irritation of sexual organs: *Ambra*.

Exalted sexual passion by intrusion of ideas: *Aloes, Graphit*.

Voluptuous fancies day and night with erection: *Digit*.

Lascivious thoughts when lying in bed, with erections: *Silic*.

Intense sexual desire without an erection, followed by ill humor and dissatisfaction: *Calc. ostr*.

Lascivious, voluptuous fancies and sexual excitement, with weakness and impotence: *Ignat*.

Lascivious thoughts without erection: *Calad., Sepia;* in the night: *Aurum*.

Sexual excitation during the night; delirium: *Stramon*.

Nightly voluptuous fancies, pollutions: *Opium*.

Lascivious dreams of disturbed coition, when awaking erection and voluptuous thoughts: *Silic*.

Sexual irritation during mental derangement: *Stramon*.

Extreme excitement of sexual parts with stupor: *Stramon*.

Decreased. Impotence, with retracted foreskin, sexual desire not extinct: *Coloc*.

Less sexual desire after lascivious fancies: *Ant. crud*.

Decreased desire, less excitation of the fancy: *Petrol*.

Suppression of sexual desire, low spirited, sad, anxious: *Conium*.

Loss of sexual power with despondency: *Spongia*.

Impotence, weak memory: *Secal*.

After Coition. Inclination to work: *Calc. phosph*.

Anxious and restless all day: *Sepia*.

Erection, followed by weakness of mind, vertigo, despondency, and lassitude; in the evening depressed and easily frightened: *Sepia*.

After exhausting coitions, weak memory: *Secal*.

Indifference, low spirits and dullness of mind after onanism: *Staphis*.

EMISSIONS.

After pollution comfortable feeling, collected: *Laches*.

Depression of spirits with spermatorrhœa, great debility: *Ferr. brom*.

Pollutions followed by anxious heat: *Petrol.;* mental and bodily prostration; anxious and apprehensive: *Carb. an*.

After nocturnal emission frightened by slight noises: *Aloes*.

After painful emission out of humor, vexatious and dissatisfied: *Natr. carb*.

Heaviness and ill humor after emission: *Thuya*.

After night emission, loud moaning: *Hippom*.

Emissions with amorous dreams, gloomy mood: *Hamam*.

Dazed feeling in head after emission: *Caustic*.

Difficulty of fixing the attention, using wrong words, with blur before the eyes, after a restless night, made so by lascivious dreams and emissions towards morning: *Lil. tigr.*

Male Parts; Prostata. Emission of juice from any emotion: *Conium;* from the slightest excitement, without an erection: *Natr. mur.*

With every stool and after urinating, semen escapes, not only prostatic fluid; is hopelessly distressed: **II***Selen.*

Drawing in testicles, with awkwardness; evenings: *Agar.*

Digging pain in the right testicle when at rest, fear of the part being struck: *Argent.*

Anxious, dull stitches in the glans penis: *Squilla.*

Delirium with inflammation of the penis and scrotum: *Plumbum.*

FEMALE INNER SEXUAL ORGANS.
Nymphomania, see Chapt. 23; Hysteria, see Chapt. 36.

After coition a feeling of great comfort, followed by irritability: *Natr. mur.*

Everything appears to be very beautiful: *Sulphur;* fits of great joy, with bursts of laughter, in hysteralgia: *Asaf.*

After excessive joy or ecstacy, metritis: *Coffea.*

Mental exaltation or ecstacy, hysteralgia: *Coffea.*

Weeps very easily about this or that thing; with almost all her sufferings there are sure to be tears and cries, she can hardly give her symptoms on account of weeping, with hysteralgia: *Pulsat.*

Sadness: *Conium;* disposed to be sad and irritable; very sensitive to impressions, in uterine cancer: *Kreosot.;* with displaced uterus: *Staphis.*

Depression of spirits in ovaritis: *Aurum;* in hysteralgia: **II***Crocus;* changing, with gaiety: *Sulphur;* with ulcers of uterus: **II***Lycop.;* and hypochondric mood in uterine cancer: *Mur. purp.*

Dread of impending evil, with bearing down: *Lil. tigr.*

Shrinking look when awaking, in metritis: *Stramon.*

In hysteralgia extremely scrupulous about the least thing: *Thuya;* fear of going crazy: *Calc. ostr.;* anxiety, as if some misfortune were impending or some bad news were about to arrive: *Ast. rub.;* anxious, sad, apprehension of dying: *Asaf.;* melancholy, anguish, dread of death: *Secal.*

Bearing down. Violent and on rectum, with vexed depression: *Magn. mur.;* after anxious constriction painless pressure in lower portion: *Platin.;* irritability of temper, anxiety and dread of impending evil, with severe dragging down sensation in the whole sexual organs, with a feeling as though the whole internal parts were being pulled downward from the breasts and umbilical region through the vagina, and an uncontrollable desire to press the hands against the vulva to prevent the parts from escaping: *Lil. tigr.*

Believes herself pregnant, looks forward to a speedy confinement, thinks she feels labor pains: *Veratr.*

Hourglass Contraction. Constant moaning, which seems to afford relief: *Bellad.;* spiteful irritability: *Chamom.;* nervous: *Nux vom.*

Metritis. After fright fear of it remains: *Opium;* anguish, fear of death; she is sure she will die: *Arsen.;* despondent: *Nux vom.*

Displacement. Anguish, fear of death: *Acon.*

Anxiety during catamenia: *Mercur.*

Malacie. Anguish, fear of death: *Acon., Arsen.;* passive disposition: *Secal.*

Uterine Symptoms are caused or aggravated by mental excitement, wounded pride and non-approval by others: *Pallad.*

Full of suppressed grief, full of grief and sighing, brooding over imaginary troubles, with which she seems to be weighed down: *Ignat.*

Indifferent to the affairs of life, even to those which used to interest her most, with ulcers of uterus: *Phosph. ac.*

Mental listlessness, with affection of uterus: *Nux mosch.*

Involuntary sighing, despondency in ovaritis: *Ignat.*

Tearful, yielding, cries at everything, sad despondency, mild; in displacement: *Pulsat.*

General unhappiness of temper, in hysteralgia: *Rhus tox.*

In all sufferings a vein of ill humor, can hardly speak pleasantly, feels like scolding about everything, gives vent to her ill humor in spite of all restraint; in hysteralgia or displacement: *Chamom.*

Headstrong, even unto quarrelling, during catamenia: *Chamom.*

Quarrelsome in displacements: *Aurum.*

Desire for things not to be had, or not wanted when offered, in hysteralgia: *Bryon.;* impatient, can hardly restrain herself to treat people civilly, in metritis: *Chamom.;* much irritability of temper, hysteralgia: *Sabin.,* and weak: *Graphit.*

Listless, apathetic: hysteralgia: *Phosph. ac.;* dissatisfied with herself when she has finished, with displacement of uterus: *Sulphur.*

Loud laughing, at appearance of menses: *Hyosc.;* quick to act: *Coffea;* wishes to do everything in a great hurry: *Sulph. ac.*

Insupportable pain near the left groin towards ovary, with lectrophilie (keeping bed unreasonably): *Alum. p. s.*

Desire to keep still: *Bryon.*

Disposed to talk, metritis: *Stramon.*

Wants to be naked, metritis: *Hyosc.*

Desires, rather than fears death: *Bellad.*

Melancholy, constantly thinks of suicide, ovaritis: *Aurum.*

Mind dwells on suicide: *Aurum;* wishes to drown herself, with cancer of uterus: *Silic.*

Uterine Congestion. Mental agitation, especially society, or musical entertainments, or excited conversation, or motion, aggravate the pain in the right ovary: *Pallad.*

Peculiar derangement of mind, nervous repetition of words, etc.: *Amyl. nitr.*

Full of ideas: *Coffea;* strange, absurd fancies; bed full of creases; she is double, lying crosswise; metritis: *Stramon.;* furious delirium, metritis: *Bellad.;* typhoid state delirium; metritis: *Hyosc.*

Feels as if she would lose her senses and die soon: *Platin.*

Emotions aggravate pain in right ovarian region: *Laches.*

Sensitive to mental impressions: *Staphis.;* with ovaritis when the mind has been dwelling too much on sensual subjects: *Staphis.;* after a fit of passion: *Chamom.*

Moral disturbances in regular paroxysms every night, morning or noon, most after dinner, with ulceration: *Arg. nitr.*

After the least excitement return of catamenia: *Calc. ostr.;* after fright: *Opium.*

Pressing pain in the genitals from sitting bent while reading: *Bellad.*

During puberty, insane depression of the mind: *Hippom.*

Great mental depression in climacteric years, with chronic uterine affections: *Psorin.*

Climaxis. See Chapter 47.

CATAMENIA TOO COPIOUS, MENORRHAGIA.

Uncommon buoyancy of mind, fears nothing, is well satisfied with herself: *Fluor. ac.*

Intolerable sadness: *Natr. mur.*

Melancholy, looks on the dark side of things: *Caustic.*

Menorrhagia. Alarmed, excited, sure she will die: *Acon.*

Sobbing, grief: *Ignat.*

Disposed to laugh in open air: *Nux mosch.*

Loquacious, strange, absurd ideas: *Stramon.*

Silly laughing and foolish manners: *Hyosc.*

Metrorrhagia. Frequent uterine bleeding, constant bearing down, great sadness: *Hamam.*

Fear of death: *Acon.;* despondency: *Ignat.*

Great irascibility: *Chamom.*

Loquacity, singing, praying and praise: *Stramon.*

Much excitability: *Acon.;* with great mental restlessness: *Apis.*

Full of strange and absurd ideas: *Stramon.*

Alternating with spells of insanity: *Cascar.*

Short time seems to be very long: *Arg. nitr.*

MODEL CURE.

After metrorrhagia over-sensitive, exalted nervous state; hasty speech, accompanied by quick gestures; eyes fiery and glistening; pulse 110. Her movements were like those of a passionate person. If she could not talk, her friends had to relate stories continually in a quick way. At times she was in the opposite state, gave short answers and desired to be alone; she was then moody and feigned sleep. The nights became more and more anxious and restless; she could not describe how terrible they were: *Sepia.*—HAYNEL.

DYSMENORRHŒA.

Sadness: *Amm. carb.;* terrible sadness: *Natr. mur.;* sad and silent, as if she would die: *Mur. ac.;* depression of spirits: *Plumbum*

Anxiety: *Act. rac., Mercur.;* anguish: *Ignat.*

Despair: *Coffea.*

Out of humor, even quarrelsome: *Chamom.;* irritable: *Senec.;* angry exclamations during sleep: *Castor.*

Loquacity: *Stramon.*

Devout, beseeching; earnest and ceaseless talking: *Stramon.*

Moaning and lamenting: *Coloc.;* sobbing, sighing: *Ignat.*

Hurried about everything: *Sulph. ac.*

Does not wish to think: *Senec.*

Almost raging: *Hyosc.*

AMENORRHŒA.

Sanguine temperament: *Acon.*

Depression, disposition to suicide: *Aurum;* looks on the dark side of everything: *Caustic.;* depression: *Crocus, Podoph.*

Melancholy during the period of development: *Helleb.*

Anguish with colic: *Coloc.*

Despairs of her salvation: *Veratr.*

Grief: *Ignat.;* after chagrin: *Acon., Coloc.;* severe indignation: *Staphis.;* has a fit if angered: *Chamom.*

Can hardly keep her temper: *Chamom.*

Loud boisterous laughing at every menstrual effort: *Hyosc.*

Loquacious: *Stramon.*

Tears, prayers and earnest supplications: *Stramon.*

Likes society: *Stramon.*

Very sensitive to mental impressions: *Staphis.*

Fearfulness, fright: *Acon., Lycop., Stramon.*

Shrinking back: *Stramon.*

Menses had not appeared for months; violent delirium: *Cuprum.*

Suppressed catamenia with mental derangement: *Pulsat.;* with screams in mania: *Cuprum.*

Climacteric years; insanity: *Hippom.*

MODEL CURES.

Suppressed menstruation with melancholy. Indifference to things she loved best. Sits alone and weeps, imagines things, especially that she might go crazy. On all parts crawling sensation as if gone to sleep, as if she had no feeling in epigastrium. Sleep unrefreshing and disturbed by dreams: *Ignat.*—GROSS.

Mental dullness with pious fanatacism. No desire to work; anxious restlessness, sleeplessness, constipation and suppression of catamenia: *Thuya.*—W. WILLIAMSON.

CATAMENIA, WITH ANXIETY, ANGUISH AND APPREHENSION, BEFORE, DURING AND AFTER.

Amm. carb.
Bellad.
Carb. an.
ı Conium.
Graphit.
Kali carb.
ı Mercur.
ı Natr. mur.
ı Nitr. ac.
Pallad.
ıı Phosphor.
ı Pulsat.
Silic.
ıı Stannum.
Sulphur.
Thuya.
Zincum.

Great anxiety and depression, bef.: *Stannum.*
Anxiety, with squalmishness, bef.: *Natr. mur.*
Fearfulness, bef.: *Natr. mur., Carb. veg.*
Two days too late, with anxious and uncomfortable feeling: *Sulphur.*
Anxiety one day before catamenia, or soon after coming on: *Nitr. ac.;* during: *Mercur., Zincum.*
Feels sore in abdomen after, with fear and apprehension that something horrible will happen: *Pallad.*
Apprehension, bef.: *Sulphur.*
Anxiety about trifles, bef.: *Conium.*

Melancholy, bef.: *Nitr. ac., Silic., Stannum.*
Melancholy, with inclination to drown herself, dur.: *Silic.*
Cardiac anxiety: *Bellad., Thuya;* with palpitation: *Nitr. ac., Phosphor.;* præcordial: *Silic.;* with trembling of all limbs: *Nitr. ac.;* with backache, dur.: *Graphit.*
Anxiety, with fainty sensation: *Natr. mur.;* anxious dreams: ııı*Kali carb.*
Heat, bef.: *Amm. carb.; Carb. an.;* dur.: *Nitr. ac.;* inner heat: *Natr. mur.*
At night and early in bed: *Kali carb.*
Forenoon: *Amm. carb.;* evening: *Nitr. ac., Stannum.*

MODEL CURES.

Irregular catamenia. Heat and congestion to head and face. Headache, præcordial weight and backache. Sleepless nights on account of great fear and anxious restlessness in the head. Despairs of her salvation, and seeks aid in constant prayers: *Pulsat.*—BETHMANN.

Anxiety during catamenia, does not know what to do. Longs for death. Indifference, even to that which she loves best. Involuntary weeping, which relieves. Inclination to commit suicide from despair, in hysteria and hypochondria: *Merc. sol.*—JOUSSEL.

CATAMENIA, WITH MENTAL CONCOMITANTS.

Sadness. Sad and doleful one day before: *Nitr. ac.*
— and melancholy, before: *Lycop.*
Unconquerable sadness, during: *Amm. carb.*
Pale face, with sadness and irritability, during: *Magn. mur.*
Sadness, thoughts turned to herself, there is no life in her, during: *Mur. ac.*
Great sadness, during: *Natr. mur., Nitr. ac.*
Dispirited, melancholy, after: *Alum., Silic.*

MIND AND DISPOSITION.

|| Acon.
  Act. rac.
|| Alum.
|| Amm. carb.
| Apis.
|| Arsen.
  Aurum.
| Bellad.
| Berber.
| Calc. ostr.
  Carb. an.
|| Castor.
| Caustic.
|| Chamom.
  Coffea.
|| Coloc.
|| Conium.
  Crocus.
|| Cuprum.
  Fluor. ac.
| Graphit.
  Hamam.
  Helleb.
  Hippom.
|| Hyosc.
|| Ignat.
|| Kali carb.
|| Kreosot.
| Lycop.
  Lyc. virg.
| Magn. carb.
| Magn. mur.
  Mangan.
|| Mercur.
|| Mur. ac.
|| Natr. mur.
|| Nitr. ac.
| Nux mosch.
| Pallad.
| Phosphor.
|| Platin.
  Plumbum.
  Podoph.
| Pulsat.
| Rhus tox.
  Selen.
  Senec.
|| Sepia.
| Silic.
| Stannum.
| Staphis.
|| Stramon.
|| Sulphur.
| Sulph. ac.
| Thuya.
| Veratr.
|| Zincum.

Ill humor. Sees dark side of everything, before: *Caustic.*
Cross, melancholic and desponding: *Lycop.*
On occurrence ill humored, intolerant, quarrelsome: *Stramon.*
After the first day out of humor: *Magn. carb.;* during: *Amm. carb., Berber., Caustic.*
Ill humored and very tired, during: *Caustic.*
With profuse discharge: *Platin.*
Heaviness of spirits, especially in morning, during: *Sepia;* in forenoon: *Magn. carb.*
Ill humor and restlessness, with toothache, after: *Magn. carb.*
Weary of life: *Berber.*
Quietude: *Amm. carb., Mur. ac.*
In the beginning ill humored, disagreeable and quarrelsome: *Chamom.*

Vexation. Before: *Sepia.*
During copious flow, with pressure in abdomen: *Platin.*
During: *Amm. carb., Zincum.*
Made worse by vexation, passes clots of blood after it has stopped: *Rhus tox.*
Before she is very sensitive, throws herself on the bed and remains lying there all day: *Sepia.*

Irritability. Some days before restless and irritable: *Kreosot.*
Very irritable day before: *Magn. mur.*
Before, attack of despair: *Sepia.*
Irritable and weak-minded, does not like to answer questions: *Amm. carb.*
Cross, everything irritates her, speaking is too much trouble, during: *Castor.*
Excitable, easily offended: *Apis.*

Conations. During catamenia, loquacity; |*Stramon.*
Before catamenia incessant loud laughing: *Hyosc.*
Weeping mood, before: *Conium,* before and the first day: *Lycop.,* during: *Arsen., Zincum.*
After catamenia whining: *Stramon.;* and hiccough: *Alum.*
Groaning and complaining: *Arsen.*
During convulsions and piercing shrieks: *Cuprum.*
Before catamenia, irresistable, almost maniacal desire for ardent spirits, has to get completely drunk, and feels afterwards distressed, wants to be brought to an insane asylum: ||*Selen.*
After, groaning: *Stramon.;* during, starts up in the night: *Zincum;* second day of, disinclination to answer: *Zincum;* speaking is too much trouble: *Cast. vesc.*
During, keeps herself close: *Mur. ac.;* before, over-sensitive: *Sepia;* frightened by trifles: *Calc. ostr.*

Exaltations. Very excitable, a day before: *Magn. mur.*

The least excitement causes return of catamenia: *Calc. ostr.*
A week before, restlessness: *Kali carb.*
Restlessness and anxiety the day before: *Sulphur.*
Moves from one side to the other, cannot bear to be uncovered; thick black blood; the night before: *Mangan.*
The night before, at midnight, chill, followed by heat, especially in face with restlessness: *Sepia;* restless and full of care: *Conium;* menstrual colic and restlessness: *Pulsat.*

Depression. Mental and bodily depression with despairing mood, after: *Alum.*
Shortly before, vanishing of thought: *Nux mosch.*
Stupid with lack of expression, during: *Lyc. virg.*
Could not collect her thoughts, during: *Calc. ostr.*
Too late, with heaviness in abdomen and dullness: *Graphit.*

Delirium. At the beginning of, delirious talk, with weeping as if going insane: *Lycop.;* copious flow with delirious talk: *Hyosc.*
Delirious with rush of blood to the head: *Apis.*

Insanity. Before menstrual flow, hiccough, mania: *Sepia.*
Before, melancholy, sees everything in dark colors: *Caustic.*
On the occurrence of catamenia, madness: *Acon.*
Before, she kisses every one; with catamenia, mania: *Veratr.*
During, insuperable melancholy: *Amm. carb.*

Rage. Day before and during first day of their appearance, raving and weeping as if she were going mad: *Lycop.*
Before catamenia, an attack of despair and wild behaviour, with sobbing; throws herself on the bed where she remains all day without eating: *Sepia.*
Neuralgic pains in teeth and head during frenzy, beats her head with her fists, before: *Arsen.;* with appearance of it, mania: *Acon.*

MODEL CURES.

With each return of the menses wildness and foolishness changing to mania. Talking, laughing, weeping, scolding, hiding herself, or attacks of rage in which she spits at people and tears her clothes. Pulse slow but accelerated during an attack. Abdomen hard and distended. Passes urine involuntarily: *Bellad.*—KIESSELBACH.

Destroys what falls in her hands; talks in a vehement, commanding tone; spits at the nurse, lifts up her clothes, and kisses hotly all who come near her. She does things wrongly and talks disconnectedly. Tongue whitish; sleeplessness. Catamenia scanty, pale and watery: *Phosphor.*—SCHMIDT.

A young lady had since three months on awaking nausea, vomituritio and constricting sensation in the throat; dullness in the head, sometimes sensation as of a piece of ice lying on the vertex. Frequent chilliness, can scarcely get warm, feet, hands and nose icy cold. Catamenia irregular, generally every three weeks. Early on the day on which menses appear diarrhœa, nausea, chilliness, four to six watery evacuations with burning pain in rectum. Irritability; sensitive, gets angry at trifles, or weeps about little things: *Veratr.*—J. C. M.

LEUCORRHŒA.

Low spirited women who sigh a great deal: *Ignat.*
Full of fears: *Acon.;* changeable mood: *Cinch. off.;* with irritability: *Acon.*
Talks much: *Laches.;* does not wish to talk nor to hear others: *Amm. carb.*
Dislike to music: *Carb. veg.*
Worse from noise and bright light: *Bellad.*
Caused by fright: *Pulsat.*
With loss of memory: *Anac.*

OUTER PARTS.

Tearing in vulva, at intervals so violent that she would like to scream: *Baryt.*

Anguish, melancholy in the week previous to catamenia; ceasing as soon as monthly flow begins, with prolapse of vagina: *Stannum.*

Strangulation of prolapse of vagina after much menstrual distress: *Acon.;* thinks she cannot get well, will die: *Acon.;* great anguish: *Arsen.;* wakens in distress: *Laches.*

Constriction of vagina; inclined to brood over her troubles; full of grief: *Ignat.;* with mild, yielding disposition: *Pulsat.;* impatient, cannot answer civilly: *Chamom.*

Induration of Vagina. Moved to tears telling her symptoms: *Pulsat.*

Vaginal Growths. Inclination to self-destruction, thinks about it even if not intending it: *Acon.;* symptoms of mind or of body appear alternately: *Platin.;* very tearful, weeps at everything, joyful or sorrowful: *Pulsat.;* feels as if she could not exist any longer: *Thuya.*

MIND SYMPTOMS DURING PREGNANCY.

Feelings. Thoughtless gaiety: *Arnic.*

Happy, imagines to be possessed of beautiful things: *Sulphur.*

Sadness: *Bellad., Laches.;* looks at the dark side of everything: *Aurum;* melancholy: *Bellad.;* better from sighing: *Laches.;* wishes to hide herself: *Bellad.;* fear of the future: *Anac.;* thinks she will lose her reason: *Nux vom.;* fears to be poisoned, betrayed, injured: *Hyosc.;* fear of death, excessive dread of it, she is sure she will die: *Arsen.;* after a fright, diarrhœa in pregnancy: *Opium;* after fright, hæmorrhage during pregnancy: *Secal.*

Periodical attacks of anguish, inquietude, tossing, inability to lie in bed: *Arsen.;* weakness during pregnancy of four months, paroxysm of indefinable terror: *Nux mosch.;* predicts the day she is to die, in pregnancy or childbed: *Acon.;* fear and presentiment of approaching death: *Acon.*

Full of grief: *Ignat.;* past events trouble her: *Platin.*

MIND SYMPTOMS DURING PREGNANCY. 183

‖ Acon.	
‖ Act. rac.	
Anac.	
‖ Apis.	
Arg. nitr.	
‖ Arnica.	
‖ Arsen.	
‖ Asaf.	
‖ Aurum.	
‖ Bellad.	
Borax.	
Bryon.	
‖ Calc. ostr.	
Canthar.	
‖ Chamom.	
Cina.	
‖ Cinch. off.	
‖ Coccul.	
Conium.	
Crocus.	
‖ Cyprip.	
Digit.	
‖ Gelsem.	
Glonoin.	
Goss. herb.	
Hyosc.	
‖ Ignat.	
‖ Kali carb.	
‖ Laches.	
Lycop.	
‖ Magn. carb.	
‖ Moschus.	
Natr. carb.	
Natr. mur.	
‖ Nux mosch.	
‖ Nux vom.	
‖ Opium.	
Phosphor.	
‖ Phosph. ac.	
‖ Platin.	
‖ Pulsat.	
Secale.	
Sepia.	
Silic.	
‖ Staphis.	
‖ Stramon.	
Sulphur.	
‖ Sulph. ac.	
Tabac.	
‖ Veratr.	
‖ Zincum.	

Feelings and Conations. Great frivolity and mischievousness: *Arnic.;* excessive mischievousness; obstinacy: *Calc. ostr.*

After vexation, hæmorrhage of clotted blood, during pregnancy: *Kali carb.*

Strange temper, laughs at serious matters and is grave over laughable occurrences: *Anac.;* sadness, with tears, alternating with gaiety and laughter: *Phosphor.*

Inclined to quarrel: *Bellad.;* reproachful and overbearing: *Lycop.;* will not be comforted: *Ignat.;* constantly worrying, fretting and crying about her real or imagined illness: *Sepia, Staphis.*

Has no confidence in herself, thinks others have none in her, makes her unhappy: *Aurum;* fears people will think her insane: *Calc. ostr.;* suspicious: *Laches.;* contempt for others: *Platin.;* erroneous, haughty notions: *Veratr.;* proud: *Laches.;* jealousy during pregnancy: *Laches.*

Conations. Excessive loquacity, with sudden change of subjects: *Laches.;* talks or prays earnestly and constantly: *Stramon.;* weeps and prays: *Aurum;* weeps even at answers and questions: *Pulsat.;* sighs and sobs: *Ignat.;* complains much, but of nothing in particular: *Moschus;* screams, curses, scolds: *Anac.;* wishes to strike and bite: *Bellad.;* bustling disposition the day before confinement: *Apis;* sluggish flow of ideas: *Nux mosch.;* desires to wander about the house: *Veratr.*

Wishes for solitude: *Ignat.;* thinks not to be fit to live, inclined to suicide: *Aurum;* wishes to run away: *Hyosc.;* worse in solitude: *Stramon.;* disposed to be taciturn: *Veratr.;* takes time to answer: *Nux mosch.*

Very sensitive to mental impressions: *Staphis.;* uneasy about her own health: *Sepia, Staphis.;* distress with inquietude: *Bellad.;* estranged from society, individually, even her husband and family: *Anac., Conium, Natr. carb., Natr. mur.*

Productions. Estranged from others and society: *Anac.;* thinks she is not at home, this is continually in her mind: *Opium.* Full of strange, ridiculous ideas: *Stramon.;* occupied with pins, counts them, hunts for them, etc.: *Silic.;* talks about rats and mice: *Calc. ostr.;* thinks and talks about murder, incendiarism: *Calc. ostr.;* thinks herself a demon: *Anac.;* inclined to jump out of a window, or from a height: *Aurum;* frightful visions: *Bellad.;* thinks all persons are demons: *Platin.;* unfortunate, harassed by enemies: *Cinch. off.;* wild look, stunned appearance: *Bellad.*

Loss of consciousness from rush of blood to the head: *Glonoin.;* loss of mental power: *Nux vom.;* loss of memory: *Anac.;* dull mind, inability to think: *Anac.;* cannot read or calculate, loses the connection of ideas: *Nux vom.*

Toothache in Pregnancy. Sensitive to mental impressions: *Staphis.,* excitement: *Calc. ostr., Gelsem.;* unbearable: *Chamom.;* insupportable, has to walk: *Magn. carb.;* unbearable, driven to frenzy: *Arsen.;* impatience: *Chamom.;* irritable temper: *Chamom.*

MIND AND DISPOSITION.

With Gastric Complaints. Great distress: *Goss. herb.;* dread of light and noise: *Bellad.;* dread of downward motion: *Borax;* fear that something untoward will happen: *Acon.;* fear of being in crowds or busy places: *Acon.;* fear of death: *Acon.;* full of suppressed grief as it were: *Ignat.;* as if she could lie down anywhere and die: *Kali carb.;* great irascibility, can hardly return a civil answer: *Chamom.;* worse after being angry: *Bryon.;* cross and peevish: *Cina;* impelled to do things hurriedly: *Sulph. ac.;* very uneasy and restless: *Arsen.;* time seems to pass slowly: *Arg. nitr.;* hears voices of absent persons: *Chamom.*

Diarrhœa. Decided indifference to external influences or surroundings: *Phosph. ac.;* despondency: *Digit.;* quarrelsome, obstreperous: *Chamom.;* apt to be quarrelsome if disturbed: *Nux vom.;* irritable, morose and sullen: *Nux vom.;* great loquacity: *Stramon.;* tearful disposition: *Pulsat.;* cannot do anything deliberately, feels hurried, as if impelled to do everything hastily: *Sulph. ac.;* sluggish flow of ideas: *Nux mosch.;* darkness and solitude: *Stramon.;* beclouded condition of mind: *Caustic.;* cannot read or study satisfactorily: *Tabac.;* constipation; sighing, full of grief: *Ignat.;* after a fright: *Opium.*

Fissure of Anus. Agony: *Arsen.*

Hæmorrhoids. Very sensitive: *Cinch. off.*

Mild, gentle women, easily controlled: *Pulsat.;* can hardly control herself, gives short answers; can hardly endure her sufferings; irritable and spiteful: *Chamom.*

Urination. Tenesmus, with agony: *Canthar.;* with pain in back previously, wild screams: *Lycop.*

Pain, especially in Lumbar and Pelvic Regions. Feels disagreeable and unhappy: *Chamom.;* distressed and unhappy: *Acon.;* fear of approaching evil: *Acon.;* spiteful irritability: *Chamom.;* will cannot command muscular movements: *Gelsem.;* excitement and sleeplessness: *Coffea;* regards pains unbearable: *Chamom.;* headache, pain unbearable: *Ignat.;* given to sighing: *Ignat.;* headache, stupor: *Gelsem.;* as if she would "go distracted:" *Coffea.*

Chorea. Excessively happy, tender or in a rage: *Crocus;* after care: *Stramon.;* after long suppressed grief: *Ignat.;* from a fright: *Calc. ostr.;* with strange, inconsistent fancies: *Stramon.;* rather stupid: *Bellad.*

Varicose Veins. Mild disposition, easily moved to tears: *Pulsat.*

Threatening Abortion. After fright: *Opium;* fear remains: *Acon.;* mild, tearful yielding: *Pulsat.;* spiteful irritability, "snappish" when speaking: *Chamom.;* talks, prays, implores, sings, constantly uttering something: *Stramon.;* weeping; sadness: *Lycop.;* sighing, sobbing; suppressed grief: *Ignat.;* unconsciousness: *Acon.*

Paroxysm of terror (in pregnancy of four months): *Nux mosch.*

MODEL CURE.

In the eighth month of pregnancy dark, suspicious and reserved manner, disturbed look on her face, sleepless. Looks for her bed in the yard, hides in a corner, to escape from a little gray man, who wants to pull out her leg: *Pulsat.*
—BETHMANN.

DURING PARTURITION.

Labor Pains. With sadness: *Ignat.;* very sad, with forebodings: *Natr. mur.;* fears she will not be delivered, but die; that something will go wrong: *Acon.;* distressed: *Gelsem., Ipec., Secal.;* a disagreeable sensation strikes through her, arresting all her thoughts; something might occur: *Asar.;* anguish with tremor: *Natr. carb.;* make her desperate, would like to jump out of the window, dash herself down: *Aurum;* most in back, after grief: *Caustic.;* spiteful, fretful, peevish, cross, cannot return a civil answer: *Chamom.;* deep sighs, with sadness: *Ignat.;* weeping, lamenting, in constant motion: *Lycop.;* shrieks out sharply, pains distressing, can hardly bear them, wishes to get away from them: *Chamom.;* distress, moaning; restless with each pain: *Acon.;* insupportable: *Act. rac., Coffea;* parturient women shrink back from fright: *Stramon.;* fear or fright suppressing them: *Opium;* drive her distracted: *Arnic.*

Os Uteri rigid. Moaning: *Acon., Bellad.;* discouraged: *Acon.;* fears will not do well: *Acon.;* pains too severe to be endured, laments, calls for assistance: *Chamom.*

Fainting. After sadness and gloom: *Laches.;* after a fright: *Acon., Coffea;* after grief: *Ignat.;* after spiteful irritability: *Chamom.;* dreading society and company: *Laches.*

Puerperal Convulsions. Preceded by mental excitement and perturbation: *Act. rac.;* anxiety, fear of death: *Acon.;* mild and tearful: *Pulsat.;* irritable disposition: *Nux vom.;* impatience and disposition to anger, excited by anger, spiteful irritability: *Chamom.;* cries with fearful visions: *Bellad.;* looks frightened, shrinks back from first objects seen after opening eyes; cries, laughter, singing: *Stramon.;* screams: *Caustic.*

After Pains. Distressing, unbearable; wishes to get away from herself, irritable, ill natured: *Chamom.;* distressing and acutely felt: *Act. rac., Coffea;* sighing, sadness, despondency: *Ignat.;* irritable: *Nux vom.;* mild and tearful: *Pulsat.*

Uterus slow in returning to its natural size, dreads insanity: *Lil. tigr.*

Retained Placenta. Anguish and distress: *Canthar.;* and moaning: *Bellad.;* mild, yielding disposition; inclined to weep about her pains: *Pulsat.*

Lochia. Fearfulness, afraid something unfortunate will occur: *Acon.;* irritable and impatient: *Chamom;* suppression from anger: *Coloc.;* thinks she is drugged or poisoned: *Hyosc.;* suppressed fear with sighing and sobbing: *Ignat.;* by fright: *Opium;* full of strange and absurd, strongly marked ideas: *Stramon.*

Lochial discharge continues too long, is profuse and excoriating; dreads insanity: *Lil. tigr.*

Pendulous Abdomen. Everything seems strange and horrible to her: *Platin.*

MODEL CURE.

Convulsions after a fright when a little girl, return after each confinement: *Sec. corn.*—HELBIG.

CHILDBED.

NOTE.—Puerperal Mania, compare Chapt. 24.

Mind. Immoderate laughing: *Apis.*
After confinement anxiety: *Cuprum.*
Eighth day, quickly following erroneous ideas: *Cuprum.*
Anxious before convulsions after confinement: *Cuprum.*
Anxiety about future and domestic affairs: *Bryon.*
Predicts the day she is to die: *Acon.*

Mind and Body. Over-excitement and over-sensitiveness of all the senses, especially after use of chamomile tea; effects of sudden joy: *Coffea.*
Constipation, with itching; dreads insanity: *Lil. tigr.*
Diarrhœa; takes a long time to answer a simple question: *Nux mosch.*
Painful hæmorrhoids, dreads insanity: *Lil. tigr.*
Painful smarting in the urethra after passing urine, dreads insanity: *Lil. tigr.*
In the night spasmodic pain in the chest, coming up from the small of the back into the region of the stomach and chest, causing dyspnœa and anxiety: *Lycop.*
Pain in back and hips, dreads insanity: *Lil. tigr.*

After Childbed. Melancholy: *Bellad.*
Does not want to go anywhere, not even to church (a young woman), since her confinement: *Angelica officinalis.*
Want of food; leucorrhœa; religious mania; imagines herself eternally damned; sees the devil coming to take her; world on fire during nights; fear, with occasional outbursts of rage; paroxysms of weeping, followed by lucid momemts, but with forgetfulness; cannot follow the course of conversation: *Pulsat.*, 3d dec., did much to relieve.—ROCKWITH.

NURSING.

Milk abundant, with derangement of mind: *Stramon.*
Milk *abnormal*, breasts knotted; discouraged, anxious: *Acon.;* cross, irritable, not easily satisfied: *Cina.*
Milk *blue;* disconsolate and sad on awaking: *Laches.*
Milk *thin;* dissatisfied, unhappy; long-standing mental trouble: *Laches.*
Milk *scanty;* very sad and depressed, says she will die, despairing sadness: *Agn. cast.;* after anxious night-watching: *Caustic.;* great apathy: *Phosph. ac.;* mild and tearful: ❙❙*Pulsat.;* anxiety and despondency after each trouble: *Caustic.;* insulting, cross, uncivil: *Chamom.;* mental derangement, thoughts of suicide: *Rhus tox.*

Breasts tender, nipples inflamed: suffering unbearable, fretful, cross: *Chamom.;* fear, anxiety, restlessness, mastitis: *Acon.;* dull, stupid feeling: *Bellad.*

Cancer of Mammæ. Becomes furious about the pain: *Chamom.*
Agonizing pain: *Calc. ox.*
Climacteric Period, see Chapters., 24 and 47.

LARYNX AND WINDPIPE.

Choking from contraction of glottis while weeping; from anxiety: *Lact. vir.*
Constriction of glottis and furor uterinus: *Gratiol.*
Spasm of the glottis, with agony: *Amm. carb., Ipec.*
Suddenly something runs from the neck to the larynx and interrupts breathing completely; it wakens at night (spasm of the glottis): *Laches.*
Constriction in the region of the larynx, as from persimmons, going from side to side, and extending to the articulations of the jaw: *Mercur.*
Pressure of swelling of throat on windpipe causes anxiety: *Natr. sulph.*
Touch of throat causes anxiety: ‖*Laches.;* in mania: *Canthar.*
Larynx much affected, voice weak and hoarse; anxiety and the greatest irritability: *Hepar s. c.;* tickling in larynx, as from dryness, and burning in throat, with anxious constriction; raises but little mucus: *Mezer.*
Croup, with anxiety: *Spongia,* and all other croup medicines.
Heat and dryness in windpipe, with irritability: *Petrol.*
Inclination to burst into tears, with choking in the throatpit: *Cotyl.*

VOICE.

Voice louder and speech bolder: *Angust.;* with bold speech and bright eyes, cold sweat on the forehead and imperceptible pulse: *Acon.*
Speaks little and says single, disconnected words with difficulty in a higher pitch: *Stramon.*
Cannot modulate the voice, it is higher and finer, sometimes a mere sound, and he cannot utter a distinct word; anxiety: *Stramon.*
High squeaking voice, with rage: *Stramon.*
Hoarse and anxious in the evening: *Graphit.;* with crying and lamenting: *Bromum;* with stupor in the morning: *Stramon.;* and very weak: *Laches.;* with anxiety and irritability: *Hepar s. c.*
Speaks only in a low voice, is sad and dispirited: *Ol. anim.;* very soft voice after dinner, with sadness and ill humor: *Ol. anim.;* with derangement: *Phosph. ac., Viol. od.*
Voice weak: *Staphis.;* scarcely audible, refuses to talk: *Veratr.;* tremulous, with whining: *Cuprum.*
Inability to speak loud, very much affected: *Amygd.*
Loss of voice, with hypochondriacs: *Sulphur;* with anxiety: *Stramon.;* during the night hoarse, during the day —, with anxious sweat: *Carb. an.;* in the morning, after crying, with fear: *Hepar s. c., Lepid.;* with confusing thoughts: *Cannab.;* with weeping: *Mercur.;* crying: *Stramon.*
Now and then his voice fails, or he cannot find the right words: *Cannab.*
Talking. Hastily: *Acon., Mercur., Phosph. ac.;* excited: *Ambra.*
When talking, anxiety: *Ambra;* nausea: *Alum.;* — and palpitation when in society: *Platin.;* — and torment, with pain in back: *Cannab.*
Speaks hesitatingly and slowly, or hastily and anxiously: *Arsen.*

Affected by talking: *Amm. carb., Calc. ostr., Kali carb., Sulphur, Lauroc.;* makes restless: *Borax;* fatigued, weary: *Jacar.;* exhausted: *Stannum.*

Talking is difficult, dragging and low from immobility of tongue and lips: *Carb. an.*

Great heat from 10 P.M. until midnight, with short breathing; she wanted to cough but could not, and *talking* was very difficult; great restlessness, screamed on account of pains in the hands, feet, abdomen and back; she stamped her feet and would not allow herself to be touched: *Acon.*

Talks slowly because recollection is slow: *Thuya.*

Talking makes confused: *Aurum;* unconscious: *Kali carb., Nux mosch.*

<small>Acon.
Agar.
Bellad.
Cannab.
Carb.sulph.
Capsic.
Coccul.
Crocus.
Cuprum.
Hyosc.
Hyperic.
Lycop.
Mar. ver.
Natr. carb.
Natr. mur.
Opium.
Phosphor.
Platin.
Spongia.
Stramon.
Tabac.
Therid.
Veratr.</small>

Singing. Inclination to sing: *Bellad.,* 11*Crocus, Natr. carb., Natr. mur., Platin., Stramon.,* and laugh: *Crocus, Stramon.*

Cheerfulness, with inclination to sing: *Carb. sulph.*

Feels an irresistable desire to sing, with excessive hilarity for a while, thereupon absent-minded and indisposed to do any kind of work: *Spongia.*

Sings involuntarily: *Lycop.;* a single note creates the desire: *Crocus.*

Almost irresistible desire: *Mar. ver.;* amounting to mania: *Coccul.*

With insanity: *Bellad., Cuprum, Hyosc., Stramon., Veratr.*

In mania or derangement of mind, singing, incoherent speech, laughing, crying, screaming, inspired talking, and moaning: *Stramon.*

Happy, very joyous and merry: *Acon., Cuprum, Natr. mur., Spongia, Therid., Veratr.*

Obscene things: *Stramon.;* love songs: *Hyosc.;* love-sick songs: *Opium.*

Alternating with weeping: *Stramon., a.m.m.*

Senseless talk followed by singing, then fearful screaming and gasping for air: *Hyper.*

Sings, although the head is internally hot: *Therid.*

In fever, during the hot stage and the sweat: 11*Bellad.*1, 1*Stramon.*1, 1*Veratr.*1*;* during the heat alone: 1*Mar. ver.,* 1*Sarsap.;* the sweat alone: 1*Crocus,* 1*Kali carb.,* 11*Spongia.*

In delirium: *Bellad., Cannab., Coccul., Cuprum, Hyosc., Stramon., Veratr.;* in typhoid delirium, with whistling or laughing: *Stramon.*

All day long: *Tabac.;* most towards evening and at night: *Veratr.;* in sleep: *Bellad., Crocus, Phosph. ac.*

Warbling: *Acon., Bellad., Capsic., Coccul.;* in an undertone: *Natr. carb.;* merry: *Phosphor., Therid., Veratr.*

MODEL CURE.

A soldier had measles, exposed in camp; now had bronchitis from exposure, etc.; became delirious; got up from his bed and would put on his clothes to go home; violent talking; kept every body else awake all night; only during the night a good deal of expectoration and debility. *Cupr. ac.*[3] was given and the paroxysm did not return.—J. C. MORGAN.

LAUGHING.

On p. 71 as the expression of an emotion, with symptoms following it, here, either as a function of the respiratory organs and its mental connections, or as a concomitant with other symptoms.

! Acon.
!! Alum.
Amm. carb.
Arnica.
!! Anac.
Asaf.
! Bellad.
Calc. ostr.
Carb. veg.
Cicut.
Conium.
!! Crocus.
!! Cuprum.
Eleis.
Graphit.
Hura.
! Hyosc.
Kali bichr.
Kreosot.
Laches.
Lepid.
Lycop.
Merc. per.
!! Natr. mur.
!! Nux mosch.
Opium.
Pedic.
Petiv.
!! Phosphor.
!! Platin.
Pulsat.
Sabad.
Sepia.
!! Stramon.
Tabac.
Tarax.
!! Veratr.
Verbasc.
Zincum.
Zinc. ox.
Zinc. sulph.

Much inclined to: *Cuprum, Graphit., Merc. per., Natr. mur., Tarax.*

Inclined to smile and jest: *Stramon.;* frequent laughter: *Bellad.;* constantly inclined to cheerful, —; disposed to —, with gay humor: *Merc. per.;* without a cause: *Tabac.;* without occasion: *Arnic.*

Bursts out in loud laughter: *Asaf., Bellad., Stramon.*

Immoderate laughing at every trifle: *Amm. carb., Carb. veg., Graphit., Zincum.*

Laughs at everything: *Hyosc., Lycop., Sabad.;* with gaiety: *Lepid., Verbasc.;* with constant flow of ideas: *Nux mosch.;* with mocking humor: *Pedic.*

Involuntary, loud, uncontrollable laughter: *Bellad., Crocus.*

Full of fun and laughter: *Cuprum;* laughs a great deal, incessantly, improperly: *Crocus.*

Laughing and singing: *Bellad.;* could not be made to utter a word: *Crocus.*

Disposition to laughing, joking and singing: *Petiv.;* dancing: *Tabac.;* foolish tricks: *Cicut., Opium.*

At serious stories: *Arg. nitr.;* at the saddest things: *Platin.;* with sadness, spasmodic symptoms: *Phosphor.*

Great hilarity about the saddest things and sadness and weeping about ridiculous things: *Platin.*

Involuntary laughing or crying, without the corresponding mood: *Sepia.*

Against her wish, while she is sad: *Phosphor.;* very easily made to laugh, yet is not lively: *Natr. mur.*

Aversion to laughing: *Ambra.*

Now serious, now inclined to laughter: *Nux mosch.*

Inclination to weeping and laughing at the same time: *Lycop.*

Disposed to laughing and whining: *Pulsat.*

Weeping alternating with laughing: *Acon., Aurum, Capsic., Conium, Sepia.*

Rapid alternation of laughing, weeping and singing: *Stramon.*

Laughing alternating with whining: *Veratr.;* loud laughing alternating with weeping: !!*Stramon.*

Now starts up impatiently and grinds teeth, now laughs merrily and sings: *Crocus.*

Loud laughing alternating with vexation or moaning and crying: *Stramon.*

Morose humor, followed by desire to laugh loud; very great ill humor, followed by loud laughing: *Stramon.*

After loud laughing a wild passion: *Stramon.*

Laughs to himself about cheerful ideas, with difficult thinking: *Sabad.*

Laughs quietly to himself: *Laches.*
A kind of mock laughter: *Stramon.*
Even when alone, with gaiety: *Eleis;* when anyone looks at her: *Lycop.;* about her singing: *Crocus.*
With derangement of mind, or with mania: *Bellad., Cicut., Crotal., Hyosc., Opium, Stramon., Veratr.;* spasmodic laughter, with mania: *Cuprum;* in a rage: *Stramon.*
With dilated pupils: *Crocus.*
Face hot and very red: *Cicut., Veratr.*
Laughing during the time she could not speak: *Stramon.*
Hysterical laughter after meals: *Pulsat.*
From tickling in pit of stomach: *Anac.;* in throat: *Stramon.;* from an irritation in stomach or the right hypochondrium: *Conium.*
Diaphragmitis, with delirium: *Stramon.*
Incessant, loud laughter, before catamenia: *Hyosc.;* with nymphomania: *Stramon.*
Immoderate laughter, in childbed: *Apis.*
Grasping with hands in air; with spasm of chest: *Stramon.*

Spasmodic Laughing. Now spasmodic laughter, now weeping: *Alum.*
In evening in bed, alternating with weeping: ‖*Alum.;* with spasmodic affections: *Bellad.;* with the greatest exhaustion, lying down immovable: *Calc. ostr.;* from the stomach: *Conium;* in mania: *Cuprum;* and weeping, with other spasmodic affections: ‖*Phosphor., Zinc. ox.*
Weakness of muscles of arms and hands: *Carb. veg.*
With debility and dilatation of pupils: *Crocus.*
With great prostration: *Conium, Crocus.*
Laughing in sleep: *Alum., Caustic., Crocus,* ❙*Lycop., Sepia, Silic.;* very loud: *Junc. eff., Kreosot., Lycop.;* in a dream: *Kreosot., Sulphur;* in the night: *Stramon., Veratr.*
At night, and weeping during the day: *Stramon.;* at 8 A.M., with gaiety: *Hura;* laughing in forenoon, in the evening grief: *Graphit.*
Without a cause all day: *Tabac.*
Remarkable laughter in the evening: *Cuprum, Natr. mur.*
In the open air: *Nux mosch.*
Chilliness in the head and limbs after laughing: *Hura.*
In typhus delirium, with singing, whistling: *Stramon.*
Delirium, with alternate laughing and whining: *Acon.;* pointing to masked people: *Opium;* before falling asleep: *Sulphur;* smiling face: *Veratr.*
As if tickled: *Stramon.;* irresistible, with a tickling all over: *Zinc. sulph.;* after tickling in pit of stomach: *Anac.*

<small>AS ADDITIONS TO PAGE 72.</small>

Tears come into her eyes: *Natr. mur.*
She looked as if she had been weeping: *Natr. mur.*
As if cold air passed out of left ear: *Millef.*
In hypochondriac region sensation: *Kali carb., Natr. mur., Platin.;* in abdominal region: ❙*Arsen., Conium.*
Hoarseness: *Calc. fluor.*
After a hard laugh spasmodic affection of chest: ❙*Arsen.*
Stinging under the ribs, left side, with loud laughter, with inhalation on right side: *Plumbum.*
When laughing dull pressure, like from a piece of wood: *Plumbum.*

SIGHING.

Remedies (left column):
- Acon.
- Act. rac.
- Aethus.
- Alum.
- || Amm. carb.
- || Ant. crud.
- Arg. nitr.
- | Arnica.
- || Arsen.
- || Bellad.
- Borax.
- Bryon.
- || Calc. phosph.
- Camphor.
- || Capsic.
- | Chamom.
- Cinch. off.
- | Coccul.
- Coffea.
- Colchic.
- Conium.
- Cotyl.
- Digit.
- Elais guin.
- || Euphorb.
- Evon. eur.
- Gran. cort.
- Graphit.
- Helleb.
- Hura bras.
- || Hydr. ac.
- | Hydroph.
- | Ignat.
- | Ipec.
- || Laches.
- Magn. carb.
- Millef.
- Mur. ac.
- || Natr. carb.
- Nux vom.
- Nuc. v. c.
- || Opium.
- Pæon. off.
- Plumbum.
- || Pulsat.
- Ran. scel.
- | Rhus tox.
- Sassaf.
- Sarsap.
- | Secale.
- Sepia.
- || Silic.
- | Stramon.
- Sulphur.
- Tabac.
- || Thuya.
- Vip. red.
- Veratr.

Mind. Relieves oppression of chest: *Hydroph.;* relieves melancholy during pregnancy: *Laches.*

Has to take from time to time a deep, sighing breath, which relieves: *Ant. crud.*

Constant sighing, with sadness; prostration: *Natr. carb.*

Quiet sadness and inner grief: *Ignat.;* lowness of spirits with sighing: *Cotyl.*

Cannot speak aloud, much depressed: *Sulphur,* and groaning from low spirits: *Chamom.;* with anxiety: *Plumbum, Digit.;* anxious breathing: *Acon.;* cardial anxiety: *Colchic.;* fear of death: |*Rhus tox.*

Sighing deep and loud about imagined cares: *Sepia.*

Feels grieved, troubled with it: *Act. rac.*

Disposed to weep, with melancholic depression: *Natr. carb., Sassaf.;* sighing, profoundly depressed, cannot speak loud: *Sulphur.*

From ill humor: *Chamom.;* worse when consoled: *Cinch. off.*

With restlessness, drives from place to place: *Tabac.*

Involuntarily, with moaning and groaning: || *Helleb.;* without pains: *Alum., Graphit.,* | *Nuc. v. c.;* without cause: *Bellad., Nux vom.;* with apathy: *Ignat.,* || *Ipec.,* | *Stramon.;* unconsciousness: | *Coccul.,* | *Ipec.,* | *Stramon.;* stupefaction: *Helleb., Ipec., Plumbum,* | *Stramon.*

Chest and Breathing. Long sighing breathing: *Opium;* gives often a deep sigh: *Silic.;* has to take a deep inhalation, chest is too full, too narrow: *Pæon. off.*

Sighing, groaning, grasping the throat with his hands: *Stramon.*

From fulness in chest: *Ant. crud.*

From congestion of blood to lungs: *Acon.*

As if chest was too narrow: *Conium;* fulness, anxiety and constriction of chest: *Arg. nitr.*

With pain in chest: *Conium.*

Melancholy, with oppression: *Sassaf.;* with pressure on chest, in fever: *Laches.*

Anxious, difficult breathing: |*Acon.;* dyspnœa: *Elais guin.*

Sighing breathing with in and exhalation: *Bryon., Ignat., Ipec.;* with slow exhalation: *Borax.*

Desire to take a long breath, followed by sighing expiration, which relieves for a moment the oppression: *Cinch. off.*

Other Functions. With heartache: *Hydroph.*

With gnawing in stomach: *Eup. purp.*

After eating, during the afternoon: *Ant. crud.;* after dinner with precordial anxiety; feeling of being very ill: *Arg. nitr.*

With anxiety in epigastrium: |*Digit.*
After convulsions: *Plumbum.*
With whining and fainting of new-born children: *Millef.*
With prostration, constant sighing and sadness: *Natr. carb.;* with restlessness, driving about: |*Tabac.*
In sleep: *Bellad.*, and after awakening: *Pulsat.*, and murmuring: *Camphor.*, and moaning in restless sleep: *Opium.*
During anxious night-sweats: *Bryon.*
Sighing and groaning in fever, with heat as well as sweat according to B.: ||*Acon.*|, |*Arsen.*||, |*Bryon.*||, |*Chamom.*|, |*Coccul.*|, |*Ignat.*|, |*Ipec.*|, ||*Nux vom.*|, |*Rhus tox.*||, |*Sepia*|.
Heat alone: |*Arnic.*, ||*Bellad.*, |*Coffea*, ||*Pulsat.* ||*Thuya.*
Sweat alone: *Baryt.*, |*Cinch. off.*, |*Cuprum*, |*Phosphor.*, ||*Stramon.*, |*Veratr.*
And sobbing: *Secal.;* with moans: *Mur. ac.;* involuntary moaning and groaning: *Helleb.;* weeping: *Tabac.*
Deeply: *Calc. phosph.*, *Silic.*, and repeatedly: *Opium.*
Frequent sighing: *Hura, Ran. scel., Stramon.*
Involuntary sighing: *Calc. phosph., Helleb.*
Great weakness, no pain; is compelled to sigh: *Graphit.*

MODEL CURES.

After unhappy love, quiet, dreamy, no ambition to work, little desire to eat; sighs heavily as if visited by a great misfortune; at last becomes taciturn, takes no interest and refuses to eat or drink. Lies on the sofa with a painful expression on his face, sighing deeply. Nothing makes an impression on him, he scarcely says yes or no, looks drowsy and wears a sad smile on his face: *Hyosc.*—BETHMANN.

A young man, otherwise healthy, had for several months spells of sighing, deep breathing, about six deep inhalations at intervals of five minutes: *Ant. crud.*—W. W. TAFFTS.

MOANING AND GROANING.

With anxious restlessness: *Ant. tart.;* anxiousness and spasmodic laughter: *Alum.;* with anxiety and cramp in stomach at night: *Kali carb.*
With fear and hurry: *Laches.*
And tossing about in despair, with bellyache and headache: *Chamom.*
With ill humor: *Chamom.;* feels miserable: *Sarsap.;* without a cause: *Nux vom.*
Inconsolable; full of reproaches: *Nux vom.;* and beside himself: *Veratr.*
Violent weeping: *Alum.;* grunting: *Helleb.;* crying: *Eup. purp.;* and whimpering in epilepsy: *Coccul.*
Alternating with laughing: *Stramon.;* with jumping and dancing: *Bellad.*
Headache and crying for help: *Silic.;* whining from peevishness: *Zincum.*

MOANING AND GROANING.

Acon.
Alum.
Amm. carb.
Ant. tart.
Bellad.
Bryon.
I Calad.
Carb. veg.
Chamom.
Cicut.
Cina.
Coccul.
Colchic.
Cuprum.
Eup. perf.
Eup. purp.
Graphit.
Helleb.
Ignat.
Ipec.
Kali carb.
Laches.
Magn. carb.
Mercur.
Mur. ac.
Natr. carb.
Nitr. ac.
Nux vom.
Phosph. ac.
Pulsat.
Sarsap.
Sepia.
Silic.
Stannum.
I Stramon.
Veratr.
Zincum.

Eyes half open: *Phosph. ac.*
Face pale, body cool, child: *Ipec.;* — with crying and running about: *Veratr.*
Heat of face: *Chamom.*
Red hot cheeks: *Nux vom.;* hot sweat on forehead: *Chamom.*
Child will have a passage: *Pulsat.*
With every exhalation moaning: *Bellad.*
Constant moaning, with occasional shrieks, pacified only when holding chest pressed close to mother's breast: *Stramon.;* grasping throat with hands: *Stramon.*
With desire to take a long breath: *Carb. veg.*
Involuntary: *Alum.,* I I *Helleb.;* during the heat in face: *Chamom.;* with the pains: *Sarsap.;* without any cause: *Bellad.*
Inclination to it when fatigued: *Graphit.*
With spasms: *Cuprum, Stramon.;* jerks in hands: *Phosph. ac.;* tossing with arms and legs: *Stramon.;* restless motions, with brain affections of children: *Stramon.*
In sleep: *Bellad., Ignat., Sepia;* in first sleep: *Alum.;* in sleep during the day: *Cina;* with whining: *Chamom.;* with whimpering: *Mercur., Nitr. ac.,* I I *Nux vom.;* with lamentations and restless, tossing about: *Stramon.*
In morning: *Bellad.*
In cold stage of fever: *Eup. perf.;* cold hands: *Mercur.*
In fever: *Acon.;* crying and running about: *Veratr.;* with fever heat: *Pulsat.;* face pale, with crying and howling: *Ipec.;* in fever, delirium, red cheeks: *Chamom.;* red hot cheeks: *Nux vom.;* hot face: *Chamom.*

At night lying unconscious, with cold sweat followed by weakness: *Bryon.;* early when getting awake: *Amm. carb.*

With the pains: *Sarsap.,* a.m.m.

When child is being carried: *Pulsat.*

Sobbing: *Magn. phosph.;* and weeping: *Nux vom.;* is overcome by hearing of cruelties: *Caustic.*

Sobbing on wakening: *Cina, Secal.;* getting awake with — and weeping in the night: *Carb. an.*

After weeping, when alone, before an attack: *Conium.*

With weeping and twitching in hands and feet: *Thuya.*

And great dejection, with exhaustion: *Lob. infl.*

With ill humor: *Agn. cast.*

Sobs from anger, after irritation: *Stramon.;* with whining, after menses: *Stramon.*

From vexation and irritability: *Sepia.*

From listening to trials of others: *Caustic.*

And screaming, with hallucinations: *Stramon.*

With headache: *Stramon.*

Attacks at night: *Sec. corn.*

MIND AND DISPOSITION.

WEEPING, WHINING.

I Acon.
II Alum.
Amm. mur.
Amygd. am.
Ant. crud.
Argent.
Arnica.
II Arsen.
I Aurum.
Baryt.
Bellad.
II Borax.
II Bryon.
II Calc. ostr.
II Camphor.
Canthar.
Capsic.
II Carb. an.
II Carb. veg.
I Caustic.
II Chamom.
Cicut.
Cina.
II Coccul.
I Coffea.
Conium.
Crotal.
I Cuprum.
Digit.
Dulcam.
Graphit.
Helleb.
Hepar s. c.
Hura.
Ignat.
Kali carb.
Kreosot.
II Lycop.
Magn. mur.
Mercur.
Mezer.
II Natr. mur.
Nitr. ac.
II Nux vom.
Opium.
Pet. tetr.
I Petrol.
Phelland.
II Phosphor.
Phosph. ac.
I Platin.
Plumbum.
II Pulsat.
Rheum.
II Rhus tox.
Ruta.
Sabina.
I Sepia.
Silic.
Spongia.
Staphis.
Stramon.
II Sulphur.
Tabac.
II Veratr.
I Viol. od.

Weeps often: *Cuprum;* much disposed to it: II *Lycop., Natr. carb., Ruta;* involuntarily: II *Natr. mur., Platin., Rhus tox., Veratr.;* with an old woman: *Stramon.;* attacks she can scarcely suppress: *Sepia;* bursting into tears against her will: *Alum.;* even in the presence of strangers in the street: *Carb. veg.;* irresistible propensity to it: *Aurum;* without a cause: II *Bellad., Graphit., Kreosot.; Lycop., Staphis., Sulphur, Viol. od., Zincum;* causeless flow of tears: *Camphor.;* for nothing: *Staphis.;* does not know why: *Kali carb., Rhus tox.*

Abundant tears: *Crotal.;* must weep profusely: *Hepar s. c.*
Cannot cease weeping: *Carb. an.*

About trifles: *Calc. ostr., Caustic., Coccul., Petrol.,* and inconsolable: *Stramon.;* children weep at the least cause: *Nitr. ac.;* the slightest word makes her weep: *Silic.;* is set to weeping for a long time by the smallest trifles; the sight of everything surrounding him moves to tears: *Ant. crud.;* even joyous, laughable things: *Platin.;* if any one but looked at him: *Natr. mur.;* when spoken to kindly, after gentle reproaches: *Platin.;* when the least word is said to him: *Staphis.;* when any one does the slightest thing contrary to him: *Nux vom.;* when improper things are refused him: *Ignat.;* at slight disagreeable things: *Sulphur;* when disturbed in his work, 4 P.M.: *Pulsat.*

Child cries when touched: *Cina.*
Weeps when telling her symptoms: *Pulsat.*
While singing: *Hura.*

Great inclination to weep, with excitability: *Natr. mur.;* with uneasiness: *Alum.;* spirits much affected: *Amygd. am.;* piteous whining: *Opium;* with home-sickness: *Magn. mur.;* receiving thanks easily moved: *Lycop., Platin.;* overcome by hearing of cruelties: *Caustic.*

From sad thoughts: *Alum., Carb. veg., Cina, Phelland., Platin.;* in the evening: *Kali carb.*

Looks at the dark side of everything: *Alum.*
Sadness, can scarcely be quieted: *Sepia.*
Violent weeping, thinking of death; very sad: *Stramon.*
Depression: II *Rhus tox.;* melancholy: II *Phosphor., Pulsat., Stannum.*

Child is restless and anxious, wants this and that: *Kali carb.*
Anxiety ending with tears: *Kali carb.; Lycop.*
Great anxiety, impelled to weep: *Natr. mur.*

With anxiety and trembling: *Carb. veg.;* with apprehension: *Alum.;* frequent fits: *Graphit.;* apprehensions several afternoons: *Tabac.*

Loud lamenting, with apprehension; despair and bitter complaining: *Acon.*

WEEPING, WHINING.

As if she must die; inconsolable on being talked to, or sitting sadly in solitude: *Platin.;* inconsolability, bursts out in loud weeping: ||*Nux vom.;* inconsolable, anxious, heartache: *Spongia.*

Weeps about her weakness of thought: *Stramon.*

With despair: *Lycop.;* anxiety and sorrowfulness: *Sulph. ac.*

Sorrowful weeping, changes into impatient, violent howling: *Bellad.*

When thinking of evils long past: *Natr. mur.*

With fearfulness, as from grief and sorrow: *Amm. mur.*

From grief and woe: *Kreosot., Staphis.,* || *Veratr.*

Tears, with ennui: *Hura.*

Tired of life: *Aurum, Carb. veg., Lauroc., Ledum, Platin., Spongia.;* discouraged: *Baryt.*

Aloud, with vexation: *Sabin.;* crossness: *Staphis., Sulphur.*

Discontented and very much given to weeping: *Ruta.*

Is annoyed at it herself: *Platin.*

With moodiness: *Pulsat.;* on account of indignation: *Arsen., Sepia.*

Weeps aloud on mildly refusing her anything she wishes: on speaking much to her in mild words; on giving advice or doing anything else she does not wish: *Ignat.*

When in the least opposed: *Nux vom.*

From anger: *Bellad.;* cross and impetuous children: *Thea.*

With irritable humor: *Calc. ostr.;* and irritable temper: *Canthar.;* for vexation over pain: *Opium;* with impatience: *Acon.;* aloud; peevishness: *Sabin.*

On being reproved: *Calc. ostr., Platin.;* if one only attempts to speak to her: *Staphis.*

On surmising to be pitied: *Natr. mur.*

Imagines to have lost the affection of others: *Aurum.*

After scolding or reproaching, howling and weeping aloud: *Nux vom.;* when alone: *Conium;* about the thoughts which crowd upon her when alone: *Natr. mur.*

Cares for no one, does not want to listen to anything: *Staphis.*

And praying at night: *Stramon.;* and longing for death: |*Aurum.;* would like to die on the spot: *Spongia;* creeps into a corner: *Camphor.;* with dislike to work: *Natr. mur.*

With restlessness: *Chamom.;* anxious restlessness, driving from place to place: *Carb. veg.*

After hallucinations: *Dulcam.;* tearful fantasies: *Acon., Dulcam., Lycop.*

Head. After mental emotions, with a feeling of lightness in the head: *Kreosot.;* headache with weeping: *Coloc., Ferr. magn., Kreosot., Phosphor., Platin., Ran. bulb., Sepia;* pressing pain in the top of the head: *Zincum.*

Involuntary weeping, hanging the head: *Veratr.*

Eyes. Weeping after affecting poetry, with pain in the eyes; *Laches.;* weeping mood, with burning of eyes, running of tears: |*Nux mosch.*

Staring, pupils dilated: *Stramon.;* red: *Borax;* sensation of dryness: *Natr. mur.;* itching after weeping: *Sepia.*

Ears. The sound of churchbells moves to tears: *Ant. crud.*
From hearing music: *Graphit., Kreosot., Nux vom.*
Nose. With nosebleed: *Nitr. ac.*
Face. Hides her face and weeps aloud: *Staphis.*
Tearful expression: *Phosph. ac.;*
Stomach. Loss of appetite after weeping: | | *Coccul.;* after dinner: *Magn. mur.*
Causes pain in cardiac region: *Spongia.*
Abdomen. Over inanimate objects not about living beings, with burning in abdomen: *Capsic.*
With rumbling: *Rhus tox.*
Catamenia. Before and first day, with raving: *Lycop.;* after, with hiccough and whining: *Alum.;* whining and sobbing after menses: *Stramon.*
Chest. Inclined to weep, with pain in forehead and constriction of the throat: *Laches.*
Tremulous voice, in mania: *Cuprum.*
Whining and quick breathing: *Cuprum;* breathing labored and short: *Ant. crud.*
With oppression of chest: *Hura;* constriction: *Tabac.*
After coughing: *Arnic.;* children, during nocturnal cough: *Sulphur;* weeping mood and screaming with the cough: *Osmium.*
Nervous Conditions. Great bodily restlessness: *Sulphur.*
Children with neuralgia: | | *Chamom.;* anxious tossing about in bed: *Camphor.*
With trembling and anxious sweat: *Arsen.;* with trembling, sighing and prostration: *Natr. carb.*
With hysterics: | *Viol. od.*
Spasmodic: *Bellad., Ignat., Laches., Natr. mur.;* tendency to start: *Hura.*
With anxiety, in chorea: | *Cuprum.*
Sleep. Weeping in sleep: | *Caustic.,* | | *Kali carb.,* | | *Natr. mur.,* | *Pulsat.;* aloud: *Rhus tox.; Thuya.*
Anxiety: *Nux vom.;* weeping, incessant; throws herself anxiously about in bed: *Camphor.*
And growling: *Lycop.;* and howling: *Chamom.*
With moaning and groaning: | | *Alum.;* moaning and howling: *Silic.*
Wakens: *Cina;* before midnight: *Alum.;* towards morning: *Kali hydr.*
With nightly cough and great restlessness: *Sulphur.*
On awaking from sleep: *Bellad.;* a long time on awaking in the morning: *Pulsat.;* with sadness when awaking: *Carb. an.*
In the morning in bed, with ill humor: *Pulsat.;* after a night of anxiety: *Spongia;* on awaking from a dream, could not stop his tears for fifteen minutes or more, in the morning: *Phosphor.;* with sadness and involuntary tears, in the morning: *Petiv.;* with inconsolable grief: *Phosphor.;* with vexation: *Kreosot.*
Time. Weeping in the morning: *Pulsat., Kreosot., Magn. sulph.;* morning and evening: *Sulphur;* in forenoon: *Sarsap.*
Anxious for the future, worse every day at 6 P.M., with sadness, weeping

does good: *Digit.;* given to weeping in the evening: *Calc. ostr.;* with grief: *Graphit.;* terrified: *Carb. an.*

All night, during the day laughing: *Stramon.*

All day: *Bryon., Lycop.*

For weeks: *Alum., Mezer.*

Goes in the open air to weep: *Hura;* worse in-doors, better out-doors: *Platin.*

With heat and anxiety: *Spongia;* with pains: *Nux vom.;* distresses herself about a pain till she weeps: *Opium.*

Weeping and Sobbing: *Carb. an., Caustic., Conium, Natr. carb.;* aloud: *Nux vom., Stramon.*

Weeping and Howling, Crying or Wailing: *Acon., Alum., Chamom., Cicut., Coffea,* ❙❙*Lycop., Natr. carb., Natr. mur., Opium, Pulsat.*

And howling, with broken sentences: ❙❙*Arsen.;* with hiding in corners: *Camphor.;* first over the past, then over future ills: *Lycop.;* sees everything in a bad light: *Natr. carb.;* after scolding or reproaches: *Nux vom.*

Alternating with Laughing: *Aurum,* ❙*Bellad.,* ❙❙*Capsic., Lycop., Nux vom.,* ❙❙*Platin.,* ❙*Pulsat., Sepia, Stramon., Sulphur.*

Spasmodic laughter and weeping: *Phosphor.*

Alternating with queer antics: *Cuprum.*

With irritability and laughing at trifles: ❙❙*Graphit.*

Children, who are now vexed, then laughing: ❙❙*Borax.*

Fearfulness: *Graphit.;* anxiousness: *Digit.;* irritability: *Platin.*

Weeping relieves: ❙❙*Anac., Digit., Graphit., Ignat.,* ❙*Lycop.,* ❙❙*Mercur., Nitr. ac.,* ❙❙*Phosphor.,* ❙*Platin.,* ❙❙*Tabac.*

Discontented with himself, dissolving into vehement weeping and relieved thereby: *Nitr. ac.;* deems the world terrible: *Phosphor.;* woful sadness: *Tabac.*

Oppression of the chest: *Anac.*

MODEL CURES.

A simple catarrhal cough with a delicate little girl, a year and a half old, became spasmodic with twitches of the fingers, *weeping and screaming,* and dryness of the larynx: *Osmium.*—LIEDBECK.

A woman, æt. 36, with insanity, has lectrophilie, red burning face, anxiety, hopelessness, despair, continual moaning and screaming without a cause. Does not eat or drink, is sleepless. Brought on by sexual excitement: *Veratr.*— —SCHUELER.

CRYING AND SCREAMING.

| Acon.
Aurum.
| Bellad.
| Borax.
Bryon.
Calc. ostr.
| Canthar.
Carb. an.
Castor.
| Caustic.
❙ Chamom.
Cicut.
Cinch. off.
Coccul.
| Coffea.
Crocus.
❙❙ Cuprum.
Elaps.
Hura.
❙ Hyosc.
Hyper.
| Ignat.
| Jalap.
Kali carb.
❙❙ Lycop.
Magn. carb.
Mercur.
Nitr. ac.
Nux vom.
❙❙ Opium.
| Phytol.
Platin.
Pulsat.
Ran. scel.
Rhus tox.
Seneg.
| Sepia.
| Silic.
❙❙ Stramon.
Sulphur.
| Veratr.

Whimpering: *Arnic., Phosph. ac.;* very loud: *Aurum;* with timidity: *Ipec.;* and bending head back: *Rheum;* head and arms in motion: *Hyosc.;* with quick breathing: *Cuprum,* during sleep in the daytime: *Anac.;* third hour after midnight: ❙*Arsen., Bryon.*

Crying and whimpering: *Aurum,* ❙*Chamom.,* ❙❙*Hyosc.,* ❙*Ignat., Mercur., Nitr. ac., Nux vom., Veratr.*

Crying like a child: *Cuprum;* irresistible desire to cry out: *Elaps;* horrible cries, in mania: *Stramon.*

Crying, singing, laughing and speaking: *Stramon.;* screams, sings and moves hands; shrieks, attempts to escape, mental derangement: *Stramon.;* children run away, with a violent, fearful scream: *Stramon.*

In attacks, with anxiety: *Cuprum.*

Lamentations and melancholy: *Stramon.*

She imagines she sees a dead person, and cries: *Hura.*

Loud shrieks, with an air of affright; body distorted: *Stramon.*

With high screeching, talked disconnectedly: *Stramon.*

Cries with bellyache, pain in limbs, headache, and after the slightest touch: *Cuprum;* cries with pain in stomach: *Phytol.*

Screaming about growling in abdomen from living animals: *Stramon.*

Shrill cries, with catamenia: *Cuprum.*

Shrieked violently during fits, voice hoarse: *Stramon.*

Would like to scream, but could not on account of phlegm: *Stramon.*

With spasms in the chest interrupting breathing, loud crying or whimpering: *Stramon.;* difficult breathing, with screams: *Hyosc.*

Screams after stinging pain in pit of stomach: *Cuprum;* had to cry loud, several violent stitches in region of heart: *Rhus tox.*

Child screams day and night, whooping cough: *Stramon.*

With spasms, periodical: ❙❙*Cuprum.*

Screaming and howling all night; uttering crowing screams, tossing about in bed; scream interrupts sleep: *Stramon.*

Crying, with fever heat and sweat: ❙*Bellad.*❙❙, ❙❙*Chamom.*❙, ❙*Cuprum*❙❙, ❙❙*Lycop.*❙, ❙❙*Opium*❙❙, ❙❙*Platin.*❙❙, ❙*Stramon.*❙; with the heat alone: ❙❙*Acon.,* ❙*Bryon.,* ❙*Capsic.,* ❙❙*Coffea,* ❙*Ipec.,* ❙*Pulsat.,* ❙*Veratr.;* with the sweat alone: ❙*Arnic.,* ❙*Calc. ostr.;* ❙*Camphor.,* ❙*Phosphor.,* ❙❙*Rheum.*

Utters a sharp cry now and then, especially when shaken: *Stramon.*

IN AND EXHALATION.

During a sort of asthma, with precordial anxiety hindering inhalation: *Ferrum.*

With every inhalation a stitch in heart, with anxiety: *Plumbum.*

Pain in the epigastrium, worse when inhaling, with anxiety in the chest: *Moschus;* anxious constriction and oppression of chest, most when inhaling; anxious and trembling palpitation: 11 *Calc. ostr.*

Slow and very difficult inhalation; exhalation relieving: *Staphis.*

Able to inspire but not to expire, with anguish; infants awaking at night with it: *Sambuc.;* quick palpitation, with anxiousness after exhalation: *Aurum;* sighing exhalation lessens anxiousness in chest: *Cinch. off.;* with every exhalation a moan: *Bellad.*

NOTE.—Dogs when getting mad have a peculiar bark ending in a howl; the same was observed after dogs had been bitten by rattlesnakes.

SHORT BREATHING.

Short and anxious: *Nux vom.;* with trembling: *Opium,* and depression: *Laches.,* and restlessness: *Prun. spin.*

With great expansion of chest: *Opium.*

Short and labored with sorrowful humor: *Ant. crud.;* with abdominal anxiousness in the morning: *Bryon.*

In all positions: *Arsen.*

In the evening until he can succeed in getting a long breath, which relieves: *Stannum.*

With crawling and thirst: *Capsic.;* with fever heat, could not cough: *Acon.;* with burning heat and starting in sleep: *Lycop.;* anxiety with profuse sweat: *Mangan.*

Breathing labored and short, sorrowful humor: *Ant. crud.*

With painful distension of the abdomen, anxious breathing, has to loosen the clothes; eructation, rumbling, difficult passage of loud flatus and chilliness, with yawning: *Mezer.*

Short breath, with anxiousness: *Bellad.*

Quick Breathing. With anxiety: *Seneg., Squilla.*

Attempting to exercise the mental faculties increases the depression and occasions rapid respiration with a feeling of great anxiety: *Plant. maj.*

Rapid, audible breathing and palpitation, with anxiety and peevishness: *Veratr.*

Respiration 140 in a minute, excitement: *Stramon.*

On awakening has to sit up and breathe quickly, as if suffocating, with weeping: *Sambuc.;* — and whining: *Cuprum;* — fretfulness: *Veratr.*

Anxious, wave-like sensation coming up from the abdomen, causing quick breathing: *Rhodod.*

SLOW, LABORED, PANTING BREATHING.

Slow, with depressed spirits and slow pulse: *Secal.;* — cannot be urged to speak: *Ignat.;* laborious, with snoring, rattling and loss of senses: *Morphin.;* stertorous, — and dull-minded: *Opium;* snoring and blue face: *Opium,* and wheezing: *Sambuc.*

Panting and anxious: *Camphor., Plumbum;* — dislike to business; irresolution; beside himself: *Pulsat.;* gasping and inconsolable: *Pulsat.*

DEEP INHALATION.

Inclined to take a long breath, with depression and sadness: *Al. p. s.*

As if the thorax could not be expanded, with inward restlessness and palpitation: *Acon.*

With dullness in head and shuddering: *Sepia;* with anxiousness: *Capsic.*

From restlessness; sighing exhalation which relieves: *Cinch. off.*

A deep inhalation relieves shortness of breath and anxiety: *Stannum;* better from deep breathing, anxiety, with weight in breast: *Rhus tox.;* breathes with difficulty, sometimes very deeply: *Rhus tox.*

With fearfulness and inner heat: *Phosph. ac.*

After stitches in chest thinks it impossible to cough or take a deep breath: *Psorin.*

Fearfulness, anxiety and pressure in the epigastrium, worse after deep inhalation: *Natr. mur.*

Breathing causes a pain in the liver, also worse from touch, with the greatest ill humor and white stools: *Calc. ostr.*

With mania after fright and mortification: *Opium.*

Deep, slow breathing and aversion to talk: *Ignat.*

Constriction of chest and anxious feeling in throat; has to take a deep breath: *Cannab.*

Better from deep inhalations: *Cinch. off., Rhus tox., Sepia,* I*Stannum.*

MODEL CURE.

Since a great fright asthmatic attacks after mental emotions or lifting arms over head, every day during catamenia; at all times short breathing, *has to take a deep breath,* walking fast or going up stairs makes her breathing short; clothing oppressive over the pit of stomach. During the attack she has to lie down; begins with hiccoughing, draws chest together, cannot speak a word, cannot get a single good breath; respiration incredibly short, sometimes *with a gasping sound,* chest does not move, convulsive motions of the muscles; face red, puffed, covered with hot sweat; mesmeric application of the hand on the pit of stomach shortens the attack, great exhaustion remaining: *Cuprum.*—W. GROSS.

IMPEDED BREATHING, WITH ANXIETY AND OTHER CONCOMITANTS.

!! Acon.
Aethus.
!! Agar.
!! Aloes.
Alum.
Al. p. s.
!! Ambra.
!! Amm. carb.
Amm. gumm.
!! Anac.
!! Arnica.
!! Arsen.
! Ars. hydr.
Asaf.
Aurum.
! Bellad.
!! Borax.
!! Bromum.
! Calc. ostr.
! Calc. phosph.
! Carb. veg.
Chelid.
Cimex.
!! Coccul.
! Crot. tigl.
Cuprum.
Gelsem.
Ginseng.
! Hepar s. c.
!! Ignat.
! Ipec.
Jatroph.
!! Jodum.
! Lact. vir.
!! Lauroc.
Lycop.
Mercur.
Mezer.
Mygale.
Natr. mur.
Nitrum.
!! Nitr. ac.
!! Nux vom.
Ol. anim.
Opium.
Phelland.
Phosphor.
Phosph. ac.
Platin.
!! Plumbum.
Psorin.
Pulsat.
Ran bulb.
! Rhus tox.
Ruta.
! Seneg.
!! Silic.
!! Spigel.
! Spongia.
Squilla.
Stannum.
Stramon.
Sulphur.
Tabac.
Thuya.
!! Veratr.

Mind. Sadness: *Tabac.*; melancholy all day: *Lauroc.*; apprehension: !! *Tabac.*; impatience: *Cinch. off.*; fretfulness: *Spongia*; relieved by weeping: *Tabac.*; much disposed to weep: *Thuya*; spasmodic crying: *Thuya*; obtuse mind: *Opium*; forgetfulness: *Guarœa*.

Headache: *Arnic.*; violent pressing together in occiput: *Nitrum*.

Eyes. Fear of the slightest darkness, it suffocates her: *Aether*; involuntary shutting of eyes (spasmodically), tears bursting out: *Spongia*; eyes broken, full of water: *Opium*.

Nose. Stopped up, can only breathe with mouth open: *Amm. carb.*

Throat. Spasmodic constriction: *Sarsap.*; impeded swallowing: *Nitrum*; oppressed breathing as from stomach upward into throat, anxiety, restlessness, bad conscience, or as if something was going to happen: *Ignat.*; anxious soreness, particularly at night: *Zincum*; attacks of anxiety: *Spongia*.

Thirst. For water: *Thuya*.

Greatest aversion to fluids: *Mercur.*

After eating, dysphagia: *Merc. subl.*; gagging: *Laches*.

Scrobiculum. Anxiety: *Ferrum, Stramon.*; pressure: *Natr. mur.*; deep in: *Rhodod., Sumbul*; often repeated: *Guaiac.*; spasmodic throbbing: *Chelid.*; sudden drawing together: *Sulph. ac.*; swollen: *Carb. an.*; the same in region of stomach: *Guaiac.*

Hypochondria. Drawing and dull stitches along the cartilages of the short ribs: *Rhodod.*

Abdomen. With pain in lower part of abdomen: *Arnic.*

Caused by incarcerated wind: *Carb. veg.*

Griping, as if the intestines were tied up in a knot: *Spigel.*

Great distention of abdomen felt in the throat: *Magn. mur.*

Difficult passage of loud flatus: *Mezer.*; emission of flatus relieves: *Spigel.*

Cough. Violent, difficult expectoration: *Carb. an.*

Chest. With insupportable sore feeling, causing spasmodic fits of weeping and screaming, returning daily from 4 to 5 P.M.: *Thuya*; with pain in the chest: *Guarœa*.

And restlessness, spasmodic sensation of fulness: *Gelsem.*

Pressure: *Sulphur*; with fearfulness: *Calc. phosph.*; lightness, with pressure and anxiety: *Laches*.

Heavy and full feeling, as if the chest could not be expanded: *Acon.*; as from a weight on the chest: *Aethus*.

With a feeling as if the chest expanded: *Stannum;* commotion of the chest: *Arsen.;* with constant nausea: *Laches.*

With throbbing in the lower right chest: *Phosphor.;* with sensation of warmth in the chest: *Ol. anim.*

Palpitation: *Acon., Cannab.*

Oppression of breath and palpitation from anxiety: *Platin.;* when going up stairs: *Nitr. ac.*

Attack in the night, as if she must die, audible beating of the heart, cold sweat and involuntary weeping: *Amm. carb.*

With fear of death and losing consciousness, trembling of limbs: *Platin.*

When taking a deep breath or holding it: *Spigel.*

As if the chest was too narrow, anxious and trembling beat: *Calc. ostr.*

Heart. With a drawing under left breast: *Nux vom.*

Cannot stay in bed, sensation as if heart was being squeezed off, objects around her seem to grow narrower and smaller, horrible visions in the dark: *Carb. veg.*

From pressure in the region of the heart: *Bellad.*

With dull stitches and pressure, relieved by motion: *Pulsat.;* with a stitch when inhaling, and rush of blood to the face: *Plumbum.*

Terrible anguish like death agony, great restlessness, ebullition, sensation as if suffocating: *Thuya.*

With sudden weakness, nausea, pallor, spasmodic closure of the eyelids through which tears force their way, will has no power over the muscles: *Spongia.*

Pulse. Accelerated, small and rapid: *Indium sulph.;* now slow, then fast: *Rhus tox.;* weak, scarcely perceptible: *Cinch. off.*

Outer Chest. With external pressure on sternum, worse when sitting bent: *Cinch. off.;* sweat: *Nitr. ac., Cina.*

Neck. Pain as if drawn by the hair, extends to shoulders: *Nitrum.*

Back. Sweat: *Nitr. ac.*

Upper Limbs. Trembling of arms and hands: *Opium.*

Motion, Rest and Position. Almost to suffocation when moving: *Calc. ostr.*

The chest is pressed together all around when sitting, moving or standing, a very unpleasant anxious feeling: *Menyanth.*

As if tightly laced, worse from walking: *Ferrum;* in the forenoon when standing: *Nitrum.*

And constriction when walking a little too fast: *Nitr. ac.*

As from fear when fatigued: *Arsen.*

Tightness when standing, with sweat on the chest: *Cina.*

A stitch between the shoulder-blades, worse while sitting: *Kali carb.*

Constriction, with restlessness, better from exhaling, worse when sitting, better when walking: *Staphis.;* cannot get breath while sitting, fear: *Aloes.*

Loses breath when climbing, gets anxious: *Aloes, Arsen.*

Sleep. With inclination to take a deep breath and yawning: *Lact. vir.;* starts from sleep and calls for help: *Hepar s. c.*

Wakes at 12 o'clock, has to take frequent deep respirations: *Ignat.;* after midnight, with anxiety: *Calc. ostr.;* with suffocative feeling, cannot breathe through the nose, pain in the chest: *Amm. carb.;* with constriction, has to sit up: *Lact. vir.;* with coldness: *Carb. an.*

Starts from sleep, with suffocative attack and trembling: *Sambuc.*

When waking in the night or in the morning anxiety, constriction and sweat: *Alum.*

Times of Day. Early in bed: *Natr. carb.;* in the morning: *Carb. an., Pulsat.;* 11 A.M. till 4 P.M.: *Nitrum;* 4 to 5 P.M. every day: *Thuya;* afternoon and evening: *Sulphur;* evening: ‖*Arsen., Phosphor., Stannum;* evening in bed: *Borax;* in the evening constriction, with restlessness: *Arsen.*

Out-doors. Has to leave the room and go into the air: *Lauroc.*

NOTE.—Anxiety and impeded breathing have no doubt been observed very often to drive out-doors, but it is neither mentioned in Materia Medica as appearing together, nor among the cures. This shows the importance of keeping an account of such cases, if any should be observed.

Heat, Sweat. Constriction, with inward anxiety and heat: *Anac.*

Attack of heat, with anxiety, as if the walls of the chest were pressed together: *Mercur.;* as if the chest was too narrow, with inward heat: *Phosph. ac.*

With warm sweat on the forehead: *Acon.*

Gradually increasing until sweat breaks out all over body: *Nux vom.*

Sweat after lying down, which relieves: *Sulphur.*

Tissues. In rheumatic fevers: *Laches.*

Difficult Breathing. With anxiety: *Acon.,* ‖*Arsen., Iodium, Mygale, Opium, Plumbum, Rhus tox.,* ‖*Spongia, Stramon.,* and constriction in chest: *Spigel.;* with fulness of it: *Crot. tigl.;* wakes with feeling of a load on it: *Phosphor.;* difficult and short, overcome by feelings to tears: *Ant. crud.*

Sensation of anxiousness in the chest: *Bromum;* around pit of stomach: *Cuprum;* with restlessness: *Asaf., Prun. spin., Rhus tox.;* with oppression and anguish: *Arsen., Asaf., Graphit., Platin.;* with anticipation of death: ‖*Lobel. infl.;* with apprehensiveness: *Rhus tox.;* from a distressing sensation in belly, with complaining mood: *Arsen.;* with expression of the deepest terror: *Gelsem.;* with fear of death: *Lobel. infl.;* despair: *Cuprum;* great alarm: *Spongia;* uneasy mind: *Rhus tox.*

With difficult comprehension: *Phosphor.;* dullness: *Kalmia.*

Sluggishness of mind and body: *Sepia;* dyspnœa, senses leave him: *Camphor.*

Mania: *Bellad., Mercur., Stramon.;* in delirium: *Hyosc.*

With cold face and hands and drops of sweat: *Opium.*

With great thirst: *Bellad., Cuprum,* ‖*Thuya.*

Worse when sitting idle: *Bellad.;* when walking and speaking: *Ferrum;* with bellyache and anxiousness: *Bryon.;* after stools colored by blood: *Kali carb.*

NOTE.—Oppression and constriction. See further on under "Chest."

THREATENING SUFFOCATION.

Anxiety. Takes the breath away: ∎*Arsen.*, *Lauroc.*, ∎*Phosphor.*, *Rhus tox.*, *Ruta;* in the highest degree: ∎*Veratr.;* as if in danger of suffocating: *Acon.; Agar.;* with a slow, difficult breathing, cannot inhale air enough, is afraid of suffocating: *Mezer.;* children with asthma: *Sulphur,* and chest as if too narrow, as if she could not get a breath: *Rhus tox.*

Choking Sensation, with fear of death: *Apis;* as if every breath was his last: *Oleand.;* as if dying, breath interrupted: *Ruta;* with great restlessness: *Gelsem.;* distraction of mind: *Camphor.;* frequent spells in mania: *Stramon.;* — in throat and out of spirits: *Iodium;* fretful and anxious: *Spongia;* with fright: *Sambuc.;* something warm rises in throat, shuts off the breath, remaining in windpipe: *Cannab.;* with anguish of heart: *Thuya.*

After eating, with a sensation of dysphagia, fear of suffocating: *Merc. subl.;* from pain in pit of throat, with distress: *Acon.;* with palpitation and flying heat: *Cannab.*

Interrupted breathing from an unbearable anxiety, an annoying sensation in abdomen; complaining bitterly: *Arsen.;* has to bend double and constantly change his position: ∎*Arsen.*

Wakening from a slumber, in which eyes and mouth had been open; could not get his breath, had to sit up, breathing then very rapid, with a whistling, as if he would suffocate, throwing about his hands, face and hands turned bluish and puffed up; body hot, without thirst; all such attacks without any cough: worst from 12 to 4 A.M., and when awake weeping before attack: *Sambuc.*

Suffocating jerks waking every few minutes from sleep, in hydrothorax: ∎*Lact. vir.;* starts, from below up as soon as he falls asleep, with cerebro-spinal meningitis, after a sun stroke in the nape of neck: ∎*Bellad.*

Gasping for air after a screaming spell: *Hyper.*

After Emotions and Exertion. With sadness: *Laches.;* hypochondric mood: *Lobel. infl., Sepia;* fear of death, as if he could not take another breath: *Apis.*

Dyspnœa after vexation: *Arsen., Chamom., Cuprum;* with icy coldness: *Thuya.*

Children extremely obstinate, throw themselves angrily on the floor when in the least opposed, and cannot get their breath: *Thuya.*

With downheartedness: *Pulsat.;* indolence: *Pulsat.;* mental inquietude: *Ambra, Hepar, Prun. spin., Pulsat.;* insanity: *Hyosc., Mercur.*

Talking, reading or writing improves constriction of chest: *Ferrum.*

When thinking, anxious breathing: *Phosphor.;* slow breathing during reflection: *Rhus tox.*

Asthma caused by mental emotion: *Cuprum, Sepia.*

Loses breath when thinking of old evils: *Sepia.*

MODEL CURE.

Fears he will be impelled to destroy his life, with asthma, midnight till morning, has to leave the bed. Eight successive nights: *Arsen.*^{2m}. One dose cured.—L. WHITING.

COUGH AND MENTAL CONCOMITANTS.

Pleasurable Feelings. Contented and cheerful in the morning: *Zincum.* Cheerfulness: *Carb. an., Cuprum, Ferrum, Verbasc.;* gaiety: *Carb. an., Cuprum, Ferrum, Verbasc.*

Painful Feelings. Gloominess: *Bromum;* sorrow: *Ignat., Staphis.;* sadness: *Ferrum, Mezer., Natr. mur.;* in the evening: *Zincum.*

With whooping cough; oversensitiveness of all senses: *Cuprum.*

Dejection: *Anac., Baryt., Caustic., Sepia;* depression: *Bromum, Cuprum, Jodum;* melancholy: *Caustic., Cepa, Digit, Jodum;* hopelessness: *Arsen., Carb. veg., Stannum,* — of recovery: *Acon., Bryon., Silic.*

|| Acon.
|| Anac.
|| Arnica.
|| Arsen.
| Baryt.
| Bellad.
|| Bryon.
|| Carb. veg.
|| Caustic.
|| Cina.
| Cinch. off.
| Chamom.
| Conium.
|| Cuprum.
| Digit.
| Droser.
|| Ferrum.
|| Hepar s. c.
| Hyosc.
| Ignat.
|| Jodum.
|| Ipec.
| Kali carb.
|| Laches.
|| Lauroc.
|| Lycop.
|| Magn. carb.
| Magn. mur.
| Mercur.
|| Mezer.
| Moschus.
|| Mur. ac.
| Natr. mur.
|| Nitr. ac.
|| Nux vom.
|| Phosphor.
| Pulsat.
| Rhus tox.
| Sabad.
|| Sambuc.
| Seneg.
| Sepia.
| Silic.
|| Spigel.
|| Spongia.
| Squilla.
|| Stannum.
|| Stramon.
|| Veratr.

Anxiety, Anguish and the Like. Apprehensions: *Caustic., Hyosc., Kali carb.*

Before attack of whooping cough, anxious: *Cuprum.*

Anxious sweat drives out of bed: *Silic.;* anxiety of pregnant women: *Conium;* fear of fainting: *Spigel.*

Full of care about household concerns: *Pulsat.;* concern about his health: *Sepia;* about the future: *Natr. mur.*

Dread of strangers: *Baryt.;* of men: *Baryt., Ignat., Lycop., Stannum.;* of ghosts: *Droser.;* of death: *Acon., Anac., Arsen., Bryon., Moschus, Nitr. ac., Pulsat., Squilla.*

Pangs of conscience: *Ferrum.*

Anguish in the chest: *Phosphor.;* in evenings: *Carb. veg.*

Whooping cough, with fear and terror: *Spongia.*

Premonition of death: *Acon.*

Seems to be beside himself: *Droser.*

Disposition to despise: *Arsen., Ipec.*

Despair: *Arsen., Bryon., Carb. veg., Silic., Stannum.;* of recovery: *Acon., Bryon., Silic.*

Grief: *Ignat., Lycop., Phosph. ac.;* weariness of life: *Silic.*

Mental Feelings. Earnestness: *Ambra;* seriousness, aversion to laughing: *Ambra;* indifference: *Cinch. off., Conium, Phosph. ac.;* complete apathy: *Cinch. off.*

Feelings and Conations. Sensibility: *Lycop.;* gentleness; yielding disposition: *Pulsat.;* irresolution, cowardice: *Baryt.;* captiousness: *Staphis.*

Despondency: *Anac., Baryt., Caustic., Sepia;* faint-heartedness: *Baryt., Silic.;* fearfulness: *Acon., Calc. ostr., Kali carb., Sambuc.,* at noise: *Sabad.*

Timidity: *Baryt., Chamom., Conium, Droser., Hyosc., Kali carb., Magn. mur., Mercur., Moschus, Phosphor., Pulsat., Sabad., Scilla, Silic.;* of pregnant women: *Conium;* during a thunder storm: *Glonoin., Phosphor.*

With a dry cough and evening fever, he worries his family with his bad humor: *Psorin.*

Aversion to business; ill humor: *Silic.;* captiousness: *Staphis.*

MIND AND DISPOSITION.

Moroseness: *Bellad., Ipec., Kreosot., Nux vom., Sepia, Stannum, Verbasc.;* in the evening: *Zincum.*

Obstinacy (especially in children): *Bellad., Calc. ostr., Droser., Mercur., Nitr. ac., Silic.,* ||*Spongia.*

Irascibility: *Anac., Baryt., Caustic., Ledum, Nux vom., Phosphor.*

Fault-finding disposition: *Arsen., Ipec.*

Quarrelsomeness: *Arnic., Caustic., Hyosc.;* peevishness, with indignation: *Staphis.;* fretfulness: *Bellad., Bryon., Carb. veg., Chamom., Kali carb., Kreosot., Natr. mur., Nitr. ac., Staphis., Sulphur, Veratr., Verbasc.;* impatience: *Dulcam., Ipec., Mercur., Sulph. ac.*

From being vexed: *Ant. tart., Chamom., Asar.*

Irritated condition: *Cinch. off., Hepar, Ipec., Kali carb., Lycop.;* irritability: *Bryon., Cinch. off., Kali carb., Natr. mur., Nux vom., Phosphor., Seneg., Sulphur.*

Irritability under insults: *Seneg.;* resentment long after insult: *Nitr. ac.*

Vehemence: *Bryon., Carb. veg., Ledum, Nux vom.*

If children get angry the coughing spell comes: *Ant. tart.*

Hatred of men: *Baryt., Ignat., Ledum, Lycop., Stannum.*

Joy at the misfortune of others: *Arsen.;* spitefulness: *Acon., Anac.*

Lack of moral feeling: *Anac.;* delight in mischief: *Arsen.* insatiability: *Pulsat.*

Conations. Loquacity: *Hyosc., Stramon.;* laughing: *Hyosc.;* humming and singing: *Spongia.*

Cough from weeping: *Ant. tart., Arnic., Bellad., Chamom., Droser., Hepar, Lycop., Phosphor., Veratr.*

Whooping cough, commencing with crying and tears, and then the paroxysms come on: *Arnic.*

Disposition to weep: *Ant. tart., Arnic., Baryt., Bellad., Calc. ostr., Carb. an., Caustic., Chamom., Conium, Digit., Hepar, Ignat., Lycop., Magn. mur., Mezer., Natr. mur., Osmium, Phosph. ac., Pulsat., Rhus tox., Spongia, Sulph. ac.*

Weeping: *Arnic., Arsen., Bellad., Cina, Hepar, Lycop., Sambuc., Silic., Sulphur, Veratr.*

During nocturnal cough, weeping, with restlessness: *Sulphur.*

Whooping cough with weeping: *Spongia;* whining: *Arsen., Cina;* complaining: *Laches.;* lamentations: *Acon., Arnic., Bromum.*

Crying out: *Ant. tart., Arnic., Bellad., Chamom., Cinchon., Ipec., Osmium, Phosph. ac., Sambuc., Sepia, Veratr.;* about bellyache before the cough begins: *Phosph. ac.*

Cough, with weeping mood and screaming: *Osmium.*

Yawning and screaming: *Opium.*

Howling: *Acon., Arnic., Bellad., Bromum, Chamom., Ipec., Stannum.*

Striking about one: *Stramon.*

Hastiness: *Hepar s. c., Sulphur;* of speech: *Hepar.*

Disposition to escape: *Hyosc.*

Will always be alone: *Baryt., Ignat., Lycop., Stannum.*

Solicitude: *Ignat., Staphis.*

Aversion to laughing: *Ambra.*

Introverted condition: *Euphras., Ignat., Lycop., Mur. ac.*
Unwilling to be alone: *Arsen., Droser., Mezer., Stramon., Verbasc.*
Cannot bear being spoken to: *Natr. mur., Silic.;* will not answer: *Ambra, Arnic., Euphras., Phosph. ac., Veratr.;* taciturnity: *Ambra, Arnic., Euphras., Phosph. ac., Veratr.*
Indisposition to play: *Baryt.;* aversion to work: *Ignat., Squilla.*
Keeping bed without necessity (lectrophilie): *Al. p. s.*
Exaltations. Intolerance of music: *Chamom., Phosph. ac.*
Excitability: *Bryon., Cinch. off., Kali carb., Natr. mur., Nux vom., Phosphor., Seneg., Sulphur.;* excitability under insults: *Seneg.;* excitement and anguish, with blood spitting: *Acon.*
Alternating states of mind: *Carb. an., Cuprum, Digit., Ferrum, Ignat., Sabad., Sulph. ac., Verbasc., Zincum;* changeable before cough, merry and gloomy: *Ferrum;* alternating states of mind every other evening: *Ferrum.*
Restlessness: *Acon., Arnic., Arsen., Bellad., Chamom., Dulcam., Laches., Lauroc., Mercur., Nux vom., Rhus tox., Sabad., Sambuc., Stramon., Sulphur, Sulph. ac.;* with tossing in bed: *Acon., Chamom., Cina, Ferrum, Mercur.;* with screaming and groaning: *Bromum.*
Terror: *Acon., Calc. ostr., Kali carb., Sabad., Sambuc.;* at noise: *Sabad.*
Full of projects: *Cinch. off.*
Cough, with tough mucus, delirium: *Veratr.*
Coughing phlegm up, with gagging and retching, in mania: *Bellad.*
Delirious talk, memory stronger: *Bellad.*
Claps her hands together above her head: *Bellad.;* and sings: *Veratr.*
Insanity: *Arnic., Bellad., Digit., Stramon., Veratr.*
Rage after insult: *Seneg., Stramon.*

MENTAL CAUSES AND CONDITIONS.

Hemorrhage of the lungs after excitement: *Acon., Opium.*
Emotions. Grief: *Ignat.;* indignation: *Arnic., Ignat., Staphis.;* after fright: *Acon., Ignat., Stramon.*
From anger: *Acon., Arsen., Bryon., Chamom., Cinch. off., Ignat., Nux vom., Sepia, Staphis., Veratr.;* with fright: *Acon., Ignat.*
Cough from laughing: *Argent., Bryon., Cinch. off., Cuprum, Droser, Kali carb., Mur. ac., Nitr. ac., Phosphor., Stannum, Zincum.*
Screaming, vexation and tossing about, with children: *Arnic.*
Consoling words displease, and excite cough: *Arsen.*
Mental excitement is followed by stitches in the throat, producing a cough: *Cist. can.*
Emotions increase coughing: *Laches.;* thinking of his cough increases it: *Baryt., Nux vom.;* brings it on: *Baryt., Ox. ac.*
Mental agitation increases the cough: *Cist. can.;* excitement: *Digit.*
Cough increased by every excitement: **Spongia.*
From reading and thinking: *Nux vom.*

PECTORAL ANXIETY.

Acon., Agar., Aurum, Calc. ostr., Lauroc., | *Lycop., Mercur.,* | *Mezer.,* | *Natr. mur.,* | *Nux vom., Phosph. ac., Plumbum,* | *Sulphur.* See pp. 83, 84.

In left side of chest: *Seneg.;* with fulness: *Merc. per.;* with a throbbing in lower right side: *Phosphor.*

Under the sternum: *Anac., Mercur.*

Rising from chest to head: *Acon.;* from abdomen to chest: *Bryon.*

Without suffering any pain, it is as if he could not remain in the room, had to go in the open air, and be very active there: *Anac.*

With vertigo, fainting and cold sweat: *Ignat.*

With pain in left occiput and neck: *Kali carb.*

With stoppage of nose: *Calc. ostr.*

With nausea: *Arnic.*

With pressure in left hypochondriac region and nausea in the chest: *Rhus tox.*

With dyspnœa: *Arsen., Phosphor., Pulsat., Rhus tox., Valer.;* after eating: *Carb. an.;* with inhalation: *Calc. ostr.;* short breath: *Bryon.*

With fulness of chest: *Capsic.;* has to take a deep breath: *Mercur.;* is worse after it: *Natr. mur.;* could not inhale deeply: *Tabac.;* feels as if suffocating: *Kali carb.*

Heart trembles: *Calc. ostr.;* pulse more frequent: *Pulsat.*

Worse from exercise, has to lie down: *Ferrum;* worse when resting: *Seneg.*

Getting better in the evening: *Zincum,* worse: *Kali carb., Phosphor.;* worse in the morning: *Bryon., Carb. an., Pulsat.;* after breakfast: *Valer.;* forenoon: *Ol. anim.;* with a cold chill: *Ol. anim.;* anxiety in attacks: *Platin.*

MODEL CURE.

A young blooming woman became, as often before, a violent attack of acute rheumatism. She was left with valvular troubles already after previous attacks. After metastasis of swelling to different joints the pains now principally affect the right wrist and shoulder; the index finger is considerably swollen. Stiffness particularly in the neck. Moaning and complaining about the pains; hopeless and despairing; gets but little sleep, which is broken by whimpering. With the attacks there is oppression and dyspnœa, with violent palpitation and inexpressible anxiety. *Acon.* relieved, but the spells returned. Before going to sleep she had a crawling and stinging sensation in the side of the throat. Soon after olfaction of *Laches.*[30] more quiet and improved. This was followed by an itching eruption on the left mammæ. Later there came a pain as if all the tendons were contracted. *Caustic.* completed the cure; she had no return of rheumatism after 1835.—C. HG.

A boy, æt. 9, after scarlet fever, during desquamation, sudden agony, has to sit straight up, can hardly breathe, pulse thread-like, vomituritio, sweats with anxiety; abdomen and particularly under the short ribs swollen: *Acon.* tinct., in water.—W. WILLIAMSON.

CONSTRICTION AND OPPRESSION, WITH ANXIETY.

Acon.
Aloes.
Alum.
Al. p. s.
Amm. gumm.
Anac.
ǁ Arnica.
Arsen.
Ars. hydr.
Ars. jod.
Asaf.
Aurum.
Calc. ostr.
Cimex.
Crot. tigl.
Cuprum.
Ginseng.
Glonoin.
Guaræa.
Ignat.
Jatroph.
Jodum.
Kali carb.
Lycop.
Mercur.
Nitr. ac.
ǁ Nitrum.
Nux vom.
Opium.
Ox. ac.
Phelland.
ǁ Phosphor.
Phosph. ac.
Platin.
ǀ Psorin.
Spigel.
ǀ Sulphur.
Tabac.
Veratr.

Oppression, with anxiety: *Aloes, Cimex, Jodum, Ox. ac., Phosphor., Psorin.;* beginning in right side of chest: *Acon.*

Chest constricted, with anxiety: *Alum., Aurum, Jatroph., Opium, Psorin., Sulphur, Veratr.;* with a sensation as if the throat was swollen: *Glonoin.;* with agony: *Ox. ac.;* with bad humor: *Cuprum.*

Oppression, with anxious breathing: *Nitr. ac.;* increasing to fear: *Asaf.;* with anxiety: *Guaræa, Phelland., Phosph. ac., Tabac.;* anguish: *Ars. jod., Jodum;* with restlessness, bad conscience and apprehension: *Ignat.*

Anxious and heavy: *Phosphor.;* oppression like a stone: *Al. p. s.;* with forgetfulness and painful chest: *Guaræa.*

After dinner: *Phosphor.,* one-half hour after: *Phelland.;* and quick pulse: *Natr. mur.*

With headache and colic: *Arnic.;* with a warm rising from pit of stomach to pit of throat: *Platin.;* a warm rising towards the heart: *Ant. tart.;* from pit of stomach upwards: *Ferrum.*

Crampy contraction: *Kali carb.;* and fear of suffocation, alternating with a cramp-like drawing in occiput and neck, has to bend the head backwards, has to scream: *Nitrum.*

In the night, with spasms of the chest, rising up from the small of the back into the region of the stomach and into chest (in childbed): *Lycop.*

Short breath, worse while sitting: *Calc. ostr.*

With fever heat: *Arnic.*

With other Mental Concomitants. Constriction, with apprehension: *Phelland., Phosph. ac.*

Oppression and apprehensiveness: *Tabac.*

Chest as if screwed together, with great fear: *Glonoin.*

Contraction of chest, with bad humor: *Cuprum.*

Oppressive feeling in chest, out of humor: *Sabin.;* and restless: *Ambra, Asaf., Psorin., Veratr.;* driving from place to place: *Staphis.*

Chest constricted, weeping: *Hura, Tabac.;* restlessness: *Ambra.*

Constriction, with delirium: *Bellad.*

Constriction, with forgetfulness: *Guaræa.*

PAIN IN CHEST WITH ANXIETY.

Painful anxiety of chest: *Arnic., Hydr. ac., Lauroc., Morph. ac., Rhus tox.;* which affects the whole body: *Natr. carb.;* pressure in pit of stomach: *Natr. mur.;* constriction there: *Arsen.*

Pain in chest, has to scream : *Kali carb.;* with the greatest anxiety, in spells : **I***Psorin.*

Pressure on chest, with anxiety: *Arnic., Calc. ostr., Capsic., Hyper., Sulphur.*

Pressure on right side of chest, causing anxiety : *Aurum, Bellad.;* near the ensiform cartilage and last true rib, with anxiety and oppression: *Hyosc.;* in the lower part of right chest, with anxiety and shortness of breath when going up stairs : *Hyosc.;* in left chest, in front : *Seneg.*

Pressing drawing pain across lower portion of chest while sitting, causing anxiety : *Cinch. off.*

Cutting pressure from within out in the chest, with anxiety: *Angust.*

Pressure and constriction in chest felt all over, with anxiety : **I***Sulphur.*

With earache and deafness : *Aloes.*

OTHER SENSATIONS IN CHEST, WITH ANXIETY.

Fulness : *Lact. vir., Carb. veg.;* heaviness : *Arnic., Laches., Phosphor., Prun. spin.;* as if compressed : *Phosphor.*

Tension and dullness in the left side of chest, with little jerks, palpitation and anxiety : *Cannab.*

Pressure and tension : *Ledum;* drawing pain : *Arnic.*

Cutting constriction: *Spigel.;* in the evening: *Stannum;* with restlessness: *Seneg.*

Cramp-like pain in the chest, with anxiety, wakens at night : *Sepia.*

Fine stitches in side of chest ; anguish : *Acon.;* stinging, with vexation : *Acon.*

Stitches as from a knife, in front into left chest and into back, in the night with great restlessness and tossing about: *Caustic.;* stitches in left side : *Phosphor.;* under the arm to epigastrium: *Caustic.;* stitches in chest cause anxious breathing : *Bryon.*

Throbbing in chest and epigastric region: *Acon., Conium, Ferr. ac., Phosphor.;* pulsation in chest, in different places : *Alum.*

Dull pulsations up the back, between the shoulder-blades, in rhythm with the heart-beats : *Calc. ostr.*

Ebullition causing anxiety: *Nux vom.;* anxious heat: *Bellad.;* ascending to the mouth, with restlessness and sleeplessness : *Nux vom.*

Blood seems to boil in his chest : *Anac.*

Burning, with dullness in head, as if he did not know where he is : *Chamom.;* with melancholy, weeping mood : *Hyper.*

Weakness in the chest: *Stannum.*

Chest as if wider, with sharp anxiety and palpitation : *Stannum.*

Emptiness, expansion : *Guarœa.*

Heat in stomach and chest: *Phosphor.;* warm ebullition : *Carb. veg., Nux vom.;* ebullition, with anxious dreams, screaming: *Pulsat.;* from the epigastrium to throat-pit : *Platin.*

SENSATIONS IN CHEST, WITH OTHER MENTAL SYMPTOMS.

Apprehensive sensation: *Glonoin.*
With pain in chest, hopeless, despairing: *Ant. tart.*
Restlessness and melancholy, with pain in side: *Kali bichr.*
Forgetfulness: *Guarœa.*
A peculiarly agreeable feeling of cheerfulness, with fulness: *Cinnab.*
Rush of blood to chest, congestion with every emotion, cramp-like contraction between the shoulder-blades: *Phosphor.*
Pain over the whole anterior wall of the chest, with marked hyperæsthesia, relieved by heat; extending next day to infrascapular spaces; imagines what is effected with regard to any object, is done in the same way to herself: *Amyl. nitr.*
Very disagreeable sensation of heat in chest, when walking out-doors: *Rhus tox.*
Congestion with excitement: *Asaf.;* with foreboding: *Anac.;* oppression and fulness: *Carb. veg.;* very much oppressed and heavy, like a stone on the chest: sadness: *Al. p. s.*
After dinner a feeling of great roughness on the chest, with a pressure in pit of stomach which makes him ill humored: *Natr. carb.*
Heavy feeling and trembling after starting up from half-slumber: *Strontian.*
Oppression and heaviness, with a feeling as if a voice within cried, "Woe! woe:" *Thuya.*
Tightness of chest, peevish about everything: *Chamom.*
Twisting or stitching pain as from a sharp instrument, in his chest, causing screams at night: *Hura.*
Speechlessness, with throbbing in the chest and an indescribable bad feeling: *Mancin.*
Restlessness and pulsation in the chest: *Bellad.*
Dull stitches in the left side of chest and abdomen, causing screams: *Chamom:, Ratanh.*
Inward trembling or shuddering in the chest, makes her irritable: *Natr. sulph.*
Burning and soreness rising from pit of stomach behind the sternum to the roof of the mouth, with great restlessness: *Mancin.*
Inward emptiness and cold sensation around the heart, with sadness: *Graphit.*
Chest-affection, with melancholy and weak feeling in head: *Hyper.*
Stitches in side of chest, morose: *Acon.*
With every breath stinging from the lowest rib on the right side to the point of the shoulder-blade, with complaining, weeping mood: *Acon.*
Stitches through the chest with moaning: *Psorin.;* through the side like knives, with loud moaning: *Conium.*
Fleeting stitches in the right side of chest, causing him to scream: *Baryt.*
Continued stitches in the left chest, causing screams, relieved by inhaling: *Sulphur.*

A violent stitch in the right side of chest, causing him to scream out: *Lauroc.*
Stitches in the side, outcries before or after, interrupting sleep: *Cuprum.*
With vexatious stitching in upper part of breast, loss of appetite and headache, feels every step in the head: *Natr. mur.*
Sudden stitches and burning deep in the left side of the chest, frightening her: *Baryt.;* acute stitches in front of left chest, startling her: *Graphit.*
Violent stitch under left ribs at dinner, has to scream: *Ratanh.*
Startling stitches in the chest: *Sulphur.*

Diseases. Catarrh, with melancholy: *Cepa;* weary of life: *Phosphor.;* ill humor: *Mercur.;* despair: *Psorin.;* irritability: *Lycop.;* whimpering: *Arsen.;* confused mind: *Arsen.*

Pneumonia and other pulmonary diseases, with great anxiety and restlessness, tossing about: *Arsen.;* delirium: *Bellad.;* with bellowing: *Cuprum;* with restlessness: *Hyosc.;* muttering, with loss of consciousness: *Sulphur;* with circumscribed redness of cheeks: *Lachnanth.;* greatest agony: *Hyosc.;* after pneumonia, sort of stupor; piercing, shrill screaming "my baby:" *Apis.*

Chronic laryngitis. Irritable, anxious, restless, loquacious: *Arsen.;* torpid, aversion to motion, indifferent, taciturn: *Kali bichr.*

Diaphragmitis. Anxious impatience: *Acon.;* anxious, with short breathing, loud complaining: *Chamom.*

Chest symptoms, in mania: *Veratr.*

Hydro-thorax. Calm: *Turpeth.;* slow comprehension, slow at answering questions: *Helleb.*

Emphysema. Agonizing dyspnœa, could not lie in a recumbent position: *Hepar.*

Tuberculosis. Every little emotion flushes the face: *Ferrum;* easily frightened: *Kali carb.;* easily affected, anxious despairing: *Merc. subl., Stannum.*

Mental symptoms of bluest remorse: *Natr. ars.*

Crossness, ill humor, desire to injure or kill: *Arsen.;* opposite condition: *Digit.*

Chest complaints of children, with anxiety: *Calc. phosph.*

MODEL CURES.

A young man has cramp-like pain in the chest; comes in stormy, cloudy weather, when walking fast, from warm, tight clothing, change of temperature, and violent laughing; has to stand still when walking against the wind. Oppression on the chest, anxiety, alternately cold and hot, raises white slimy mucus, which relieves; going into a warm room makes worse: *Arsen.*—W. GROSS.

A lady, æt. 49, stout and fleshy, had catarrh every winter, with violent coughing. After being in a draft, the cough was tormenting and dry; she had to sit straight up day and night, with horrible anxiety about a rattling in chest, with soreness as if raw on the chest; fears to suffocate. *Sepia*^{3} made an aggravation, great orgasm to the chest, sensation as if the throat was being laced; after a while expectoration commenced, and all her symptoms disappeared.—NITHAK.

ANCUISH OF HEART.

|| Acon.
Agar.
Alum.
Ambra.
Amm. carb.
Anac.
Ant. tart.
Arnica.
|| Arsen.
Ast. rub.
|| Aurum.
| Bellad.
Bromum.
|| Cactus.
| Calc. ostr.
Camphor.
Canthar.
| Carb. veg.
Castor.
|| Caustic.
Chamom.
Cina.
Cinnab.
Coccul.
Colchic.
Crocus.
Crot. tigl.
|| Cuprum.
Digit.
Evon. eur.
Glonoin.
Gran. cort.
Graphit.
Hæmatox.
Hydr. ac.
| Ignat.
Laches.
Lauroc.
|| Lycop.
Magn. mur.
| Menyanth.
Merc. per.
Natr. mur.
Nitr. ac.
|| Nux vom.
Oleander.
Opium.
| Phosphor.
Phosph. ac.
| Platin.
|| Plumbum.
| Psorin.
| Pulsat.
Rhus tox.
Sepia.
Silic.
| Spigel.
|| Spongia.
Stramon.
Sulphur.
|| Thuya.
Veratr.
Viol. od.
Viol. tric.
Zincum.
Zinc. ox.

Cardiac Anxiety. In the region of the heart and around it: *Aurum,* ||*Bellad., Calc. ostr., Canthar., Cina, Colchic., Coccul., Cuprum, Crocus, Oleand., Platin., Plumbum, Pulsat.,* and in precordiæ: *Acon.*

From congestion, in mania: *Ignat.*

Attacks of cardiac anxiety: *Laches., Veratr.*

Stronger pulsations, with anxiety in attacks: *Acon.,* ||*Nux vom., Veratr.*

Omitting beats: *Bellad.*

Suddenly violent beating of heart, with disturbed rhythm; a feeling of impending death, with terror and anxiety, slightest motion increases anxiety and palpitation: *Digit.*

With a fixed pain, in endocarditis: *Aurum.*

As if the heart was squeezed off, beside himself with anxiety, whimpering and profuse sweating: *Chamom.;* anxious constriction: *Merc. per.*

Stitches with inhalation; in hypertrophy: *Plumbum.*

Anxious sensation at the heart, murmur, throbbing, intermitting pulse: *Bellad., Digit., Glonoin.*

Mind. Melancholy, longs for death: *Aurum.*

Great alarm and agitation: *Spongia.*

As if something untoward was to happen: *Menyanth.*

With irritability: *Platin.;* sadness: *Lycop.;* melancholy: *Caustic.*

Suicidal disposition: ||*Aurum, Plumbum, Pulsat.,* ||*Nux vom., Rhus tox.;* by stabbing: *Calc. ostr.;* by drowning: *Ignat.*

Anxious dread of heart disease: *Calc. ostr.*

With restlessness: *Opium;* while sitting, has to get up and move around: *Caustic.;* driving from place to place: *Aurum.*

Around the heart, with fretfulness: *Platin.*

As if she had done wrong: *Coccul.;* while walking in the open air: *Cina.*

Religious melancholy, compunctions of conscience: *Aurum.*

Fearful visions, despairs of salvation, wants to stab himself: *Calc. ostr.*

An inward oppression affecting the mind: *Evon. eur.;* as if she had done wrong: *Cina.*

Oppression about the heart worse after vexation: *Lycop.*

Palpitation worse after emotions, in valvular disease: *Phosphor.*

When thinking of it: *Baryt., Ox. ac.*

Head. With heat in the head, drives out of bed and room: *Thuya;* with headache and flushed face: *Bellad.*

The attacks begin before the headache and increase with it until 10 P.M., several days at the same hour: *Platin.*

Abdomen. Great thirst and internal heat in carditis: *Carb. veg.;* nausea: *Plumbum, Spongia;* in pit of throat: *Plumbum;* in epigastrium: *Pulsat.*
Vomiting in the night of food and bile: *Lycop.*
Catamenia. During catamenia: *Bellad.;* tempts him to sigh: *Colchic.;* necessitates a deep breath: *Sepia;* increases by taking or holding breath: *Spigel.*
With anxious oppression: *Nitr. ac.;* stopping breathing: *Ambra, Veratr.;* with flying heat: *Ambra.*
When lying down, undulating throbbing of heart: *Viol. tric.*
With fear of dying, and constriction, with attacks of pain in the chest: *Psorin.;* driving from place to place: *Aurum;* restlessness: *Arsen.*
With trembling: *Aurum, Bellad.;* trembling all over without anxious ideas: *Oleand.*
With fear of fainting: *Nitr. ac.;* a weak sinking sensation down through abdomen to feet: *Crocus.*
After violent exercise: *Lycop.;* when lying on the left side: *Phosph. ac.*
Night. Keeping her awake half the night, worse in the afternoon than morning: *Rhus tox.;* wakes at 4 or 5 A.M., feeling as if sweat would come, which is not the case; anxiety disappears after getting up: *Alum.*
At night: *Arsen., Calc. ostr.*, and in the morning: *Ast. rub.;* at noon and most in the evening: *Bellad.;* afternoon: *Canthar., Rhus. tox.;* evening: *Bromum.*
With anxious thoughts, drives out of bed and room at night: *Thuya.*
After midnight with violent palpitation and inclination to commit suicide: *Nux vom.*
When walking in the open air: *Cina;* after exercise in the open air, with weakness and nausea: *Spongia.*
Flying heat, with impeded breathing: *Ambra;* internal heat: *Carb. veg.*
Copious sweat: *Chamom., Plumbum;* cold sweat: *Phosph. ac.*
In attacks: *Veratr.*
Diseases. Endocarditis. Fixed pain and great anxiety: *Aurum;* carditis, anguish, internal heat, great thirst: *Carb. veg.*
Valvular diseases, anguish at night: *Calc. ostr.;* great alarm, agitation, anxiety: *Spongia;* easily frightened: *Cactus.*
Hypertrophy; anguish about heart, cold sweat: *Plumbum;* stitches with inhalation, anxiety: *Plumbum.*
Aneurism. Frightened when examined: *Spigel.*
Heart disease with fear and terror: *Spongia.*

MODEL CURES.

Since a nervous attack five months ago, a kind of insanity with ecstasy and despair of salvation, his heart troubles him. Any exciting or elating thought causes palpitation more than emotions. *Indescribable bad feeling about and below the heart,* with soreness and pains, flying stitches all over: *Badiag.*—JAMES B. BELL.

In rheumatic endocarditis, valvular insufficiency, attacks of severe oppression and pain in the region of the heart, all the symptoms are aggravated by lying with the head low, or inability to lie down at all: *Spongia.*—JAMES B. BELL.

HEARTACHE, WITH MENTAL SYMPTOMS.

Acon.
Act. rac.
Ambra.
Amm. carb.
Anac.
Argent.
Arsen.
Ars. met.
Aurum.
Badiaga.
Baryt.
Bellad.
Calc. ostr.
Carb. veg.
Chamom.
Cicut.
Crotal.
Daph. ind.
Gelsem.
Helleb.
Hydroph.
! Laches.
Lycop.
Mercur.
Millef.
Naja trip.
Nitr. ac.
Petrol.
Platin.
Psorin.
Rhus tox.
!! Spongia.
Thuya.

Kind of Sensations. Pressure in region of heart, with anxiety: *Rhus tox.*, with inhalation: *Kali carb.*; and pressure in scrobiculum, with inhalation: *Ignat.*, *Pœonia*; takes breath away and makes anxious: *Bellad.*; anxious feeling, followed by sadness: *Lycop.*; dull stitches, anxiousness, impedes breath, better from walking: *Pulsat.*

Constrictive feeling in region of heart, with anxiety; ceases after a strong beat of heart: *Nitr. ac.*

Painful contraction, like a jerk of the heart, with apprehension: *Argent.*

Grasping sensation at heart, with restlessness: *Rhus tox.*; squeezing, with anxiety: *Arnic., Cactus.*

Fear of sudden death, with spasmodic pains in cardiac region: *Lauroc.*

Urging sensation in the heart towards abdomen and region of the liver, with great anxiety at night: *Act. spic.*

Stitches about the heart, with anxiety: *Nitr. ac.*

Severe stitches in region of heart synchronous with the pulse, has to scream, worse when sitting: *Rhus tox.*

Anxiety, with stitches over the heart, fancies he talks wildly, inclination to fall: *Nitr. ac.*

With inhalation stitches in heart: *Lauroc.*; with anxiety, rising heat and red face: *Plumbum*; better from stooping: *Valer.*; with exhalation, shooting in heart: *Ignat.*

Pulsating stitches in heart while sitting in the evening, has to scream: *Rhus tox.*; shooting pain in region of heart, has to scream: *Capsic.*

Stitches through heart, as if they would kill him if repeated: *Psorin.*; horrible shooting in region of heart, with apprehension: *Argent.*

Scraping sensation in the heart, with uneasiness: *Rhus tox.*

Acute flying pains near the heart, with trembling and timidity: *Daph. ind.*

Mental Concomitants—Feelings. With sadness: *Crotal., Petrol., Spongia*; sadness after pressure: *Lycop.*; melancholy: *Crotal.*; depression, ill humor, wants to be alone: *Ars. met.*

Hypochondric mood: *Lycop., Platin.*

With anxiety: *Baryt., Carb. veg., Chamom., Cicut., Millef., Nitr. ac., Spongia.*

Anxiety, taking her breath away, pressure: *Bellad.*; causing pressure: *Pœon. off.*; pressure, followed by sadness: *Lycop.*; inexpressible anxiety, with pressure: *Rhus tox., Pulsat.*; with stitches over the heart: *Nitr. ac.*

With spells of heat and sweat: *Spongia.*

Apprehensive feelings rise from the abdomen to the heart, with restlessness, inward trembling and confusion: *Thuya*; apprehension: *Aurum*; with jerking and horrible shooting pains: *Argent.*

Anxious and inconsolable: *Spongia.*

Feelings, with Conations. Despondency: *Chamom., Petrol.;* thinks she will not recover: *Cactus.*

Timidity and trembling, flying pains all over: *Daph. ind.*

Actions. Sighing: *Hydroph.;* weeping: *Spongia;* very much: *Cactus.*

Has to scream loud, with stitches over the heart: *Rhus tox.;* screaming with pain, or complete loss of consciousness: *Cactus.*

Conations. Palpitation, with depression of spirits, thoughts of suicide: *Aur. mur.;* would like to die on the spot: *Spongia.*

Exaltations. After excitement heart aches: *Cactus.*

Uneasiness, scraping in heart: *Rhus tox.;* restlessness: *Amm. carb., Anac., Arsen., Bellad.*

Points to it, restlessness: *Helleb.;* anxiety and restlessness: *Hydroph.;* with grasping: *Rhus tox.*

Fears it would kill if returning: *Psorin.*

Intellect. Imagines she is delirious, with stitches: *Nitr. ac.*

Great pain near heart and wandering of the mind, with swelling of the whole body: *Naja trip.*

Pain intense all over left chest, down left arm, red face and unconsciousness: *Act. rac.*

MODEL CURES.

Heaviness and dullness in the head, particularly in the occiput; sensation of heat in the head; hands numb. The heaviness is worse from motion, better when sitting still. If her head is placed ever so high, she thinks it is too low; drowsiness in the afternoon every other day; starting on falling asleep; heat in the head and arms at night, with weakness in the epigastrium. Sleeps little, and the fulness and heaviness in the head and body are worse in the morning. Restlessness, driving from place to place. Symptoms change place; now more in the left arm, now in the foot, which is cold as ice. Every cold gives her a sore throat; swelling and stiffness, painful when swallowing and to the touch. Now and then *a sudden stitch in the region of the heart*, which makes her weak. Hemorrhoidal tumors, which she had once before in childbed, are very painful during stool; frequent urging. Menses too late and profuse, with throbbing headache. *Bellad., Hepar, Sepia* and *Magn. mur.* failed. *Hepar* caused a diarrhœa which lasted two weeks; when it stopped, the night attacks returned. *Laches.* cured.—W. WESSELHŒFT.

Painter, æt. 43. Great anxiety of conscience; any crime he reads of he imagines to have committed once himself; worse at night, with palpitation of the heart; has to be kept by force in the room; great fear to be left alone; despairs of ever getting well; loss of appetite; whitish-coated tongue; flatulency; constipation: *Arsen.*[3], every evening one dose, for ten days. Much better. Eight more doses. Entirely well since one year.—STENS, JR.

Sarah H., æt. 66. Palpitation of heart originated in *grief. Pain in left part of chest* and in left arm; enlargement of heart: *Digit.*[3] restored her.—J. H. NANKIVELL.

OTHER SENSATIONS IN HEART, WITH MENTAL CONCOMITANTS.

Sorrowful feeling at the heart without cause, a voluptuous tremor in the body: *Calc. ostr.*

Soreness about the heart: *Gelsem.*

It presses on the heart, with anxiety and tearing in the sacral region: *Rhus tox.*

Nervous excitement affecting the heart: *Hura.*

Oppression of heart, heart feels pressed down, overwhelmed with anxiety: *Chamom.*

A momentary but fearful stitch in the region of the heart, as if in the pleura; frequent spasmodic contraction of the muscles of the heart, worse when lying on the back; he has an idea that he will have a stroke of apoplexy, but which causes him no anxiety: *Argent.*

Soft, low music causes tensive heart-cramps: *Thuya.*

Constriction in region of heart, sensation of scraping in heart: *Rhus tox.*; with anxiety, relieved when a strong pulsation comes: *Nitr. ac.*

Confused, the heart is dragged downward towards the left side: *Thuya.*

Restlessness, with anxiety, grasps at the heart, dyspnœa: *Rhus tox.*

Squeamish feeling around the heart, sad ideas: *Ambra.*

Attack in the evening, rising to the heart, nausea with anxiety, trembling, likes to bend forward and rest his head on the table: *Nux vom.*

Sensation of coldness around the heart after mental exertion: *Natr. mur.*

Anxiety, with heat: *Acon.*

Attack after midnight, crawling in hands and feet, rising to the heart, flushed face, burning and pressing in the epigastrium, rising to the throat, nausea and anxiety, mounts to the head, dullness and ringing in the ears: *Nux vom.*

A weakness as if falling from heart down through abdomen, to the feet, anxious: *Crocus;* stupefaction and sense of falling: *Calc. ostr.*

Sad and despondent, a sick and weak feeling at the heart: *Petrol.*

Sinking at heart, melancholy thoughts: *Ambra;* sinking feeling is most distressing: *Digit.*

Pulsating sensation in region of heart, with restlessness and anxiety: *Carb. veg.*; jerks in region of heart, with anxiety: *Calc. ostr.*

Does not know where to turn: *Amm. carb.*; with melancholy: *Caustic.*

Stitches, with anxiety, heat and flushed face: *Plumbum.*

As if something rested on her heart: *Thuya.*

Easily moved to laughing or crying: *Calc. ostr.*

MODEL CURE.

A French milliner had a jealous quarrel with her lover. With the words: "O, my heart!" putting both her hands to it, she fell down and was nearly twenty-four hours in an asphyctic state; no pulse could be felt, breathing was hardly perceptible; was laid out on her back. *Laches.*[30] was followed in a few minutes by a loud sighing, turning on her side, and recovery.—C. Hg.

MIND AND DISPOSITION.

PALPITATION, WITH MENTAL SYMPTOMS.

a signifies anxiety.

‖ Acon.	a
Aesc. hipp.	a
Agar.	a
Alum.	a
Al. p. s.	
Amm. carb.	a
Amyl. nitr.	
Anac.	
Angust.	a
∣ Ant. tart.	a
‖ Arsen.	a
Arnica.	a
Asaf.	a
Aspar.	a
Ast. rub.	a
∣ Aurum.	a
Aur. mur.	
∣ Badiag.	
Baryt.	
Bellad.	a
‖ Borax.	a
Bovist.	a
Bromum.	a
Bryon.	a
Calc. ars.	
‖ Calc. ostr.	a
Calc. phosph.	a
Camphor.	a
∣ Cannab.	
∣ Carb. veg.	
‖ Caustic.	a
∣ Chamom.	
‖ Cinch. off	
∣ Coca.	a
‖ Coccul.	a
Codein.	
Colchic.	a
Coloc.	a
Crocus.	a
Cuprum.	a
Cyclam.	a
‖ Digit.	a
∣ Ferrum.	a
‖ Gelsem.	a
‖ Graphit.	a
Helleb.	a
Hyosc.	
∣ Ignat.	a
Ipec.	
∣ Kali carb.	a
∣ Laches.	a
Lauroc.	a
∣ Lycop.	
‖ Magn. carb.	a
Menyanth.	
Merc. per.	a
Merc. sol.	a
Merc. subl.	
Mezer.	a
∣ Moschus.	a
‖ Natr. carb.	a
∣ Natr. mur.	a
‖ Nitr. ac.	a
Nitrum.	a
Nux mosch.	
‖ Nux vom.	a

Cheerful, contented, confident, alternately with palpitation and anxious oppression: *Spigel.*

Palpitation from pleasant emotions, any exciting or elating thought: ∣*Badiag.*

Sadness: *Natr. mur., Nux mosch.;* dejection: *Natr. mur.,* low spirits: *Cactus.*

Depression of spirits, with frontal headache and spinal pain: *Naja trip.*

Apprehension: *Aurum, Natr. mur.;* fear of dying: *Platin.*

Oppression: *Gelsem.;* anxious oppression: *Psorin.*

Palpitation after anxiety: *Acon.;* during anxiety, or soon after: *Nitr. ac.;* as from anxious expectation: *Moschus.*

Almost constant palpitation, with slight anxiety and apprehension: *Sarsap.*

Fear: *Sarsap.;* of apoplexy: *Argent.;* of everybody: *Pulsat.;* of being left alone: *Arsen.*

Nervousness in company, can scarcely talk: *Platin.*

Anxious fear of getting a heart trouble: *Calc. ostr.*

Despairs of ever getting well: *Arsen.*

After the loss of a relative; worse when speaking of his loss: *Gelsem.*

Pangs of conscience, as if he had committed every crime he ever heard of: *Arsen.*

Vexatious occurrences of long ago come back and torment him so he does not know what to do with himself; anxiety, palpitation and sweat: *Sepia.*

After vexation, weak and trembling: *Lycop.;* weary of life: *Nux vom.*

Ill humored: *Ant. tart.;* vexed: *Phosphor.,* and fretful: *Veratr.;* suicidal inclination: *Aurum, Nux vom.*

Better from diverting talk: *Gelsem.*

Subdued manner: *Gelsem.*

Faint-hearted and anxious after meals: *Thuya.*

Peculiar anxiety and ill humor: *Aspar.*

Very peevish at slightest cause: *Phosphor.;* quick-spoken: *Sepia.*

Weeping, coldness and weakness: *Mezer.*

With starting in the night: *Bellad., Nitrum, Phosph. ac.*

Easily frightened: *Mezer.*

Violent palpitation on seeing a woman, has the greatest aversion to them: *Pulsat.*

Anxious restlessness: ‖∣*Aspar., Bovist., Calc. ostr., Crocus.*

BODILY SYMPTOMS, WITH MENTAL CONCOMITANTS. 219

I Oleander.	a	
Opium.	a	
Ox. ac.		
Petrol.	a	
II Phosphor.	a	
Phosph. ac.		
II Platin.	a	
Plumbum.	a	
Podoph.		
II Psorin.	a	
II Pulsat.	a	
Rhus tox.	a	
Ruta.	a	
! Sarsap.	a	
Secale.	a	
Senega.		
II Sepia.	a	
I Silic.	a	
II Spigel.	a	
Spongia.	a	
Staphis.	a	
II Sulphur.	a	
Sulph. ac.		
Terebinth.	a	
I Thuya.	a	
Valer.	a	
II Veratr.		
I Viol. od.	a	
I Viol. tric.		
Vip. torv.		
II Zincum.	a	
Zinc. ox.	a	

Embarrassed: *Carb. veg.*

After Emotions or Exertions. Slightest emotion or thought causes forcible pulsation of the heart, with fluttering and vibrating: *Badiag.*

After the slightest mental emotion: *Calc. ars., Nitr. ac., Phosphor., Podoph.*

The slightest thing vexes him, which causes palpitation and anxiety: *Veratr.*

Heart beats violently after mental excitement: *Al. p. s.*

In the epigastrium, with anxiousness from the slightest cause: *Ferrum.*

On attempting to study or write, painful pulsations of the heart: *Codein.*

More after exertions than emotions: *Badiag.*

When thinking of it: *Al. p. s., Ignat., Ox. ac.*

Anxious palpitation when writing: *Natr. carb.;* after talking: *Pulsat.*

MODEL CURE.

An elderly man with chronic asthma and proctalgia; sudden attacks of fluttering, disappearing as quickly as they came: *Al. p. s.*[30]—NEUMANN.

PALPITATION OF HEART, WITH OTHER BODILY AND MENTAL SYMPTOMS.

Sensorium. As if all the senses would leave him: *Platin.;* as if going to faint: *Nitr. ac.*

It mounts to the head, feels as if stupefied: *Acon.*

Head. With lassitude and stitches in the forehead: *Platin.;* frontal headache: *Naja trip.*

Eyes. Sparks before eyes: *Coca.*

Ears. Humming in ears: *Coca.*

Face. Sad, discouraged look: *Pulsat.;* flushed: *Gelsem.;* with anxiety: *Acon.;* pale: *Pulsat.*

Tongue. Whitish-coated tongue: *Arsen.*

Thirst. No thirst, no appetite: *Pulsat.*

Eating. With great anxiety before dinner, has to lie down: *Mezer.;* after dinner with anxiousness: *Silic.*

Bitter eructation: *Phosphor.*

Gastrics. Nausea without inclination to vomit: *Nitr. ac.;* in the morning with empty stomach: *Baryt.;* can not remain up on account of great nausea: *Phosphor.;* vomiturio: *Laches.*

Stomach. Pinching across stomach: *Phosphor.;* pressure in pit of stomach with painful constriction: *Sulphur.*

MIND AND DISPOSITION.

Hypochondria. With anxiety, has to remove his clothing: *Pulsat.*

Abdomen. Anxious palpitation, with rhythmic contractions of the abdomen: *Caustic.;* pulsations in different places: *Alum.*

Flatulency, constipation: *Arsen.*

Female Parts. Voluptuous crawling in the vagina and abdomen, with anxious oppression and palpitation: *Platin.*

Catamenia. Soon after setting in, attacks of palpitation, heat, anxiety and trembling: *Nitr. ac.;* during palpitation and anxiety, lassitude, has to lie down: *Phosphor.*

Breathing. With anxious, quick, audible breathing: *Veratr.*

Great anxiety, with violent beats, breathing scarcely perceptible: *Viol. od.*

Anxiety, with short breathing, no particular dread: *Caustic.;* anxiety, necessitating deep breathing, no particular influence on the mind: *Sepia.*

Anxious shortness of breathing in the evening: *Caustic.*

With anxiousness and quick breathing: *Veratr.*

Terrible anxiety and restlessness, oppression of chest, with every breath she utters a sound as if it was her last: *Calc. ostr.*

With great anxiety, oppressed breathing and lassitude, blood mounts to the face: *Acon.*

Palpitation, with anxious constriction: *Spigel.*

When lying on the left side, anxious, quick palpitation, taking away her breath: *Pulsat.;* taking away his breath, with anxiety: *Nitr. ac.*

Pressure on chest with anxiety, without a cough: *Laches.*

Anxious, with slight stitches in left chest: *Cannab.*

Great and inexpressible anxiety from dyspnœa and weight on the chest, with acute rheumatism: *Laches.*

Severe palpitation, with feeling as if a large box were inside: *Amyl. nitr.*

Almost audible, pressing, constricting beats, with anxiety and spasmodic pains in the sternum and under the ribs, worse when leaning forward: *Digit.*

Palpitation, with cramp-like pains in belly, chest and hip-joint, after anxiety, which wakes at night: *Sepia.*

Anxiety, with pulsations in different places in the chest and abdomen: *Alum.*

Painful anxiety, weakness, with weak and intermitting pulse, numbness of fingers, palpitation and restless sleep: *Tereb.*

Several strong pulsations, with increasing anxiety about $12\frac{1}{2}$ A.M.: *Agar.*

Heart. Anxiety in the region of the heart, with quicker and stronger pulsations: *Acon.*

Stronger pulsations of heart, with anxious feeling: *Cinch. off.*

Pulsations in chest, with anxious restlessness: *Carb. veg.*

Strong pulsations moving the arms and hands, with anxiety: *Graphit.*

Attacks of anxiety, causing palpitation and heat: *Veratr.*

Soreness from pain in heart: *Badiag.;* soreness about it: *Gelsem., Baryt.*

Fine dartings, palpitation and anxiety: *Acon.*

Indescribable bad feeling about and below the heart: *Badiag.*

Fluttering of the heart after mental emotion: *Lith. carb.;* with great anxiety and trembling of the fingers and legs: *Sepia.*

Fluttering, with sad weeping: *Natr. mur.;* after rising, with anxious oppression: *Spigel.*
Heart beats anxiously and tremblingly: *Calc. ostr.*
Nervous fluttering of the heart, with anxiety: *Cinnab.*
Single beats omit: *Ox. ac.;* with anxiety: *Sepia;* with timidity: *Natr. mur.*
Pulsations interrupted, without bodily sickness; dejected: *Natr. mur.*
Irregularity of the heart's action: *Sanguin.*
Anxiety, trembling: *Chamom.;* trembling, with anxious oppression: *Spigel.*
Wave-like pulsations, with anxiety: *Viol. tric.*

Back. Spinal pains: *Naja trip.*

Hands. Trembling, with anxiety: *Bovist.;* numbness of fingers: *Tereb.*

Feet. Anxiety, with weakness and trembling in the feet: *Borax.*

Limbs. All the limbs tremble: *Nitr. ac.;* great anxiety, lassitude in all the limbs, with sleepiness: *Aurum;* limbs asleep: *Pulsat.*

Motion. Palpitation varying in intensity, worse after slight motion, with lassitude and anxiety, as if he was going to faint: *Nitr. ac.*
Anxious palpitation when taking a walk: *Platin.;* when stooping, or when writing: *Natr. carb.*
From motion and going up stairs anxious restlessness: *Aspar.*

Position. Peculiar palpitation when lying down: *Viol. tric.*
When lying on the back, wakes at midnight with anxiety, has to sit straight up: *Nitrum.*
Cannot lie on the left side on account of ebullition and violent pulsations, sensation of soreness in the heart and great anxiety: *Baryt.*
Palpitation so violent in the evening, when lying on the left side, that the covers are moved, with anxiety; better when changing position: *Graphit.*
From lying on the left side, with anxiety and dyspnœa: *Pulsat.*

Weakness and Trembling. Trembling anxiety: *Chamom.;* anxiety, with weakness: *Aurum;* trembling and restlessness of the whole body: *Bovist.;* and anxiety: *Phosphor.*
Weak, sinking feeling from the heart down through the abdomen to feet: *Crocus.*
Great lassitude in all the limbs: *Acon.;* lassitude and anxiety: *Aurum;* can scarcely walk across the room: *Mezer.;* tired and weak, can scarcely keep on the feet: *Phosphor.;* has to lie down before dinner: *Mezer.;* as if he would faint: *Nitr. ac.*

Sleep. Cannot sleep on account of anxiety: *Pulsat.;* no sleep till the latter part of night: *Gelsem.*
When turning in bed, anxious palpitation: *Lycop.*
Violent, with extreme anxiety after midnight: *Nux vom.*
At 3 A.M. irregular but violent audible palpitation, with anxiety: *Arsen.*
Could not stay in bed, feeling as if she had done wrong, the palpitation cannot be felt with the hand: *Nitr. ac.*
After waking from an anxious dream, anxiety and audible palpitation: *Silic.;* half-waking dream, as if spirits would grasp him, cannot move a limb, with sweat and anxiety: *Silic.*

With anxiety, waking from sleep: *Nitrum;* after midnight: *Nux vom.*

Daytime. In the morning when awaking, with anxiety: *Phosphor.;* after midnight: *Spigel.;* with sudden anxiety, forenoons: *Natr. mur.;* severe at noon before eating: *Mezer.;* in the evening very ill with the catamenia: *Phosphor.;* in the evening in bed: *Calc. ostr.;* evening and morning: *Phosphor.*

Out-doors. When taking a walk: *Platin.;* after drowsiness, the veins in the hands enlarge: ı*Nux vom.*

Fever. Cold all over and cold sweat, with great anxiety, restlessness and backache: *Calc. ostr.*

Fever heat, anxious in the night: *Ignat.;* with anxious palpitation: *Petrol.*

Periodic. Great anguish, with severe periodic and frequent palpitation of the heart: *Aesc. hip.*

Has to throw the clothes off, with great anxiety: *Pulsat.*

Without Anxiety. Almost without any: *Ipec., Pulsat.;* in the evening: *Carb. an.*

Visible, but without anxiety: *Thuya, Zincum.*

At all times of the day, without anxiety: *Sulphur.*

Anxious palpitation, without anxious thoughts: *Natr. mur.*

Trembling: *Calc. ostr., Nux mosch.*

Fluttering. Sad and weeping; consolation aggravates, a fluttering of the heart follows: *Natr. mur.;* after emotion; *Lith. carb.;* and vibrating from slightest emotion: *Badiag.;* with trembling of fingers and legs: *Sepia.;* after rising: *Spigel.;* nervous: *Cinnab.;* trembling anxiety: *Calc. ostr.;* headache: *Formic.*

MODEL CURES.

Mr. F., a wealthy man, had now and then an omission of one beat, felt as "a stopping." Fearing a heart disease, and according to coroners' pathology, sudden death, he travelled to consult European celebrities. Only one confirmed his fears, but was wisely mistrusted. After an attack of cholera, cured by quinine, this omission appeared as soon as he was talking or thinking of it. After one dose of *Ox. ac.*^{30}, given as an experiment, it happened never to return for years.—C. Hg.

PALPITATION FROM EMOTIONS.

Acon.
Aur. mur.
Badiag.
Calc. ostr.
Chamom.
Coccul.
Coffea.
Ignat.
Nitr. ac.
Nux mosch.
Nux vom.
Opium.
Phosphor.
Phosph. ac.
Podoph.
Pulsat.
Thea.
Veratr.

The slightest mental excitement: *Coccul., Nitr. ac.;* the slightest emotion of mind: *Aur. mur., Nitr. ac., Phosphor., Podoph., Pulsat.*

Exaltation: *Acon., Coffea;* after exciting talk: *Thea.*

After sadness: *Nux mosch.;* grief and sorrow: *Opium;* after long grieving: *Phosph. ac.*

In the morning, after fear: *Nux mosch., Veratr.*

Great vexation from slight cause: *Phosphor.*

Vexation: *Acon., Chamom., Ignat., Nux vom.*

After alarming events, causing fright: *Opium.*

Fright: *Acon., Coffea, Nux mosch., Opium.*

PALPITATION AFTER MENTAL EXERTIONS.

Al. p. s.
Badiag.
Baryta.
Ignat.
Natr. carb.
Ox. ac.
Thea.

When thinking about his disease he feels the heart beating: *Al. p. s.*
Renewed by thinking of it: *Baryt.*
When thinking about the painless omission of single beats he is subject to, the heart stops for one beat: *Ox. ac.*

As soon as he turns his attention to any one thing his heart palpitates: *Natr. carb.;* when thinking deeply: *Ignat.*

RUSH OF BLOOD TO THE HEART.

Congestion, Orgasm and Ebullition. Ebullition, with anxiety: *Nitr. ac.*

Rush of blood to the heart, falls down unconscious: *Glonoin.*

Oppresion, anxiety, quick circulation, congestion to the heart of short duration: *Indig.*

Rapid circulation, cheerfulness, mental excitement, followed by lassitude and inability to work: *Phosphor.*

The blood boils, with prickling, at the least contrariety: *Elaps.*

Blood seems to boil in chest, anxiety: *Anac.*

Ebullition, blood boils in arteries: *Aurum.*

Great excitement in the blood: *Sepia;* restlessness, is beside himself: *Phosph. ac.;* does not know what to do with himself; as if he had done wrong, as if he had no power over his senses: *Mercur.*

Agitated, as if he had been frightened: *Mercur.*

Very much excited in the evening, with distended veins: *Carb. veg.*

Great circulatory excitement: *Acon.*

Ebullition in the evening, with oppression: *Kali carb.*

MODEL CURES.

After catamenia which came at the right time, symptoms of insanity. She believes herself married and pregnant, is tormented by remorse for imagined crimes; seeks constantly to escape and drown herself. Terrible anxiety from *rush of blood to the head and heart.* Is only quiet when lying undisturbed and brooding over her troubles which she rehearses in a doleful tone. If disturbed, she screams, strikes and tears things, crying all the while " I am neglecting my duty, breaking my oath !" Face pale and distorted: *Ignat.*—GROSS.

Rheumatism had left the lumbar muscles and seized the heart (the second similar metastasis). Was awakened between 1 and 2 A.M. by a sense of suffocation, accompanied by violent, loud cough, great alarm, agitation, anxiety, and difficult respiration. *The action of the heart was violent and rapid, each beat was accompanied by a loud blowing, as of a bellows: Spongia*[20] (J.).—P. P. WELLS.

ORGASM.

With Anxiety: *Aloes, Amm. mur., Baryta, Bryon., Kali carb., Laches., Nitr. ac.;* during the night: *Amm. carb., Mercur.*

Restlessness of mind: *Calc. ostr., Laches.; Sulphur;* starts when going to sleep, from rush of blood: *Sepia.*

From disagreeable news or disagreeable fancies: *Laches.*

Is nervous, faints: *Bellad.*

With weariness of life: *Platin., Spongia.*

With mental excitement: *Graphit.*

Orgasm and other affections of blood, after vexation: **I***Acon.,* **II***Chamom.,* **I I***Coloc.,* **I***Ignat.,* **I I***Mercur.,* **I***Petrol.,* **II***Sepia,* **I I***Staphis.*

Anxiety, with beating of all the pulses: *Arg. nitr., Carb. veg.*

After emotions in general: **I***Acon.,* **I***Apis,* **I***Aurum,* **I***Bellad.,* **I I***Bryon.,* **I I***Calc. ostr.,* **II***Chamom.,* **I***Coffea,* **I***Colchic.,* **I***Coloc.,* **I***Conium,* **I I***Cuprum,* **II***Hyosc.,* **II***Ignat.,* **I***Kali carb.,* **I***Laches.,* **I***Lycop.,* **I***Magn. carb.,* **I I***Mar. ver.,* **I***Natr. mur.,* **I***Nitr. ac.,* **I***Nux vom.,* **I***Opium,* **I***Petrol.,* **I***Phosphor.,* **I***Phosph. ac.,* **I***Platin.,* **II***Pulsat.,* **I***Sepia,* **I***Staphis.,* **I***Stramon.,* **I***Thuya,* **I I***Veratr.*

During relaxed state of mind, mental prostration; heart and circulation of blood affected: **I I***Acon., Asar.,* **I***Bellad., Bismuth.,* **I I***Cicut.,* **I***Cinch. off., Digit., Magn. carb.,* **I I***Natr. mur.,* **I***Petrol.,* **I I***Phosphor.,* **I I***Spongia, Stannum,* **I I***Stramon.*

From nervousness: **I I***Ambra,* **I***Bellad.,* **I***Calc. ostr.,* **I I***Ferrum,* **I***Mercur.,* **I***Nitrum,* **I***Nitr. ac.,* **I***Phosphor.,* **I I***Phosph. ac.,* **I***Sepia.*

MODEL CURE.

Screaming "hold me, hold me, the storm whirls me deeper and deeper into the fire, I burn, I burn!" Clings nervously to her bed or friends. Appears like one stricken with fright or terror, not furious and raving. Sweat over the whole body; throat and face bloated; throbbing carotids; distended jugular veins; eyes injected; pulse very frequent, large, not hard: *Bellad.*—LINDNER.

PULSE AND MENTAL STATES.

Pulse unaltered, with warmth and anxiety in head: *Lauroc.;* with restlessness: *Bellad.;* 50 beats, with difficult comprehension: *Cicut.*

Full. In delirium, talkative mania: *Bellad.*, and irritable, with anxiety: *Camphor., Rhus tox.*, and tense in delirium: *Stramon.*, and strong: *Cuprum;* 80 beats, with senselessness: *Stramon.;* with heat, thirst and exhilaration: *Opium*, and hard; vivid delirium: *Stramon.*, and quick: *Bellad., Cuprum,* and slow: *Stramon.*

Quick, strong, in mania: *Cuprum, Sulphur.*

Frequent. 90, pleasant warmth, but with a trembling, anxious feeling coming from the abdomen: *Valer.;* 12 beats increased, with reddened face and great serenity: *Clemat.;* increased 20 beats towards evening, with excitement: *Mezer.;* one-third more frequent, playful and mirthful: *Ox. ac.;* towards evening 20 beats more, with increased temperature of body, and sweat: *Mezer.*

100, small and soft, violent delirium: *Cuprum;* 120, in delirium: *Stramon.;* rose to 134, in the height of delirium; able to express his feelings in writing: *Coca.*

Very frequent, large but not hard, with mental derangement, attacks of anxiety: *Bellad.;* hard: *Acon., Coccul., Natr. mur., Opium,* and soft, with maniacal illusions: *Hyosc.;* small and soft in rage: *Stramon.;* weak in melancholy and delirium: *Stramon.*

Feeble and unequal, mental exhaustion: *Cuprum;* single beats intermitting, with stupor: *Stramon.*

Quick. With wanton gaiety: *Valer.*

With anxiety: *Pulsat., Thuya;* after dinner: *Natr. mur.;* when thinking of past ills: *Sepia.*

Cold skin and unconnected answers: *Crotal., Laches.,* and unconscious: *Glonoin.*

And irritated, with mania: *Stramon.*

With nervous perturbation: *Ananth. mur.*

And small, with a strong memory: *Bellad.;* small and hard, deranged mind: *Arsen.*

And full, with anxious derangement of mind: *Bellad.*

And strong, with attacks of mania: *Cuprum.*

And small, hard; insensibility: | | *Arsen.,* and small while raving: | | *Bellad.*

And unequal, with quick, erroneous ideas: *Cuprum.*

Tense. And more frequent: *Ox. ac.,* and full in delirium: *Stramon.*

Irritable. With hypochondric mood: *Platin., Sepia;* in mania: *Arsen., Crotal., Cuprum.*

And full, with anxiety: *Camphor., Rhus tox.;* small and quick, with confused talk: *Menyanth.;* and quick, with mania: *Stramon.*

Slow. With less liveliness: *Opium.*

With great anxiety: *Chin. sulph.*

In delirium: *Hyosc.;* with stupefaction: *Morph. ac.;* mental derangement, unconsciousness, rage, or insensibility: *Stramon.*

And weak, with melancholy: *Helleb.;* with unconsciousness: *Plumbum.*

Now slow, now quick, with anxiety: *Rhus tox.*

Hard. And small: *Arsen.;* and quick: *Arsen., Bellad.*

Strong. With a wild look: *Cuprum.*

Soft: *Cuprum, Stramon.;* and large: *Bellad.*

Irregular. With insensibility: *Sanguin.*

Small. And soft, with violent delirium: *Cuprum;* and weak, with uneasiness to despair: *Cuprum.*

And quick, with confused talk; *Menyanth.*

Hardly to be felt: *Bellad., Conium, Pulsat., Veratr.*

Feeble, with despair: *Vip. red.;* and unequal: *Cuprum;* and restless: *Jatroph.*

Weak. With stupefaction: *Hydr. ac.;* and despair: *Vip. red.*

And frequent: *Stramon.;* and slow, with melancholy: *Helleb.;* and intermitting, with anxiety: *Tereb.;* and changeable, with anxious restlessness: *Arsen, Cuprum;* hardly perceptible: *Arnic., Crotal.;* with anxious impatience: *Cinch. off.*

Almost no pulse, becomes dumb: *Stramon.;* pulse could not be felt on right wrist, with rage: *Stramon.;* pulse not to be felt: *Acon.*

Pulselessness and unconsciousness: *Mercur., Stramon.*

MODEL CURES.

A crippled girl who fell down suddenly with an attack of convulsions, was brought to bed and had a shaking chill. She sat up in bed in a semi-conscious state, refusing assistance, food or drink. Anxiety, with groaning and sighing all night long. Chides her father for taking part in the revolution; thinks she hears the drum which proclaims his execution. This is followed by silent brooding and occasional starts. Menses checked, the abdomen tense, face pale, arms cold, eyes fixed with contracted pupils. *Pulse slow and almost imperceptible: Veratr.*—WOOST.

Imagines she has to die, even after confinement, with violent congestion to the chest and constriction as if she would suffocate; pulse intermitting: *Acon.* W. GROSS.

OUTER CHEST.

Pressure on the sternum, with busy, anxious manner, as if anticipating a great pleasure: *Aurum.*

Anxiety in the region of the sternum, without pain; gives him no rest in the house, has to go into the open air and be active: *Anac.*

Anxiety under the sternum, has to breathe deeply: *Mercur.*

Pressing pain in the middle of the sternum, with anxiety; afterwards stinging pain in the sternum: *Coccul.*

Warm about breast and anxious: *Ol. anim.*

Several successive short stitches in sternum, has to scream: *Canthar.*

Gnawing and heat in the walls of the chest, with itching and anxiety: *Calc. phosph.*

Cannot sleep on account of restlessness, with pain in the chest, cannot touch it: *Laches.*

Large painful blisters on the left side of the chest and back, which break with fever heat, sweat and anxiety: *Caustic.*

Miliary itching eruption, with derangement of mind: *Bellad.*

MODEL CURES.

Unquiet look, lips bluish-red; weak memory; pangs of conscience about religion and the female sex. Violent palpitation when in the presence of a woman; abhors and hates the whole sex; has to go out of their way for fear of injuring them; he looks upon them as evil beings and is afraid; considers their presence injurious to *his soul.* Respiration short and difficult; *painful pressure in the chest: Pulsat.*—MALAISE.

A girl, æt. 24, of healthy constitution, catamenia regular, suffered from nervousness to such a degree that the approach of a stranger gave her sudden twitches; when spoken to she answered with tears and sobbing. *The skin on the chest and right side of abdomen was deep yellow: Thuya.*—HAYNEL.

NECK AND BACK.

Neck. Pressing pain in left side of neck, with exhilaration: *Formic.*
Spasmodic contraction in the neck so violent she has to scream: *Nitrum.*
Drawing pain in neck when reading, with ill humor and impatience: *Natr. carb.*

With pain in the neck illusion as if the head were not a part of the body: *Psorin.;* tearing and tension in the left side of the neck, as if too short, has to scream when moving: *Sulphur.*

Stiff neck, complains loudly when going to move it: *Rhus tox.;* with dullness in the head, the muscles seem too short: *Cicut.*

Throbbing Carotids. With desire to run away: *Glonoin.;* shunning mental labor: *Agar.;* inability to find the right expression: *Arg. nitr.*

Jugular veins overfilled, with mental derangement: *Bellad.*
Neck or throat feels as if swollen, with great fear: *Glonoin.*

Back. Continued stinging pressure under the shoulder-blade, excited and cheerful: *Laches.*

Restlessness starting in the back: *Sulphur.*
Wave-like sensation going up the back with heat and anxiety: *Lauroc.*
Loud moaning about unbearable pain in the back: *Ars. hydr.*
Pinching from belly to the lumbar region, with anxious sweat: *Sulph. ac.;* from loins to spine, with anxiety: *Nux vom.;* tearing from back into belly: *Chamom.*

Pain in back, with disposition to weep: *Lil. tigr.*
Dull pain in lumbar region; mood gloomy, depressed: *Hamam.*
Throbbing pain in back from slight emotions: *Baryt.*
Biting pain in the back causing him to start: *Phelland.*
Symptoms in the back, with melancholy after unhappy love: *Ignat.*
Great pain in the back, with anxiety; impeded speech improves: *Cannab.*
Restlessness and anxiety, with pain in the back: *Arsen.;* without pain: *Carb. an.*

Stitches in spine, while sitting, with sudden anxiety: *Ruta.*
Stinging as from needles in the middle of the spine, can hardly keep from screaming, worse when walking in the open air, better when standing: *Calc. ostr.*

Stitches in the lumbar vertebræ causing screams: *Phosphor.*

Sacrum. Great pains in back and sacrum in the morning, with melancholy: *Petrol.;* loud complaining of pain in the back and loins: *Arg. nitr.*

Vexation and ill humor, with drawing pains in back spreading through the whole pelvis, worse in the evening: *Aloes.*

Lameness in lower part of back, could hardly walk, with religious mania after abuse of alcohol: *Veratr.*

Lameness, with cramp-like drawing forward above the hips, with anxious forebodings: *Coccul.;* weakness in lower part of back; fears she will be unable to move: *Agar.*

Heavy feeling in sacrum with anxiety: *Rhus tox.;* pain in sacrum with anxiety: *Nitr. ac.;* stitches which take away the breath, with anxious feeling around the pit of the stomach: *Sulphur;* repeated stitches and tearing in os coccygis which startle her: *Canthar.*

Pinching pain in the sacrum with melancholy: *Caustic.;* ill humor: *Aloes;* restlessness: *Laches.;* vice-like, or as if beaten and crushed; sudden screams from the least motion: *China.*

Unbearable pain in small of back: *Psorin.*

Cold. Chilliness in the back after vexation: *Nux vom.*

Cold creeps with anxiety: *Natr. mur.;* running down the back, vexatious, taciturn: *Borax;* shuddering, with anxiety: *Natr. mur.;* with starting in the night from noises: *Carb. veg.;* after heat in face with anxiety: *Pulsat.;* coldness in the night with restlessness: *Natr. mur.;* cold chills in back, most after going to bed with hot flushes towards morning, and depression of spirits: *Lil. tigr.*

Sweat on back at night, followed by heat and uneasiness, which prevents her from going to sleep: *Petrol.;* sweat on back after 3 A.M., with anxious restlessness: ‖*Rhus tox.;* sweat, with rash on the back, with dullness of all the senses and anxiety: *Stramon.*

UPPER LIMBS.

Shoulder and other Joints. Pain causing screams; in the neck and shoulders when bending the head forward; she cannot raise her arms to the head: *Graphit.;* shoulder-joint as if torn out: *Sepia;* anxiety and sweat, with pain in the shoulder-blade: *Cimex;* pain as if beaten, in the shoulder-joint after vexation: *Coloc.;* in the left shoulder-blade, with stinging and tension, worse when turning head, has to weep and scream: *Mercur.;* stitches in the elbow-joint after a fright: *Phosphor.;* restlessness and anxiety in the articulations of the arm and hand: *Calc. ostr.*

Motions. Could not keep the limbs quiet, especially the arms, had to stretch them, with anxiety: *Natr. carb.*

Uneasiness in the arms with restlessness: *Bellad.;* restlessness with pain in the forearms, sensitive to the slightest touch: *Colchic.;* arm is drawn backward with anxiety: *Alum.*

Lifts the arms above the head, with screaming: *Stramon.*

Spinning and weaving motions with hands and arms, senseless: *Stramon.;* spasms in arms, with unconsciousness: *Bellad.*

After vexation, twitches in arms and hands on falling asleep: *Conium.*

Sensations. Violent tearing pain in wrist, elbow, axilla, shoulders and chest, with restlessness: *Laches.;* jerking, tearing in the right upper arm, now in one place then in another, with anxiety: *Amm. mur.*

Stinging in the upper limbs after fright: *Phosphor.*

Pain in right arm, wakens from sleep with whining: *Cast. equ.*

Early in the morning felt as if going out of her mind, elevated, careless

state, lasting five minutes, followed by a sensation as of blood trickling down the left arm, from the shoulder to the finger-joints: *Cotyl.*
Tingling in right arm and hand, with difficult comprehension: *Natr. carb.*
Crawling pain in the right arm, particularly in the hand and tips of the fingers: *Natr. carb.*
Crawling in the arms, with anxious fear and the like: *Natr. mur.*
Chilliness running over the arms, with anxiety: *Pulsat.*
As if arms were stretched, restlessness: *Natr. carb.*
Weakness in the muscles of the arms and hands after excitability with laughter: *Carb. veg.*
Anxiety, with restlessness in the arms, with cheerful mood, heaviness, has to move them constantly: *Mur. ac.;* anxiety, with heaviness and sensation, as if beaten in the forearms: *Sabin.;* arms fall asleep and feel as if dead, with anxiety: *Natr. mur.;* ill humor, with lameness of the left arm: *Bromum.*
Swelling of arms while raving: *Bellad.*

HANDS.

Sensations. Tearing, stinging and swelling of the left wrist, with weeping; beside himself: *Sabin.*
Stitches in palms, with melancholy: *Clemat.*
Crawling in hands, unable to think: *Thuya.*
A kind of anxious feeling in the hand, has to take hold of things: *Sulphur.*
Hastiness and awkwardness, with weak feeling: *Chlorof.*
Motions. Grasping with the hands and screaming: *Calc. phosph.*
Claps his hands together in mania: *Stramon.;* catches at bystanders with his hands, delirium: *Stramon.;* grasping with the hands toward the nose, ears and head, stupor: *Stramon.;* wrings the hands and throws them wildly about, with derangement of mind: *Bellad.;* endeavors to grasp imaginary visions in the air, on the clothes and bed: *Pastinaca sativa.*
Hands constantly active, with derangement of mind: *Morph. ac.*
Delirium, with picking and motions of the hands as if they were in contact with real objects: *Atrop.*
Constant motion of the hands to catch imaginary little bodies in the air: *Bellad.;* grasping about in the air, in delirium or unconsciousness; catching imaginary things, unconsciousness without fever; picking at her clothes or things near her; searching with hands on bed-covers, delirium: *Stramon.;* picking at flocks in delirium: *Hyosc., Rhus tox.;* stretched out his hands as if he would lay hold of something; senseless: *Stramon.;* moving hands as if keeping off what they fear: *Stramon.*
After working with hands, anxious: *Jodium.*
Trembling. With uneasiness of mind: *Magn. carb.;* anguish: *Coffea;* anxiousness: *Amm. carb., Cicut., Platin., Pulsat.;* with flushes of heat: *Platin.;* with sweat in the face: *Cicut.;* with apprehension and restlessness: *Psorin.:* with violent burst of anger about trifles: *Sepia;* with excitement and talkative-

ness: *Argent.;* after fright: *Sambuc.;* with inner restlessness and absentmindedness cannot write a letter: *Magn. carb.;* cannot hold the pen: *Coffea;* with wantonness, as if intoxicated, after meals: *Tabac.*

Weakness. Lets every thing fall, light-minded, in young girls: *Apis.* So weak during the attack, she cannot raise a cup to her lips: *Silic.* Weakness of hands with irritability: *Carb. veg.*

Cold. With anxiousness: *Graphit.*, ǀǀ*Pulsat.;* with anxiety and flying heat: *Pulsat.;* dislikes to be alone: *Calc. ostr.;* afraid of ghosts: *Pulsat.;* with great peevishness: ǀǀ*Nitr. ac.;* vexed and fretful: *Phosphor.;* icy cold hands, with heat in the head when talking much: *Phosph. ac.;* starting in sleep, whining, with anxious expression: *Ignat.*

Heat. Excitable; gets hot hands from talking: *Graphit.;* by day, with mental excitement: *Sepia;* congestion to the hands, with cheerful, clear mind: *Phosphor.;* careless humor: *Veratr.;* flying heat mostly in hands, as from fear after a fright: *Calc. ostr.;* with anxiety: *Carb. veg., Phosphor.;* with shuddering and tearful anxiety: *Ignat.;* with hypochondric mood: *Nux mosch.;* heat in right hand, with very ill humor: *Pulsat.;* easily frightened: *Veratr.*

Sweat. With anxiety: *Chamom., Mercur.;* cold sweat on hands, stupid: *Coccul.;* in palms of hands with inability to think: *Calc. phosph.;* with anxious heat: *Lamium;* cool sweat in palms of hands, with anxiety and irresolution: *Chamom.*

Outside of Hands. Redness from congestion, with great brightness of mind: *Phosphor.;* anxiety, with trembling and red spots, no heat: *Pulsat.;* distended veins on arms and hands, with lassitude and ill humor: *Strontian;* a scurf on the back of the hand which came over night brings him all out of humor: *Psorin.*

FINGERS.

Greater mobility in the fingers with brightness: *Spigel.*

Grasping with fingers, in mania: *Stramon.;* twitching with the fingers and anxiety: *Pulsat.*

Cannot hold the pen, anguish: *Coffea.*

Stitches in the little finger running upwards, with anxiety and sadness: *Caustic.*

Pains in the fingers with mental dullness: *Moschus.*

Tingling in point of fingers, especially the thumb, with difficult comprehension: *Natr. carb.*

Crawling in points of fingers, in hands and arms, with great anxiety: *Natr. mur.*

Crawling in fingers causes anxiousness: *Veratr.*

Drops of sweat hang on the points of the fingers, with anxiety: *Sepia.*

Pains in sore finger, makes him frantic: *Cepa.*

Tetters on fingers with weakmindedness: *Ran. bulb.*

LOWER LIMBS.

Thighs. Cramp-like pain in the hip-joint, after anxiety, waking at night: *Sepia;* twitching of the muscles in inner thigh, with anxiety and faint feeling: *Mangan.;* periodical, nervous (spasmodic) drawing, from the hip to the knee, causing screams: *Arg. nitr.;* tearing stitches causing screams, in the left thigh when at rest: *Sepia.*

Great weakness in the muscles of the thighs with anxiousness: *Spigel.*

Motions of Lower Limbs. Raises the feet up high in walking, as in gressus gallinaceus, because all objects seem larger: *Agar., Euphorb.;* anxiety, with spasmodic drawing in the right leg: *Thuya;* spasms in lower limbs, with or between attacks of mania: *Cuprum;* stamping of feet, with senselessness: *Stramon.*, with restlessness: *Dulcam.*, in rage: *Veratr.;* trembling of the legs after talking, has to go by herself to rest: *Ambra;* jerking of the legs with anxiety: *Hepar s. c.;* starts from sleep, with involuntary jerks of the left leg: *Zincum.*

Sensations and Conditions. On seeing anything to vex her, feels it in the limbs: *Nux vom.*

Restlessness in the legs when standing, with anxiety: *Anac.*, when in a close room, with desire for air: *Asterias.*

Lower limb gets asleep, feeling in the joint as if dead, most towards evening, with great anxiety: *Natr. mur.*

Heaviness, as of lead in the legs after vexation: *Lycop.*

Lassitude and fatigue of the lower extremities, with dazed feeling as if drunk: *Arg. nitr.*

Weakness of lower limbs, as if unable to support the body, uses wrong words when speaking: *Lil. tigr.*

Great weakness in the feet and joints after walking in open air, cannot do mental work: *Borax.*

Feeling of anxiety and weakness in the right leg when walking: *Sulphur.*

Weakness in the feet, with melancholy: *Nitr. ac.;* with vexation: *Ant. crud.;* after abdominal anxiety: *Sulphur.*

Unable to stand on her feet, delirium: *Stramon.*

Tired feeling in the thighs and knee-joints, ill humor, no inclination to think: *Clemat.*

Heaviness of the legs, with ill humor: *Calc. ostr.*

Pain in the legs, with sadness· *Graphit., Nitr. ac.*

Stiffness of the legs: *Ignat.;* lameness: *Chamom.*, with stupor: *Stramon.*, with anxiety: *Bellad.*

Immobility of left leg, unconsciousness: *Nux mosch.*

Tearing in the bones, causing loud moaning: *Nitr. ac.*

Jerks in the legs, waking from sleep: *Magn. carb.*

Shuddering in the legs with inclination to laugh: *Hura.*

Trembling of legs, with anxiety: *Borax, Rhus tox., Sarsap.*

Knees. Knocking together of knees after a fright: *Cinnab.*

Unsteadiness in the knees, compels to lie down after a fright, caused by sudden surprises: *Mercur.*

Trembling in the knees, with anxiousness: *Hepar s. c.*
Trembling of one knee and foot, with eager expectation: *Nux vom.*
Tired feeling in the knees, with mental activity: *Mezer.*
Knees give way, with indifference and depression: *Rhodod.*
Knees give way after the least vexation: *Caustic.;* after a fit of rage: *Glonoin.;* in delirium: *Stramon.*
Pain in knees, with restlessness: *Arsen.;* moaning: *Canthar.*
Pain, as if beaten in left knee, with anxious heat: *Conium.*
Terrible pain in knees, with moaning and whimpering: *Canthar.*
A terribly disagreeable feeling of short duration in the knee: *Ars. hydr.*
Boring pains in knees, with loud screaming: *Canthar.*
A stitch in the knee when falling asleep: *Mercur.;* startling stitches: *Sulphur.*

Legs and Calves. Restlessness in legs, with anxiety: *Calc. phosph.*
Cramp-like feeling in the calves, with lassitude: *Arg. nitr.*
Hardness of the calves, as if flattened, with unbearable pain, cramp-like feeling: *Arsen.*
Painful stitch in the right leg when rising from kneeling posture, which frightens her: *Carb. an.*
Lassitude and tired feeling in the legs, with hypochondric mood: *Arg. nitr.*
Restlessness and anxiety at night, with coldness of legs and cold sweat on them: *Thuya.*
Malignant ulcers, with marked indifference: *Crotal.*

FEET.

Sensations. Pain in the joints, with despair and thoughts of death: *Acon.*
Pinching, cutting pains in the feet, cause weeping: *Hyosc.*
Itching, boring stitch in the dorsum of right foot, has to scream: *Spigel.*
Pain, as if beaten in the outer side of the foot, has to scream, better from rubbing: *Hepar s. c.*
After vexation, feels it in her feet: *Nux vom.*
Has to look down when walking, to assure himself that the left foot which he turns in when walking, is not twisted: *Psorin.*
Restlessness in the feet, with crawling and heat: *Sulphur.*
Has to move the feet continually and walk about: *Alum.*
Trembling of feet, and weeping from music: *Thuya;* with anxiousness first in head: *Sarsap.*
Weak feeling in the feet, with trembling after anxiety in abdomen: *Sulphur;* lassitude, beside herself, with fear of death: *Magn. sulph.*
Tired feeling in the feet at twilight, with quiet mood: *Ignat.*
Languid feeling in the feet, not well humored: *Zincum.*
Heaviness. With anxiety: *Ignat., Nitr. ac.;* with dejection: *Graphit.*
When walking in open air, followed by ill humor when in doors: *Ignat.*

Sadness: *Calc. ostr.*, *Graphit.;* timidity: *Spongia;* irritability: *Calc. ostr.;* aversion to labor: *Calc. ostr.;* to mental labor: *Clemat.*

Melancholic weeping mood, with heaviness: *Clemat.; Cyclam.*

Cold feet, with mental excitement: *Magn. carb.;* with anxious trembling: *Pulsat.*

Coldness. With anxiety: *Cuprum, Graphit., Sulphur;* impatience: *Sulphur;* with mental excitement: *Magn. carb.;* with anxious trembling: *Pulsat.*

With hot head and dislike to talk: *Laches.*

Worse when alone: *Calc. ostr.;* in mania: *Stramon.;* sitting at the table, with itching of nostrils: *Sulphur.*

And heat in head, forgets every moment what he was to do: *Sulphur.*

Better warming the feet, became heated; stupefaction: *Laches.*

Soles. A burning stitch at the inner border of the sole of the left foot, has to scream: *Ratanh.*

Violent stitches in soles and palms of hands: *Clemat.*

Burning in the soles, with anxiousness: *Hepar s. c.*

Toes. Violent tearing in the right big toe, has to scream: *Paris.*

Tearing and stitching in the left big toe, with vexation: *Baryt.*

Toes ache, with mental dullness: *Moschus.*

Stinging in the corns, has to scream: *Sepia.*

ALL THE LIMBS.

Pain. With exaltation of mind, "going to sleep:" *Natr. mur.;* tension: *Angust.;* sore aching, with excessively low spirits: *Cotyl.;* as if bruised after surprise: *Mercur.;* drawing, with anxiety about it: *Rhus tox.;* anxiety causes sleeplessness: *Bellad.;* tearing, with anxiety: *Arsen., Bellad.;* in the points of the fingers and toes: *Amm. mur.;* anxious and restless: *Canthar.;* tired of life: *Lycop.;* disposition to weep: *Phosphor.;* as if beaten: *Chamom.;* with crying: *Cuprum;* restless mind: *Arsen., Rhus tox.*

Dullness and depression, with pain in limbs: | | *Gelsem.*

When thinking of it: *Ox. ac.*

Other Sensations. Fixed idea that the body and limbs are of glass, and will break easily: *Thuya.*

Hands and feet feel as if loosened from the joints, which fills him with despair: *Stramon.*

After being irritable, it goes to the limbs: *Nux vom.*

Greater mobility with mental excitement: *Cinch. off., Coffea, Stramon.*

Throws the limbs about at night as if anxious, lies like one bereft of senses, with cold sweat on the forehead: *Bryon.*

Anxious feeling in the limbs, can find no rest: *Sepia;* restlessness with eructation: *Calc. ostr.*

Restlessness, does not know what to do with himself: *Bellad.;* with twitching in the limbs: *Cuprum;* unbearable restlessness in the evening: *Caustic.*

Restlessness particularly in the bends of the elbows, can bear no covering: *Asterias.*

Great restlessness and anxiety, driving from place to place, with trembling of the limbs: *Lam. alb.*

Trembling. With anxiety: **|** *Arsen.*, *Aurum*, *Calc. ostr.*, **|** *Carb. veg.*, *Caustic.*, **|** *Chamom.*, **|** *Coffea*, *Crocus*, *Cuprum*, *Graphit.*, **|** *Laches.*, *Magn. carb.*, *Mezer.*, *Moschus*, **|** *Natr. carb.*, *Phosphor.*, **|** *Pulsat.*, *Rhus tox.*, *Sarsap.*, *Sepia*; and restlessness: *Lam. alb.*

With anxiety in the evening: *Mezer.*; in afternoon: *Carb. veg.*

With vexation: *Sepia*; vehemence: *Aurum*, *Sepia.*

Hands and feet tremble, out of sorts, sad and inclined to weep: *Thuya.*

With disinclination to speak: *Sulphur*; excitability: *Mar. ver.*, *Nuc. v. c.*, *Petrol.*, *Valer.*; sudden out-cries: *Bellad.*; starting in sleep: *Petrol.*; mental dullness: *Aurum*; idiocy: *Opium.*

Twitching and starting in sleep with anxious heat: *Alum.*; sobbing· *Thuya*; uneasiness: *Cuprum*; loss of consciousness: *Stramon.*

Shaking of hands and feet, followed by anxiety: *Kali carb.*

Striking about with hands and feet in mental derangement: *Stramon.*

Strange movements with hands and feet in mania: *Bellad.*, *Stramon.*

Spasms with piercing screams: *Cuprum.*

Cramp and stinging in the limbs with agitation: *Ananth.*

Limbs go to sleep after excitement: *Natr. mur.*

Heaviness. Of all the limbs, with great clearness of mind: *Carb. veg.*; and relaxation, indisposed to work, but not ill humored: *Spigel.*; pain in joints and muscles, with anxiety: *Caustic.*; with ill humor and headache in morning: *Silic.*; dejection: *Graphit.*; and thoughtlessness: *Thuya.*

And occiput; trembling and anxious, forenoon: *Caustic.*

Pains in the limbs, with anxiety: *Magn. carb.*; sadness: *Graphit.*

Want of Strength. Sluggish, depressed: *Sarsap.*; lassitude in all the limbs, with ill humor: *Acon.*, *Petrol.*; after fits of weeping: *Conium*; with excitability: *Laches.*; with anxiety: *Acon.*

After waking from siesta, dissatisfied and angry: *Ciemat.*

Stretching with lassitude and drowsiness, vexatious and taciturn: *Borax.*

Lassitude after rising, no inclination to work: *Lact. vir.*

Lassitude in all the joints, which feel as if stretched, with anxiety: *Mangan.*

Weakness in all the limbs, with aversion to all work, constant desire to rest: *Arsen.*; with toothache driving to despair and anxious sweat: *Clemat.*; with anxiousness: *Aurum*; dejection: *Sabin.*

Limbs tired, anxious: *Acon.*; exhausted, faint-hearted: *Sabin.*

Lameness. With anxiety: *Aloes*; dejection, indifference, dispirited, as if a heavy burden weighed him down: *Conium*; with mania: *Hyosc.*; unconsciousness: *Stramon.*; after a fright: *Stannum*; irresolute: *Bellad.*, *Coccul.*

Cold, Heat, Sweat. Chilliness, with restlessness and anxiety: *Lam. alb.*; with mental derangement: *Stramon.*; with apprehension: *Arsen.*, *Sulphur.*

Coldness, with insensibility: *Aethus.*; stupor: *Nux mosch.*

Cold hands and feet, with anguish: *Graphit.*; with anxiety in the evening:

Graphit.; with mental depression, one cheek red, the other pale: *Ipec.;* from talking much and hearing conversation: *Amm. carb.;* does not like to be alone: *Calc. ostr.*

When standing, cold sweat on the back of hands and feet, with apprehension: *Lil. tigr.*

Burning of hands and soles, with anxiety: *Copaiv.*

MOVEMENTS.

Better from Motion. Trembling anxiety worse in rest: *Pulsat.*

Ill humor and drowsiness, with lassitude, better from exercise: *Cyclam.;* has to move, even rocking the chair relieves: *Angust., Carb. an.*

Better from Walking. While walking sensation as if carried on wings: *Thuya.*

Cheerful, inclined to work, walks with greater ease, as if the muscles had more elasticity: *Cicut.*

Dullness and heaviness in head, better from walking: *Sulphur.*

Sadness and lassitude in the morning which leaves one while walking: *Amph. ver.;* forsaken mood: *Rhus tox.;* unsteadiness: *Graphit.*

Worse while Walking. Desire to walk more than is good for her: *Arsen.*

Sad: *Sulphur;* and gloomy: *Sepia;* and grave: *Phosph. ac.;* anxiousness: *Nux vom.*

Fear of some one behind: *Anac., Bromum;* dejection: *Conium, Therid.;* depression: *Acon.;* low-spirited: *Thuya;* restless: *Caustic., Mercur.;* hypochondric: *Petrol.*

Morose: *Pulsat.;* uneasy: *Thuya.*

Whilst walking in street, suspicious about talk of people: *Baryt.;* afraid people suppose her to be crazy: *Calc. ostr.;* weeping: *Carb. veg.*

When walking after dinner absence of thoughts: *Rhus tox.;* walks about absorbed in himself: *Stramon.*

Mental dullness: *Rhus tox.;* stupefaction: *Carb. an.*

When walking fast anxiety or fear: *Staphis.*

Feeling as if drunk, obtuse intellect: *Lil. tigr.;* faint, giddy: *Arnic.*

In walking she imagines she is walking backwards: *Paull. pin.*

When walking fear of falling: *Coca, Natr. mur.;* faint and giddy: *Arnic.*

When beginning to walk painful concussion of the brain, with impatience: *Platin.*

Pressing headache in right temple aggravated by walking: *Helleb.*

Burning bellyache and cutting around navel, with ill humor: *Capsic.*

Pain in hemorrhoidal tumors becomes unbearable from walking: *Caustic.*

Anxiety in the afternoon, with heaviness; it is an exertion to walk: *Carb. an.*

NOTE.—In open air see hereafter.

Worse after Motion. Indolence, with dread of the slightest motion: *Arsen.;* shunning labor, no desire to move: *Nux vom.*

Becomes more excited and passionate after motion: *Sulphur.*

Anxiety and oppression from violent exercise in the evening: *Ox. ac.*

Anxiety: *Magn. carb., Niccol.;* ill humor: *Capsic., Sulphur;* difficult comprehension: *Arg. nitr.*

Motions, especially driving produces unconsciousness: *Gratiol.*

Headache, anxiety and bad conscience: *Rheum.*

Nausea, as if she had to belch, with anxiety: *Nitr. ac.*

When moving, bellyache; a burning deep in and cutting around the navel, with ill humor: *Capsic.*

Easily heated by exercise, irritable, inclined to anger: *Caustic.*

Anxious heat and sweat from the slightest motion: *Stannum;* anxious from the least motion, as if sweat would break out: *Niccol.;* anxious, with sweat: *Magn. carb.*

Rising. From the seat increases restlessness: *Caustic.;* from bed, anxiety, with shooting pains: *Magn. carb.*

Stretching. Inclination to stretch, more eventempered: *Calc. phosph.*

Cannot keep the limbs quiet, has to stretch them, particularly the arms, with anxiety and hasty restlessness: *Natr. carb.*

Dull and stupid feeling, with an inclination to stretch and yawn frequently, with oppression in the chest and aversion to mental and physical labor: *Plant. maj.; Sabin.*, see Model Cure, page 237.

When lying stretched out on the sofa sadness: *Hepar s. c.*

On Stooping. Worse from stooping, headache, anxiousness, bad conscience: *Rheum;* does not know where she is: *Calc. ostr.;* dullness in head: *Valer.*

Inability to think, indifference: *Natr. mur.*

Heaviness in head: *Lauroc.;* stitches in ear, irritability: *Chamom.;* burning bellyache, with ill humor: *Capsic.*

Dazed feeling after rising from stooping: *Lauroc.*

Great anxiety relieved by bending forward: *Bar. mur.*

Upper body bent backwards, semi-conscious, in mania: *Stramon.;* without unconsciousness or loss of mental faculties: *Kalmia.*

Worse after Exertion. More excited and passionate after exertion: *Sulphur.*

After working, apprehension: *Iodium.*

After exertion in open air gloomy, lachrymose humor: *Kali carb.;* pressure in the region below the heart, followed by sadness in-doors: *Lycop.*

After slight exertion weary, irritable, dejected: *Calc. ostr.;* after overexertion complaining: *Cuprum.*

After overlifting, vanishing of thoughts: *Psorin.;* after violent motion, forgetfulness: *Mezer.;* after overexertion, mental and bodily exhaustion: *Cuprum.*

On going down stairs vertigo, as if losing consciousness: *Borax, Ferrum, Merc. per.*

Flying heat, especially when busily engaged (also when sitting) or when walking fast; he gets very hot in the face, with stinging as of needles: *Oleand.*

When Working. Anxiousness: *Graphit., Iodium;* had to stop work for anxiety: *Aloes;* during every occupation anxious: *Anac.;* irritable: *Berber., Borax.*

Aversion to work or think, indifference, weak memory: *Aster.*

Excited: *Angust., Mur. ac., Oleand.*

After a short work oversensitive: *Calc. ostr.;* sees strange persons: *Magn. sulph.;* intrusion of ideas: *Mur. ac.;* thoughts of former events hover before him: *Mur. ac.;* distracted: *Hura.*

MODEL CURE.

A transitory tensive pain in the forehead, with a sensation as if the skin had grown fast, with tension in the eyes; redness of the skin around the alæ nasi, painful to the touch; dryness of the mouth and œsophagus, without thirst; collection of white frothy mucus, filling the corners of the mouth when talking; sensation of a body in the throat, which he tries to swallow but cannot, it offers no impediment to the swallowing of food; heart-burn and sour eructations, especially *when sitting bent over, which likewise aggravates the other symptoms; amelioration from sitting erect, from moving and stretching the limbs,* for which he has an involuntary desire; rumbling and gurgling in the abdomen, especially in the evening, in a warm room; great tiredness and laziness, with a feeling of deep-seated inward trouble, which makes him melancholy and sad: *Sabin.*[30].—AEGIDI.

POSITIONS.

Standing. Better when standing, anxiety and heat in head: *Phosphor.;* anxiety and burning in belly: *Calc. ostr.;* anxiety and nausea: *Tarax.*

While standing fear of some one behind: *Anac.;* auxious oppression in the epigastrium: *Mar. ver.;* great anxiety, as if he could not live, with a pressure in the hypochondria: *Phosph. ac.;* oppression and anxiety: *Cina;* anguish: *Agn. cast.;* ill humor: *Tax. bacc.*

Standing he cannot bear: *Chin. sulph.;* has to deliberate long; when standing and thinking pain leaves him: *Bryon.*

In erect posture, cessation of mental faculties: *Rhus rad.;* stands absorbed in thoughts: *Bryon.;* absent-minded: *Guaiac.*

Dazed feeling, does not know where he is: *Thuya;* stupefaction, staggering: *Valer.*

Unsteady: *Nitrum.*

Mental dullness increases: *Bryon., Guaiac.;* stupid feeling: *Bovist.*

Lassitude of mind and body: *Spigel.*

Sitting. Better while sitting down: *Crocus, Iodium;* anxiousness: *Iodium;* restlessness: *Caustic.*

Better when sitting up, fixed idea: *Phosph. ac.*

Has to sit straight up in agony: *Acon.;* anxiousness, after talkativeness: *Ambra.*

Inclination to sit down, with slow comprehension: *China;* with languor and indolence: *Ol. anim.*

Anxiousness, with flushes of heat when at work while sitting: I *Graphit.;* flying heat: *Oleand.*

Cannot sit on account of anguish: *Graphit., Silic.*

Anxiousness when sitting: *Phosphor., Tarax.*

When sitting bent over anxiety, with fear of death: *Rhus tox.;* anxiety, with spasmodic pain in the rectum, has to get up and walk: *Calc. ostr.*

Anxiousness in upper part of chest like from sedentary habits: *Arsen.*

When sitting has to take hold of something not to fall; restlessness: *Rhus tox.*

Whilst sitting at the table fear he should fall down insensible: *Carb. an.*

Sexual excitement with restlessness, cannot sit long: *Ant. crud.*

Restlessness when at work, has to get up and walk about: *Arsen.;* uneasiness: *Taxus;* ill humor: *Calc. ostr.*

Dizziness, dullness and drowsiness: *Pulsat.;* dull feeling in head as if drunk; dizziness when getting up: *Rhus tox.*

Vertigo while sitting: *Taxus;* while sitting at the table stupefaction: *Carb. an.*

When sitting up in bed senses leave him: *Natr. mur.;* stares without thinking: *Guaiac.;* vertigo and sudden loss of consciousness: *Silic.;* unconsciousness: *Taxus;* when sitting and thinking, cannot recollect: *Argent.*

From sitting bent after reading pressing pain in genitals: *Bellad.*

Hypochondria from sedentary habits: *Nux vom.*

Leaning. Disposition to lean against something; slow thinking, has to look at objects a long time before knowing them: *Gymnocl.*

Kneeling. Kneels or stretches arms as if searching, confused mind: *Stramon.*

Lying. Better when lying; dullness in head: *Gratiol.;* inability to work: *Zincum.*

Inclination to lie down after dinner, with inability to think: *Natr. mur.*

Lying on the left side causes anxiety: *Baryt., Phosphor.*

Anxiety when lying down: *Silic.;* worse when lying on the side: *Baryt., Kali carb., Phosphor., Pulsat.*

When lying did not know what she was about: *Bryon.*

Anxious pressure in the epigastrium when lying down: *Stannum.*

Pains in the bones of the head when lying down, with depression: *Aurum.*

After lying down, in evening, anxiety: *Nux vom.;* sadness: *Stramon.;* after stretching on the lounge sadness: *Hepar s. c.*

When lying in bed roaring in ears, with impatience: *Platin.*

Cannot get a comfortable position at night, which vexes to tears: *Lycop.*

Dyspnœa worse when idle or when lying down: *Ferrum.*

Lectrophilie. Morbid inclination to keep in bed, with gastric symptoms; burning down œsophagus into stomach, tender to the touch in scrobiculum, pain in region of left ovary with lectrophilie, will not leave her bed: *Al. p. s.*

Inexpressible feeling of an inward unbearable trouble, with which he is silent and keeps his bed: *Mercur.*

Quiet but complete despair of ever getting well: *Psorin.*

Lectrophobia. Shunning the bed, abhorring it while being very sick: *Cannab., Caustic., Lycop., Mercur., Natr. carb.*

Great dread of going to bed: *Cannab.*

NOTE.—Worse in bed, see "Night."

II Alum.	
I Baryt.	
Calc. ac.	
Calc. ostr.	
Cepa.	
Cinch. off.	
I Conium.	
II Crocus.	
II Ferrum.	
I Ignat.	
I Lycop.	
I Magn. mur.	
I Natr. carb.	
I Natr. mur.	
I Nux vom.	
I Petrol.	
II Plumbum.	
II Sepia.	
II Silic.	
II Tarax.	
II Veratr.	

Worse from being Idle. Idlers become foolish. *Cepa.*

When sitting idle ill humor and drowsiness, has a disgust for everything: *Calc. ac., Calc. ostr.*

When sitting idle dyspnœa: *Ferrum;* when unoccupied dizzy pain in left forehead: *Cinch. off.*

Worse in Rest. Nostalgia, grief for lost friends, unhappy love: *Phosph. ac.*

Violent pressing pain in the region of the loins: *Nitrum.*

Inclined to Rest. Suffering, weak, listless condition, inclination to rest: *Laches.*

Aversion to all occupation, wants to rest: *Arsen.*

Has to lie down, with anguish: *Mezer., Phelland.*

Feels comfortable when at rest in cool air: *Ant. crud.*

When sitting still all anxiety disappears: *Jodum.*

SOMNAMBULISM, CLAIRVOYANCE.

See Margin List and compare Night Walking.

I Acon.
II Agar.
I Alum.
II Anac.
I Ant. crud.
Atrop.
Bellad.
I Bryon.
Cicut.
Cyclam.
Hyosc.
Kali brom.
Laches.
Moschus.
I Natr. mur.
I Nux mosch.
II Opium.
II Phosphor.
I Silic.
Sol. nigr.
Spigel.
II Spongia.
I Stannum.
Stramon.
II Sulphur.
Veratr.

Ecstasy. Sensation as if the soul had no connection with the body: *Anac.*

Ecstasy, with pleasant warmth and lightness: *Jatroph.*

Desire to make no motions, with a feeling of serenity: *Coca.*

Longing or languishing of mind and body with oversensitiveness: *Cinch. off.;* serenity, with pleasant lassitude, smiling, contented face: *Lauroc.;* unusual serenity and vivacity after supper: *Colchic.;* the same for fifteen minutes, then followed by drowsiness: *Bellad.*

Lightness. Lightness, cheerfulness and mental activity alternate with fullness and tension after eating: *Ant. crud.*

Clear mind and comfortable feeling: *Carb. veg.*

Mental and bodily exhilaration, everything feels so light: *Alum.*

Great lightness of all motions, with cheerfulness: *Cocc. cact., Gambog.;* light and cheerful: *Petrol.;* merry: *Thuya.*

Great mobility of body in mania: *Opium.*

240   MIND AND DISPOSITION.

Excitable, Agitated. Mental and physical exaltation: *Alcohol, Alum.*
Excitement of body and mind: *Aloes.*
Great agitation with nervous irritation: *Ananth.*
Overexcitability, prepared for pleasant or unpleasant emotions, no bodily weakness: *Arnic.;* hypersensitive condition of nervous system, nerves are "on the stretch:" *Cinch. off.;* overexcitability of all senses, especially after using chamomile tea: *Coffea.*
Great excitability and restlessness: *Colchic.*
Nervous excitement; every impression on mind or body excites inward trembling: *Hepar;* with mental excitement trembling of the body: *Petrol., Rhus tox.*
Great excitement, moves around so fast it gets dark before his eyes: *Stramon.*
Mobility of limbs, howling and crying about trifles: *Bellad.*
Walking is much easier, feeling as if her body was carried on wings: *Thuya;* walks fast; impulsive mind: *Arg. nitr.*
Cannot think; acts without thought; keeps walking fast as if by instinct; feels hurried, does not know why; is forgetful; cannot decide for herself; must depend upon others: *Lil. tigr.*
Involuntary hastiness in taking hold of things and walking: *Sulphur;* takes things hastily with trembling: *Rhus tox.*
Hastiness in all his ways as if driven by inward fear, with lassitude: *Viol. tric.;* does every thing hastily, cannot do anything fast enough to satisfy himself: *Aurum, Sulph. ac.;* anxious restlessness and desire to accomplish much in which she fails; suffers from lassitude: *Calc. ostr.*
Greater facility in performing motions, with cheerful humor: *Cocc. cact.;* increased muscular mobility: *Iodium;* liveliness, with red face and glistening eyes in mania: *Opium.*
Feeling of strength and cheerfulness: *Opium, Platin., Sarsap.*
Increased physical strength, with inclination for bodily exercise: *Zizia.*
Very courageous and strong, wants to fight everybody: *Bovist.*
Feels an irrisistable desire to sing with excessive hilarity, for a while, thereupon absentminded and indisposed to do any kind of work: *Spongia.*
Merriness, singing and dancing, making rhymes, telling love-tales, exploits of battle and hunting stories; increased physical strength: *Agar.*
Great strength in mania: *Bellad., Canthar., Hyosc., Stramon.*
Irresistible strength in his fury: *Hyosc.*
Strongest muscular power, with senselessness: *Stramon.*
Great cheerfulness and activity: *Aloes.*
Mental and bodily activity increased: *Bromum.*
Comfortable, easy feeling: *Cocc. cact.*
Feels fresher and more active: *Lauroc.*
Comfortable feeling, with increased cheerfulness: *Valer.*
Comfortable body, merry mind: *Aurum.*
Feeling refreshed in body, high humor: *Lauroc.*
Alternating States. Vexation and ill humor alternating with cheerful-

ness, felt like a slight tremor in the joints: *Cyclam.;* vexation and lassitude changing with cheerfulness and lightness of limbs: *Natr. mur.*

Overactivity followed by anxiousness: *Benz. ac.;* lassitude, bodily fatigue, and getting better in rest: *Cinnab.*

Bodily suffering and cheerful mind, alternating with the reverse: *Platin.*

Contradictions. Feels strong but has no will: *Calc. ac.*

Increased physical strength with aversion to mental labor: *Colchic.*

Ill humor and anxious mind, coming it seems from the abdomen, but mental activity not impeded: *Asaf.*

Vexatious all day, dissatisfied, apprehensive and yet not averse to mental activity: *Caustic.;* contemplative, taciturn, apprehensive yet desire to be active: *Mur. ac.;* vexatious, yet desire to work: *Natr. carb.;* anxious, vexed by every thing that comes in her mind, yet keeps at her work diligently: *Phelland.;* ill humor, with inclination to work: *Sarsap.*

Cheerful and communicative in spite of disagreeable fullness: *Laches.*

Would like to work, but has neither the proper attention nor the strength: *Helleb.*

Bodily weakness, with mental activity: *Thuya;* the body emaciates in the same ratio as the mind increases: *Digit.*

Feels well bodily, but ill-humored: *Phosphor., Phosph. ac.*

Imagines to be sick: *Calc. ostr., Nitr. ac., Stramon.*

MODEL CURE.

Mrs. B., æt. 29, a miner's wife with four children. At the time when menses ought to appear, violent congestions to the chest and neck; felt as if her head would burst and her heart be squeezed off; violent stitches, as if a knife was plunged into her chest and head; frequently unconsciousness and epileptic convulsions; was bled once a month, which made her so weak that she could scarcely attend to her household duties. After mental excitement, especially a short time before catamenia, slight vertigo, vanishing of thoughts and fainting, from which she recovered in a few moments, without, however, being fully conscious; the outer world had no existence for her; automatically she attended to her household duties, and on awaking from this condition, she had not the slightest recollection of what she had done. If forcibly aroused she had violent convulsions. At times she was in a *clairvoyant state*, and answered questions accurately on subjects entirely out of her sphere; on returning to consciousness she was perfectly ignorant of what she had said. Pulse small and weak; in the carotid a slight nun's murmur. *Bellad.* relieved the congestions, but did not change the main symptoms. General lassitude; tired feeling in her knees as from a long journey; great sleepiness, with dizziness as if drunk; does not know where she is; dreaminess, with closing of the eyes; weak memory; forgetfulness; absence of mind; gradual vanishing of thoughts when reading; does not carry out resolutions, but remains standing thoughtlessly on one spot; appears to herself as if chained to her surroundings: *Nux mosch.* In three months she was free from all symptoms.—LORBACHER.

RESTLESSNESS.

||Acon.
|Agar.
|Ambra.
|Amm. carb.
|Anac.
Apis.
Arg. nitr
Arnica.
||Arsen.
Asaf.
|Aurum.
|Bellad.
|Bismuth.
|Bryon.
Calad.
||Calc. ostr.
|Calc. phosph.
|Cannab.
Camphor.
||Canthar.
Carb. an.
|Carb. veg.
Caustic.
Cepa.
Chamom.
|Chelid.
Cicut.
||Cina.
|Cinch. off.
Cinnab.
Colchic.
Coloc.
Conium.
Crocus.
Crotal.
Cuprum.
Cyclam.
Digit.
Elaps.
Graphit.
|Helleb.
Hippom.
|Hydroph.
||Hyosc.
|Ignat.
|Iodium.
Kali carb.
||Kobalt.
||Laches.
|Lam. alb.
Lob. infl.
|Lycop.
||Magn. carb.
|Magn. mur.
Mancin.
|Mangan.
Mar. ver.
||Mercur.
|Merc. subl.
Moschus.
Mur. ac.
||Natr. carb.
|Natr. mur.
Niccol.
||Nitr. ac.
||Nux vom.
Opium.
Petrol.

Frequent change of Position: *Arsen., Bellad., Canthar., Chamom., Cuprum, Iodium;* from uneasiness: *Rhus tox.*

Cannot sit still, must sway herself in all directions and move all her limbs, internal uneasiness: *Rhus tox.;* cannot sit quiet, nor lie quietly in bed: *Rhus tox.;* every position becomes annoying; fretful: ||*Bismuth.*

With anxiety: *Arsen.;* anxious weeping: *Camphor.;* apprehensions: *Aurum, Helleb., Merc. subl.;* ill humor: *Bismuth.;* impatience: *Acon.*

As if being hurried: *Laches.;* unsteadiness: *Natr. carb.;* gets up, lies down: *Mancin.;* ease nowhere: *Mercur.*

Weakness, has to lie down, but does not know where for unsteadiness: *Hydroph.;* up and down, with anguish: *Apis;* bending in all directions and complaining: *Arsen.*

Can find rest nowhere, changes his position in bed conconstantly, wants to get out of one bed into the other: *Arsen.;* uninterrupted restlessness, changes position constantly, does not know what he wants: *Acon.*

Mental and bodily restlessness, takes up a book and throws it down again, changes his seat continually; with anxiety during the chill, cannot find rest in any position: *Lam. alb.*

Tosses greatly, raises himself up in delirium: *Chamom., Cina, Helleb., Stramon.*

Great restlessness in the legs in the evening, cannot keep them still: *Calc. ostr.;* cannot keep the limbs still with anxiety: *Natr. carb.*

Frequent change of Place: *Arsen., Bellad., Canthar., Crotal.,* a.m.m.; from anxiety: *Arg. nitr., Bryon., Carb. veg.;* with anguish: *Arsen.;* with despair: *Cepa;* with apprehension: *Aurum;* with inability to persevere: *Asaf.;* discouraged: *Anac.;* great depression, sets him to weep: *Chelid.;* uneasiness: *Amm. carb.*

Anxious feeling towards evening, cannot sit still, has to walk about: *Nitr. ac.;* cannot sit still long in one place: *Bellad.;* much walking: *Thuya.*

Has to keep in constant motion, regrets that he cannot accomplish anything: *Aurum;* with anxiety and dyspnœa: *Carb. veg.*

Driven from place to place: *Asaf.*

Cannot work while sitting still, has to get up and walk about: *Arsen.*

Incessant motion, unconsciousness: *Stramon.*

Restless, cannot stay long in one place: *Mercur., Stannum.*

Thinks she must move around: *Calc. phosph.*

‖ Phosphor.
Phosph. ac.
Platin.
╷ Plumbum.
╷ Prun. spin.
‖ Pulsat.
Sambuc.
Sarsap.
‖ Sepia.
Silic.
Spigel.
╷ Stannum.
╷ Staphis.
‖ Stramon.
‖ Sulphur.
Tabac.
Therid.
Thuya.
Valerian.
Veratr.
Ver. vir.

Feels as if he had committed a great crime: *Mercur.*
Tossing about in bed with great rage: *Stramon.*
Seeks one corner after another, finds rest no where: *Agar.*
Driving out of Bed. Compare *Bryon., Carb. an.,* ❙*Carb. veg., Chamom., Conium,* ❙*Graphit.,* ❙*Lycop.,* ❙*Magn. carb., Magn. mur., Natr. carb., Natr. mur., Niccol., Nitr. ac., Pulsat.,* ❙❙*Rhus tox., Sepia, Silic., Therid.;* anguish driving from one place to another, and at night out of bed; wants to go from one bed to another, lies now here now there: *Arsen.*
Desire to run away. Has to walk all the time: *Acon.*
Would like to run from one place to another: *Apis.*
He wants to run away, to leave: *Arsen.;* fear of imaginary things, wants to run away from them: ❙*Bellad.*
Wishes to go out of the house at bed-time: *Elaps;* runs about in his room at night: *Hyosc.;* wants to run out of the room; frightening illusions: *Hyosc.;* running about, with mental derangement: *Iodium.*
Runs from house to house: *Moschus.*

NOTE. See Typhoid Fevers.

Restlessness as a Concomitant. Anticipation of happiness: *Valer.*
General nervous uneasy sensation: *Cinnab.*
Does not know what to do with himself: *Petrol.*
Excitability as after an insufficient narcotic, restless and weak: *Mar. ver.*
Anxiety: *Acon., Arnic., Arsen., Lam. alb., Stannum;* fear of death: *Arsen.*
Sleeplessness and anxiety: *Cuprum.*
Anxiety, feels like a criminal: *Graphit.*
With anxious and sad dreams, restless sleep: *Lob. infl.*
Anguish: *Asaf., Bellad., Caustic., Carb. veg., Magn. mur., Nux vom., Opium, Phosphor.*
Bodily restlessness, with anxiousness: *Arsen., Natr. carb.,* ❙❙*Phosph. ac., Platin.;* apprehensiveness: *Spigel.;* ill humor: *Natr. carb.*
Uneasiness of mind and body: *Agar;* uneasiness, apparent discontent amounting often to restlessness of a distressing kind: *Acon., Ver. vir.*
Restless ill humor, with no desire to work: *Aloes.*
No rest and unsuccessful: *Amm. carb.;* displeased with everything: *Graphit.;* fretfulness: *Natr. carb.;* impatience: *Sepia;* has to move the limbs: *Colchic.;* screaming and running about: *Veratr.;* after eating: *Petrol., Phosphor.*
Great anxiety, throws himself down in despair and gets up to walk about again, with colic: *Cepa.*
A week before catamenia: *Kali carb.;* a day before, with anxiety: *Sulphur.*
And lassitude: *Cyclam.;* after lying down in evening with painful twitching of the limbs: *Hepar;* before midnight: *Sarsap.*
In all the limbs like a crawling, with anxiety; only in the day time: *Ambra.*
Weeping: *Sulphur;* hastiness: *Aurum;* disinclined to work: *Arnic.;* fear of being left alone: *Arsen.*
Mental and bodily restlessness, as if prevented from doing something that should be done: *Arnic.*

244   MIND AND DISPOSITION.

Cannot contain himself: *Calad.;* does not know where to turn: *Hydroph., Veratr.;* as if tormented: *Mangan.;* fright: *Sambuc.;* delirium: *Stramon.*

With heaviness in head, cannot speak in proper connection: *Merc. subl.;* unconsciousness: *Stramon.*

Irritable and crying children: *Arsen., Chamom.;* tossing about also when awake: *Cina.*

TREMBLING.

See Hands, pages 229 and 230; Limbs, 233, 234 and 235.

Ambra.
Anac.
I Arg. nitr.
II Arsen.
I Aurum.
I Baryt.
Bellad.
Borax.
I Calc. ostr.
Canthar.
I Carb. veg.
II Caustic.
Chamom.
Cina.
Clemat.
II Coffea.
II Crocus.
Cyclam.
Daph. ind.
Ferrum.
I Graphit.
I Hura.
Iberis.
Iodium.
Laches.
Lamium.
Lycop.
Magn. carb.
II Mercur.
Mezer.
Moschus.
II Natr. carb.
I Niccol.
II Nitr. ac.
I Nux mosch.
Nux vom.
Opium.
Origan.
II Petrol.
Platin.
Phosphor.
I Phosph. ac.
I Psorin.
II Pulsat.
Ran. bulb.
I Rhus tox.
Sambuc.
I Sarsap.
I Sepia.
Stannum.
Sulphur.
Tabac.
Thuya.
I Valer.
II Zincum.

After Emotions. Inwardly after the slightest emotion: *Zincum;* all over from every moral impression: *Psorin.;* long-lasting, like a chill: *Zincum.*

Very much affected by little surprises; trembles all over and feels as if lame: *Mercur.*

Mind much agitated, every event (music) causes trembling: *Natr. carb.*

In every limb after being frightened by a noise: *Baryt.;* all over, after noise in the street: *Caustic.;* from a door opening or a chair pushed: *Hura, Moschus;* fright from a noise in the street: *Baryt.*

Tremulousness, startled by noise: *Tabac.*

Trembling of the limbs from vexation: *Ran. bulb.;* when he cannot give vent to his rage: *Aurum;* when quarrelling: *Nitr. ac.*

Trembling from thinking deeply: *Aurum, Borax.*

Feelings. Joyful feeling: *Cyclam.;* exuberant spirits, overexcitement: *Petrol.*

Tremor in the nerves as when anticipating happiness: *Aurum, Valer.*

After a kind of voluptuous trembling of the whole body, dolefulness: *Calc. ostr.*

Trembling, with weeping (nostalgia) and anxiety: *Clemat.;* melancholy, sad weeping mood, with sighing and lassitude: *Natr. carb.;* sadness: *Petrol.;* low spirited: *Natr. carb.;* depressed: *Phosph. ac.*

Peculiar melancholy, especially in women, with subsultus tendinum: *Iodium.*

With apprehensions: *Arg. nitr., Aurum, Magn. carb., Rhus tox., Sepia;* fearful forebodings: *Psorin.*

With anxiety: I*Arsen., Ambra, Borax, Canthar., Carb. veg., Caustic.,* I*Coffea, Crocus, Graphit., Lam. alb., Magn. carb., Mezer., Natr. carb., Nitr. ac., Nux mosch., Phosphor., Platin., Pulsat., Rhus tox., Sarsap., Valer.*

With fear: *Magn. carb., Niccol.;* of apoplexy: *Thuya;* of

ghosts: *Pulsat.;* of murdering some one: *Arsen.;* anguish: *Arsen., Canthar., Carb. veg., Coffea, Graphit., Lycop., Magn. carb., Natr. carb., Platin.;* and fear of death: *Pulsat.*

With ennui: *Laches.;* apathy: *Arg. nitr.*

And timidity: *Chamom.;* fearfulness: *Niccol.;* irritability: *Arg. nitr., Daph. ind., Natr. carb.;* after ebullition of anger: *Sepia;* vehemence: *Aurum, Sepia.*

With sighing: *Natr. carb.;* weeping: *Carb. veg.;* whining and complaints: *Cina;* sudden screams: *Bellad.*

Fearfulness, desire to be alone: *Niccol.;* great desire for activity: *Psorin.*
Feels as if frightened; an indefinable dread: *Iber. am.*
With feverish restlessness and anxiety: *Ruta.*
With excitability and hypochondriacal anxiety: *Valer.*
With derangement: *Arsen., Natr. carb.;* delirium: *Arsen.;* fierceness: *Petrol.;* mania: *Arsen.*

As if senses would leave: *Platin.;* lying insensible: *Arsen., Opium;* want of consideration: *Petrol.*

Of Local Parts or whole Body. Inner: *Crocus, Natr. carb.,* ||*Petrol.,* ||*Thuya,* ||*Zincum;* hands: *Coffea, Platin., Psorin., Pulsat., Sepia;* knees: *Cinnab., Mercur., Psorin.;* feet: *Borax, Sarsap.;* hands and feet, with sudden cries: *Bellad.*

Limbs: *Baryt., Lamium, Nitr. ac., Mezer., Platin.;* of the whole body: *Arsen., Canthar., Crocus, Graphit., Laches., Mercur., Mezer., Natr. carb., Nux vom., Opium, Phosphor., Rhus tox., Therid.*

Head. In attacks: *Laches.;* pain in forehead and crown: *Sepia;* heaviness: *Sulphur;* followed by nosebleed: *Sepia;* cold sweat in face: *Arsen.;* pale face: *Nux vom.;* blue lips: *Cina;* cannot speak clearly: *Thuya.*

Abdomen. With nausea rising from pit of stomach: *Nux vom.;* vomiting: *Sulphur.*

Soon after dinner: *Nux vom.;* after supper: *Caustic.;* nausea: *Nitr. ac.;* anxiety in scrobiculum: *Sepia;* tearing pain in bowels: *Arsen.;* urging to stool: *Sulph. ac.;* after stool: *Carb. veg.*

Chest. Pain: *Cina;* ebullition of blood: *Sambuc.;* palpitation: *Chamom.*

Body. With pains in the limbs: *Cina;* waving sensation in nerves: *Natr. carb.;* weakness in arms: *Anac., Arg. nitr., Calc. ostr., Sulphur;* has to lie down: *Nux vom.;* as if tired out: *Ferrum;* as if a disease was threatening: ||*Petrol.;* involuntary motions: *Carb. veg.*

Sleep. Better after going to bed: *Magn. carb.;* wakened by dreams: *Origan.;* from 3 A.M., without sleep: *Rhus tox.*

Time of Day. Morning, after rising: *Arg. nitr.;* all day: *Magn. carb.;* afternoon: *Anac., Pulsat.;* evening: *Mezer., Sambuc., Sulphur;* lasting from ten to twenty-seven days: *Rhus tox.*

Out-doors. Continuing: *Canthar.*

Sweat. *Sulphur, Thuya.*

Sensations. During the pains: *Daph. ind.;* as from anxiousness, but without: *Laches.*

STARTING FROM FRIGHT.

‖ Acon.
Aether.
❘ Alum.
❘ Amm. carb.
❘ Ant. crud.
❙ Arsen.
Atrop.
❘ Baryt.
‖ Borax.
❙ Calc. ostr.
Cannab.
Card. mar.
Cicut.
Conium.
Hura.
❘ Hyosc.
❙ Ignat.
‖ Laches.
❘ Ledum.
‖ Magn. carb.
❙ Mercur.
❙ Natr. carb.
‖ Narc. mur.
❙ Nux vom.
❙ Rhus tox.
❘ Sabad.
‖ Silic.
❙ Stramon.
Tabac.
Therid.

Starts at a little noise: *Ant. crud., Cannab., Sabad.;* at the least noise: *Borax, Laches.,* ❙*Natr. carb., Narcot.;* at every noise: *Card. mar., Hura;* at every near noise: *Calc. ostr.*

Every little noise in the street he supposes to be an alarm of fire: *Baryt.*

Oversensitiveness of hearing: *Conium;* hearing a scream: *Borax;* from a crackling in the ear: *Rhus tox.*

When a door is opened; at every word spoken: *Cicut.;* at the smallest thing falling: *Alum.;* at a distant shot: *Borax.*

Wakes from sleep: *Nux vom.;* sets him crying: *Aether;* with desire to weep: *Hura;* from a dream; delirium: *Atrop.*

Worse in the mornings: *Calc. ostr.*

After a fright: *Hyosc., Ignat.;* in affright, rage: *Stramon.;* in an unconscious state: *Cicut., Stramon.*

MODEL CURE.

A little girl had, after a great fright which almost produced convulsions, copious diarrhœa, worse at night, painless with much wind; emaciated, great *nervousness: Ignat.*—GROSS.

Twitching. Excited about it: *Al. p. s.;* followed by senselessness: *Cuprum;* in sopor: *Opium.*

With deranged mind: *Indig.;* delirium: *Stramon.*

Subsultus Tendinum. In delirium: *Iodium, Stramon.;* jerking, gesticulating with the fingers, in delirium: *Bellad.;* muscles moving automatically in unconscious states: *Stramon.;* ludicrous gestures in mania: *Stramon.;* limbs contorted, in delirium: *Hyosc.;* convulsed, in derangement: *Bellad.;* all muscles convulsed, with insensibility: *Stramon.*

Wringing hands, with lamentations: *Sulphur;* raising arms, with crying: *Stramon.*

Spasms. After vexation: *Cuprum;* even after the slightest: *Bellad.;* after anger: *Chamom.;* after a fright: *Stramon.;* after emotional or moral disturbances: *Kali brom.;* after the least hurt: *Hyper.*

With anxiety: ‖*Alum.,* ❙*Bellad.,* ‖ *Caustic., Chamom.,* ❙ *Coccul.,* ‖ *Cuprum,* ❙*Hyosc.,* ❙*Ignat., Lycop., Natr. sulph., Veratr.;* with ill humor and hysteria: *Conium;* with groaning and moaning: *Cuprum;* screaming; *Opium;* penetrating screams: *Cuprum.*

In the hands and feet, can scarcely refrain from screaming: *Secal.*

With mania and rage: *Aethus., Canthar., Crocus, Mercur., Stramon.;* with derangement: *Stramon.;* difficult comprehension: *Arsen.;* speechlessness: *Cuprum;* stupor: *Stramon.;* with great agitation and excessive thirst: *Anath.*

Inflammation of bowels; anxiety and twitching: *Plumbum.*

Spasms alternating with fainting: *Acon.;* after spasms he awakes with paralyzed limbs; he cannot spell his name: *Thuya.*

CONVULSIONS; EPILEPTIC AND OTHER SPASMS.

With great weariness: *Bellad.;* spasmodic laughing: *Calc. ostr.;* hysterics, spasmodic motions and chill: *Conium.*
Convulsive thrashing with right arm and foot, loud screaming: *Opium.*

MODEL CURES.

Spasmodic attack in the morning in bed, with heat; after rising, cold sensation in the arm, then a jerk, with violent twitching in the trunk and arms; anxiety: *Caustic.*

Toward evening she suddenly fails to recognize her friends, screams out loud, laughs, weeps, talks disconnectedly, now as if in fright, then of her death; thinks she is surrounded by strange persons who insult her, seeks to fly. Twitching in the face and all the limbs, wrings her hands and throws them wildly about in the air: *Bellad.*—BICKING.

CONVULSIONS; EPILEPTIC AND OTHER SPASMS.
With loss of consciousness; with consciousness * according to H. Gross.

|| Acon.
|| Bellad.
|| Calc. ostr.
|| Camphor.
  Canthar.
|| Caustic.
| Chamom.
| Cicut.
* Cina.
|| Coccul.
|| Cuprum.
| Glonoin.
* Graphit.
* Helleb.
|| Hyosc.
|| Ignat.
|| Ipec.
* Kali carb.
|| Laches.
  Lauroc.
* Lycop.
* Magn. carb.
* Menyanth.
* Moschus.
* Natr. mur.
* Nitr. ac.
|| Nux mosch.
* Nux vom.
|| Opium.
* Phosphor.
* Platin.
* Plumbum.
  Secale.
  Sepia.
|| Silic.
| Stannum.
|| Stramon.
|| Sulphur.
  Thuya.
| Veratr.

With or without Consciousness: *Kali carb., Lycop., Nux vom., Platin., Plumbum;* losing it gradually: *Bellad.*

After Fright or Fear. See page 75, adding: *Cuprum, Secal., Veratr.;* starts at trifles and gets irritable: *Bellad.*

After Shock of Injury. With commotio medullæ spinalis: *Opium.*

Homesickness, love-pangs, jealousy: *Hyosc.*

Grief: *Hyosc., Ignat., Opium;* child being punished: *Ignat.;* vexation: *Bellad., Ignat., Nux vom., Sulphur;* attacks return after the slightest vexation: *Calc. ostr.*

After getting angry: *Chamom., Sulphur;* the nursing mother: *Opium.*

After emotions: *Bellad., Cicut., Hyosc., Ignat., Secal.*

After exertion of mind: *Bellad.;* of body by quick running: *Sulphur.*

With Feelings. Excessive cheerfulness: *Hyosc.*

Not sensitive to pain: *Coccul.;* overcome by sexual desire: *Laches.;* smiling before attack: *Bellad.*

Sad: *Cicut., Lycop.;* melancholic: *Psorin.;* depressed: *Lycop.*

Apprehensive about getting well again: *Calc. ostr.;* fear of falling: *Lycop.;* fear in his eyes: *Zincum;* anxiety before attack: *Lauroc.,* with it: *Bellad., Calc. ostr., Chamom., Hyosc., Sulphur,* in scrobiculum: *Coccul.,* in præcordia: *Bellad.,* with breathing: *Coccul.;* indifference: *Cicut.*

Feelings and Conations. Timid: *Bellad.;* irritable: *Nux vom., Zincum;* discontented: *Nux vom.;* wild, dark look: *Valer.;* wilful, obstinate: *Calc. ostr.;* sensitive mood: *Zincum;* malicious disposition: *Cuprum.*

Actions. Spasmodic laughter: *Stramon.;* loud laughing: *Zincum;* screaming, laughing, singing, weeping: *Bellad.;* crying without being angry: *Cuprum;* whimpering: *Laches.*

Sighing and moaning: *Chamom.*

Screaming: | | *Bellad.,* | | *Calc. ostr.,* *Canthar.,* | | *Cicut.,* **I** *Cuprum,* | *Hyosc., Ignat., Laches., Lauroc., Lycop.,* | | *Nux vom., Opium, Plumbum, Stramon., Zincum;* sudden: *Cuprum, Opium;* loud, violent: *Bellad., Cicut., Cuprum, Opium, Plumbum;* piercing: *Cuprum;* mournful: *Bellad.;* crying when approached: *Ignat.;* for help: *Lauroc.;* at the slightest noise: *Cicut.;* during catamenia: *Cuprum;* striking about with arms and legs in a rage: *Canthar.;* with cardiac anxiety: *Lycop.;* one foot goes up and down: *Opium;* in sleep: *Zincum;* with starting: *Bellad.*

Hastiness in all motions, with fear: *Arsen.;* tries to escape: *Bellad.*

Desires. Strays from one subject to another in conversation: *Valer.*

Anxious restlessness: *Calc. ostr., Zincum;* wanders about: *Bellad.;* restless, desire to escape: *Caustic.;* restlessness and anxiety towards evening: *Bellad.;* looks around shyly, with anxiety: *Zincum.*

Depression: *Zincum;* lies as if dead after the convulsion: *Cicut.;* lassitude after convulsions: *Ignat.;* misunderstands questions: *Valer.;* difficult comprehension: *Cuprum;* mental dullness: *Calc. ostr.*

Idiotic condition before the attacks: *Caustic.*

Productions. Delirium: *Bellad., Ignat., Kali carb., Opium, Stramon.;* before: *Opium;* after: *Bellad.;* bites himself, tears clothes: *Bellad.;* sees ugly people: *Kali carb.*

With mania: *Bellad.;* in alternation, with mania: *Stramon.;* after it: *Cuprum;* with furor: *Bellad., Canthar., Crocus, Hyosc., Stramon.;* after furor, uterinus and hydrophobia: *Gratiol.*

Mental derangement: *Calc. ostr.;* confused, absentminded: *Laches.*

Reproductions. Speechless: *Bellad., Calc. ostr., Cuprum;* stupor. *Bellad., Cuprum, Œnanth.;* weak memory: *Bellad., Cuprum, Hyosc.*

Convulsions if forcibly aroused from half conscious state: *Nux mosch.;* frightened appearance: *Stramon.*

Convulsions of facial muscles; stupefied: *Acon.;* loss of senses: *Camphor.*

MODEL CURES.

Called in consultation to a case of cerebro-spinal meningitis, I found the patient, a woman, æt. 35, unconscious and in spasms. Her head was bent backwards, arms and limbs rigid; pulse very quick; breathing slow. A short time before she was taken ill, she had lost suddenly and in quick succession, two of her children. This mental shock producing almost a stunning effect, I considered as main indication, and proposed *Opium*[200]. She grew better at once and recovered in a short time.—C. G. RAUE.

A man, æt. 30, insane on religion, had frequent attacks of epilepsy from childhood. *Psorin.*[10], in water, improved the mental condition and epilepsy.— TIETZE, SEN.

MIND AND BODY WEAK, FEEBLE AND RELAXED.

Agar.
Alum.
I Anac.
Anath.
I Arsen.
Baryt.
II Bellad.
Berber.
Cinch. off.
Clemat.
Coffea.
Colchic.
Conium.
Convolv.
I Cuprum.
I Digit.
Gelsem.
Gratiol.
II Hippom.
Janiph.
Kali carb.
I Laches.
Lauroc.
Lepid.
Lycop.
Magn. carb.
Magn. sulph.
II Mercur.
I Natr. carb.
Natr. mur.
Nitr. ac.
Nitrum.
Nux vom.
Oleander.
Opium.
Phosphor.
Ptelea.
Rhus tox.
II Senega.
I Spongia.
Stannum.
Vip. torv.
Xiphos.

Agreeable sense of lassitude, with relaxation of muscles: *Gelsem.*

Body and mind exhausted after ecstasy: *Laches.*

Mental activity is followed by mental and bodily relaxation: *Clemat.*

Mental and bodily prostration after overexertion of mind and loss of sleep: **I I** *Cuprum.*

Mental infirmity, weak minded: *Anac.*

Bodily and mental infirmity: *Natr. carb.*

Mentally and bodily indisposed: *Opium;* weak and dispirited: *Oleand.;* attacks of mental and bodily prostration, has to lie down: *Mercur.;* with drowsiness: *Stramon.*

Stupefied and weak, has to lie down: *Opium.*

Aversion to move: *Natr. carb.;* getting tired soon, lazy: *Nux vom.;* fatigued, morose, unable to work: *Magn. sulph.;* weary, tired, relaxed, dislike to work: *Laches.*

Lassitude, no ambition to work, irritable, frequent flushes of heat to the face: *Lycop.;* after irritability: *Cinnab.*

Great languor and indisposition for either mental or physical labor: *Ptel. trif.*

Lassitude in the limbs, with indisposition to work: *Amm. carb.;* indisposition for mental or physical labor: *Lauroc.*

With sluggishness: *Alum., Canthar., Chamom., Chelid., Cinch. off., Crocus, Laches., Lactuc., Nux vom., Staphis.;* and general lassitude: *Seneg.*

Tiredness throughout the whole body, cannot do mental work: *Spongia.*

Prostrated and indisposed to think: *Nitrum.*

Great languor and weakness, with indisposition for mental labor: *Colchic.;* indisposed for any motion or mental occupation: *Kali carb.*

Exhausted, speaking is difficult: *Rhus tox.;* lassitude, also when speaking: *Digit.*

Weakness of body and mind; does not talk: *Arsen.*

Irritable sadness: *Natr. carb.;* suicidal ideas: *Ananth.*

Bodily C.C.C. Mental and bodily prostration, with great desire to eat: *Natr. mur.*

After dinner indisposition to work, with mental dullness: *Agar.*

After eating, hypochondriac depression, with mental and physical prostration: *Anac.*

On waking in the morning mental and bodily prostration: *Berber.*

Mental and physical prostration in the morning: *Laches., Phosphor.*

After catamenia mental and physical prostration, with despondency: *Alum.*

Contradictions. Lassitude, would like to rest all the time, with active mind: *Lycop.;* with cheerfulness: *Lauroc.*

Great prostration, with inclinition to joke and laugh: *Conium, Crocus.*

With foolish singing: *Crocus;* talks to himself: *Hyosc.*

Weak, exhausted, excited, talks much: *Ambra;* with weakness of arms and hands: *Carb. veg.*

Exhausted and talkative: *Hyosc.;* weakness, corporeal exhaustion and loquacity: *Laches.*

Exhaustion, with tranquil thoughts of death: *Zincum.*

Sudden relaxation of muscles with full consciousness: *Helleb.*

Bodily weakness, with full mental power: *Thuya;* weakness especially in the knees, with mental activity: *Cyclam.;* general prostration as if not enough sleep, with mental activity: *Veratr.*

No ambition; prostration, yet not ill-humored: *Cocc. cact.*

Sluggishness, yet not fatigued by walking: *Mur. ac.*

Mental dullness, indisposed for mental labor, but likes to do mechanical work: *Iodium.*

Ill humor, but disposition to work: *Sarsap.*

Indisposed to work, but inclined to deep thinking: *Natr. mur.*

Disposition for mental labor, with physical prostration: *Cicut.*

Alternations. Lassitude alternating with activity: *Aloes.*

Cheerfulness and feeling of great strength, alternating with despondency and weakness: *The North Pole of the Magnet.*

Great weakness after good humor: *Mercur.;* weakness causes her to think deeply: *Aurum.*

When the mind is cheerful the body suffers, and vice versa: *Platin.*

With Irritability: *Ambra, Calc. ostr., Carb. veg., Caustic.*

Nervous irritability, with prostration of the whole system: *Iris vers.*

Continual agitation, with tiredness and debility: *Anath.*

Great prostration, with increased sensibility: *Iodium.*

Weakness of body, irritable: *Calc. ostr., Phosph. ac.*

Oversensitiveness, nervous excitability, with general weakness: *Chin. sulph.*

Unusually irritable, next day weak and lazy: *Cinnab.;* fatigued and nervous feeling: *Hydroph.*

Sadness, with excitability: *Hyosc.*

Bodily relaxation and fatigue, with mental excitability: *Laches.*

Lassitude; the nerves are affected: *Natr. carb.*

Every event makes a violent impression, faintness: *Natr. carb.*

Hypersensitive condition of the nerves, music is unbearable, with prostration: *Sabin.*

Mania alternating with melancholy, irresolution; weak digestion: *Digit.*

In cases of great weakness of body and fainting, especially with pregnant and parturient women, we have made use of nutmeg and wine, applied to the epigastrium and palms of hands, with the best and quickest effect, also after parturition. —M. F. BLUFF. Old school. 1835.

Weakness of mind, comp. symptoms 20—28; and pages 304 and 305, Materia Medica, Vol. I.

WEAKNESS, WITH OTHER MENTAL CONCOMITANTS.

Amphisb.
Arsen.
I Bovist.
Carb. an.
Clemat.
Crotal.
I Ignat.
I Kali carb.
Laches.
I Lauroc.
I Mercur.
I Natr. carb.
I Natr. mur.
Phosph. ac.
Rhus tox.
Secale.
II Sepia.
Zincum.

Weak and Sad. Tender sadness which disposes one to be weak: *Amphisb.*

Great exhaustion, with sadness: *Bovist.;* weeping: *Arsen.*

Prostration, with great melancholy: *Clemat.;* sadness, indifference, and disgust for everything: *Ignat.*

Very tired after rising, with sadness; inclined to weep: *Carb. an.*

All strength gone, inconsolable: *Natr. mur.;* sad, heavy spirited: *Natr. carb.;* prostration of strength, and sadness: *Laches.;* loses her strength, with sad, fearful thoughts: *Rhus tox.*

Grief and Gloom. Everything grieves: *Mur. ac.;* very weakening grief: *Natr. mur.;* exhaustion, weariness of legs, and gloomy: *Arg. nitr.;* laziness; gloomy, dull: *Nuc. v. c.*

Ambra.
Apis.
II Arg. nitr.
Ars. met.
Calc. hyp.
I Calc. ostr.
Camphor.
Caustic.
Cinnab.
Crotal.
II Eriger.
II Hydroph.
Kali brom.
II Lob. infl.
Lycop.
Myr. cerif.
Natr. mur.
II Phosph. ac.
II Sabin.
I Secale.
Strontian.
Sulphur.

Depressed, dejected, dispirited. Body weak, mind depressed: *Phosph. ac.*

Weak all over: *Ars. met.;* general languor: *Myr. cerif.;* nervous prostration: *Calc. hyp.;* powerlessness, loss of all strength: *Secal.*

Weariness and unhappiness: *Caustic.;* weary and dispirited: *Lycop.*, and lazy: *Camphor.*

Lowness of spirits, with a feeling of great languor: *Erig. can.*

Desponding, ill-humored, melancholy, joyless, with weariness in all the limbs: *Sabin.*

Sudden weakness, with melancholy: *Crotal.;* all strength gone, no hope: *Natr. mur.*

With feeling of approaching death: *Kali brom.*

Melancholy, sits quietly for days and weeps, with sexual weakness: *Ambra;* sudden weakness, with melancholy: *Crotal.*

With apathy and trembling: *Arg. nitr.*

Depressed and weak as after a severe illness: *Cinnab.;* with diarrhœa: *Apis;* weak, ill-humored, with qualmishness: *Strontian.*

Depressed and weak in the afternoon: *Sulphur;* all day: *Hydroph.*

Hypochondric mood: *Arsen., Moschus, Nux mosch., Platin., Sepia.*

Exhausted, weak as if lamed, after a short walk: *Conium.*

MODEL CURE.

Feeling of weakness extending from forehead into nose; restlessness, mental depression; weeps a great deal, especially when alone; feels as light as if she could float or hover in the air; full of fear of getting crazy: *Mancin.*
—G. BUTE.

|| Acon.
|| Agn. cast.
Alum.
| Amm. carb.
Angust.
Ant. tart.
Arg. nitr.
Arsen.
| Aurum.
|| Borax.
| Calc. ostr.
Carb. an.
Carb. veg.
|| Caustic.
Chin. sulph.
Cicut.
Clemat.
Coloc.
Digit.
Ginseng.
|| Gratiol.
Ignat.
|| Magn. carb.
Mur. ac.
|| Natr. mur.
Nitr. ac.
| Nitrum.
Phosphor.
Platin.
| Ran. bulb.
Ratanh.
|| Rhus tox.
Sepia.
Silic.
Thuya.
Veratr.
Viol. tric.
Vip. torv.
Zincum.

Weakness with Anxiety, Anguish, Fear or Apprehension. Great weakness, with anguish: *Agn. cast.;* loses all his strength, with anguish: *Rhus tox.*

Gloomy and apprehensive, with weakness: *Crot. tigl.*

Weakness and apprehension: *Arsen., Arg. nitr., Sepia;* as if near death: *Aurum.*

Very weak, imagining sickness: *Arsen.*

Melancholy, fear of death, with great weakness: *Ant. tart.*

Extreme weakness, which the patient fears will carry him off: *Digit.;* loss of strength, anxious, as if dying: *Rhus tox.*

Constant thoughts of dying, with increasing prostration: *Thuya.*

Faint, with anxious hastiness: *Viol. tric.*

Exhaustion; thinking of death: *Zincum.*

General weakness, with melancholy and anxiety: *Clemat.*

Weariness and uneasiness: *Ambra, Anthrac., Calc. ostr., Viol. tric.;* full of sad thoughts, anxious and fearful, with loss of strength: *Rhus tox.*

General exhaustion and despair: *Arsen.;* despondency: *Anac.*

Great prostration, with anxiety: *Chin. sulph.;* weakness, with anxiety; while eating: *Ran. bulb.*

Great weakness, with anxiety and trembling: *Platin.;* with dread of work and walking bent over on account of colic: *Coloc.;* fear, with weakness, as if lamed: *Mur. ac.*

Sudden weakness, with anxiety, has to lie down: *Caustic.;* general weakness, with anxiety and heat: *Carb. an.;* fatigued and anxious: *Gratiol.;* weak and prostrated, with anxiety and sweat: *Ratanh.,* on the head: *Mur. ac.*

Anxious heat all over, with weakness, better in open air: *Gratiol.;* weak, depressed and anxious in the day-time, better in open air: *Calc. ostr.*

Weakness, as if going to faint, with anxiety in the morning: *Nitr. ac.*

Indifference, Apathy. Great debility with aversion to occupation and general indifference to his surroundings; relaxed and tired feeling: *Rumex.*

Indifference, with relaxed condition, easily fatigued when walking: *Fluor. ac.*

Indifferent mood, with sick feeling: *Argent.;* not well disposed, wanting action of body and mind: *Bellad.;* prostrated and indifferent: *Merc. per.*

Melancholy, dread of men, indifference, with sudden weakness: *Laches.*

Despondency, indifference, bordering on idiocy, with weakness: *Mezer.*

Faint-heartedness: *Caustic., Lycop., Oleand., Petrol.;* no ambition, great prostration: *Caustic.;* weakness and fearfulness: *Amm. carb.*

MODEL CURE.

A lady, worn out with solicitude and care of a sick friend, had delirium followed by convulsions. After *Laches.*^{2m}, the convulsions abated; she fell into a soft slumber, awoke conscious, and with the exception of feeling weak was quite comfortable.—FINCH.

WEAKNESS, WITH OTHER MENTAL CONCOMITANTS.

Ant. crud.
Apis.
Arsen.
Baryt.
Bryon.
Calad.
Calc. caust.
Calc. phosph.
Capsic.
Carb. veg.
Chin. sulph.
Cinnab.
Conium.
Cyclam.
Gratiol.
Magn. mur.
Mercur.
Moschus.
Mur. ac.
Natr. carb.
Natr. mur.
Nitr. ac.
Nux mosch.
Nuc. v. c.
Petrol.
Phosph. ac.
Sabin.
Spongia.
Terebinth.
Thuya.

Weak and Irritable, Ill-humored, Morose. Weakness, with ill humor: *Arsen.*, *Apis*, *Natr. mur.*, *Spongia;* irritability: *Chin. sulph.;* with sluggishness and fatigue; dark, gloomy mood: *Nuc. v. c.;* tiredness, with ill humor: *Calc. caust.*

Lazy and morose: *Petrol.*

Tired in the whole body, and morose: *Spongia;* with anger: *Moschus*, *Natr. mur.*

Great irritability from weakness; better from motion: *Cyclam.*

Fretfulness, with relaxed condition: *Mur. ac.;* greatest weakness: *Natr. mur.;* whole body fatigued: *Spongia.*

Body weak, mind depressed and irritable: *Phosph. ac.*

Lassitude, talking vexes him: *Nux mosch.;* headache: *Chin. sulph.*, *Cinnab.*

Irritable, vexatious humor, with lassitude and abdominal complaints: *Terebinth.*

Sick and weak in morning in bed, with ill humor: *Conium.*

Weak and irritable in forenoon: *Gratiol.*, *Magn. mur.*

Conations. Weeping: *Arsen.;* weakness of hands, lets everything fall, while busy: *Moschus;* and hastiness: *Viol. tric.;* weakness, with listlessness: *Crotal.*

Weakness, no ambition, indifference: *Bellad.*, *Cinnab.*, *Gelsem.*, *Bromum.*

Weak, indifferent and uneasy in the morning: *Magn. carb.*, general uneasiness, with nausea: *Asar.*, with diarrhœa: *Mercur.*

Uneasiness: *Opium;* after supper: *Petrol.*

Intellect. Lassitude and great weariness; semi-conscious: *Stramon.;* weakness, loss of consciousness: *Hydr. ac.;* excessive want of strength: *Opium.*

Bodily weakness; with its increase memory declines: *Nitr. ac.;* and giddy stupefaction: *Zincum;* prostration and stupor: *Secal.*, *Stramon.*

Torpor of the mental faculties, with physical languor: *Menisp. can.*

Weariness, not disposed to think: *Merc. per.;* relaxation and difficult comprehension: *Cinch. off.*

Prostration, cannot grasp an idea nor answer a question: *Laches.*

Mental dullness, with prostration: *Alum.*, *Anac.*, *Aurum*, *Digit.;* head and body weak, with dullness: *Ran. bulb.*

Weariness, inclined to sleep, does not feel like studying, cannot think; when writing thoughts vanish: *Glonoin.*

Relaxed, weak and drowsy after dinner, mental dullness, cannot think: *Magn. carb.*

Looks disturbed, with great weakness, which she tries to hide: *Thuya.*

Weakened by tormenting ideas: *Natr. mur.;* loss of strength, with delirium: *Stramon.*

Mania and delirium, with hallucinations, convulsions and great prostration after the attacks: *Hyosc.*

Exertion of Intellect. Weak from thinking: *Aurum;* exhausted from talking and writing: *Cannab.;* mental work tires soon: *Aloes, Thuya.*

Bodily exhaustion after mental overexertion: *Cuprum.*

Weakness, with Mental and other Bodily Concomitants. Lazy and tired, with no appetite: *Arg. nitr.*

Shuns labor, with drowsiness and loathing of food, even when hearing it mentioned: *Cinch. off.*

Sluggishness after eating; everything, even writing and talking affect him: *Cannab.*

Fatigue after eating, gets very tired from walking, with ill humor: *Phosphor.*

Heaviness after eating, with fullness and no desire to work: *Digit.*

After eating, indolent and disposed to lie down: *Ant. crud.*

Indolent and drowsy after dinner: *Zincum;* yawning and stretching: *Magn. carb.*

Weariness after dinner, unable to do the usual work: *Ignat.*

Indolence and dullness, with nausea: *Asar.*

Anxiety, with prostration, nausea, distension, yawning and stretching: *Bovist.*

Prostration, with weakness in the knees and irritability after unsatisfactory coition: *Calc. ostr.*

Weary and ill-humored during catamenia: *Caustic.;* depressed: *Sepia.*

Lassitude and drowsiness, cannot study: *Gelsem.*

Weak and tired after rising, has to sit down to dress: *Caustic.*

Discomfort, Indisposition. Uneasiness, no ambition: *Gratiol.*

General discomfort, without pain: *Natr. carb.;* feeling of general discomfort: *Sabin.;* feeling of great and indescribable discomfort: *Amm. carb.*

Bodily suffering from a wretched forsaken feeling: *Clemat.*

General discomfort, with anguish: *Asaf.;* displeased with everything: *Arsen.;* hypochondria: *Zincum;* with absentmindedness: *Magn. carb., Stannum.*

Greatest bodily discomfort, quiet, silent: *Stannum;* aversion to move: *Zincum.*

Uncomfortable, no desire to work: *Ruta.*

Indisposed to all mental and bodily occupation: *Hyper.*

Great discomfort, with pale, discolored appearance: *Magn. carb., Sulphur.*

Discomfort and irritability: *Opium.*

Nervous Weakness, Irritability. Very irritable, mind depressed, body weak: *Phosph. ac.*

Nervous affection, with mental listlessness: *Nux mosch.*

Talking, even that of persons dear to him, affects his nerves and makes him irritable and impatient: *Zincum.*

Irritability, with ill humor and lassitude: *Carb. veg.;* it runs through the whole body, irritability: *Nux vom.*

Ill humor and anxiety about every trifle, from nervous weakness: *Silic.*

Sadness, feels as if he was ill: *Digit.*

Fatigued. Unusual fatigue of body and mind: *Coca;* easily frightened, whining: *Petrol.;* vexed: *Gratiol.;* exhausted, and out of humor: *Crotal.;*

WEAKNESS, WITH OTHER MENTAL CONCOMITANTS.

very tired feeling and ill humor during catamenia: *Caustic.;* weariness and grumbling: *Calc. caust.*

Weariness after little exertion, with irritability: *Calc. ostr.*, hypochondria: *Moschus*, hastiness: *Sulph. ac.*

Fatigued from playing the piano: *Angust., Natr. carb.;* from thinking: *Aurum, Chamom., Pulsat.;* affected by mental work: *Aurum, Laches., Pulsat.*

Indolence, Shunning Work, Incapacity. The ability and desire for work diminish: *Plumbum.*

When returning from a walk, every step is an exertion; longs impatiently for rest and solitude: *Conium.*

Great lassitude of mind and body, longs to be inactive and at rest: *Spongia.*

No ambition, tires soon: *Nux vom.;* disinclined to bodily or mental occupation: *Cinch. off.;* indisposed to work or walk: *Zincum;* does not want to move, shuns labor: *Ignat.;* feels lazy all day long: *Sulphur.*

Lassitude and feeling as if beaten, mental dullness, in the forenoon: *Laches.*

Joyless, dull and indisposed to manual or mental work: *Droser.*

Idle, no inclination for mental or physical occupation: *Mar. ver.*

Unable to work, with ill humor and mental dullness: *Phosph. ac.*

As if lamed or beaten after anger, unable to work, can scarcely walk: *Calc. phosph.*

Inability to think in the morning, with uncheerfulness and bodily inactivity: *Gelsem.*

Aversion to mental or bodily labor: *Agar., Cyclam., Kali bichr., Mar. ver., Oleand.;* too weak: *Arsen., Opium.*

Indolent, no ambition to work or study: *Laches.;* disinclined to move or talk: *Gratiol.;* tired and lazy: *Hura.*

Indolent, no inclination for mental work, in the morning: *Ran. scel.*

Quiet and depressed, indolent and sad: *Bromum.*

Indolent, no ambition, the slightest motion is too much: I*Psorin.*

Sluggishness, in the afternoon, walking is an exertion: *Silic.*

Shuns labor, with ill humor: *Chin. sulph.*

Dullness, no desire to work, indolence; every forenoon: *Psorin.*

Very much tired by headwork, feels exhausted: *Aurum.*

Indisposed to work, indifferent and sad, fatigued: *Laches.;* irritable and lazy: *Petrol.*

Indolence and ill humor, particularly with phlegmatic constitutions: *Laches.*

Disinclined to exertion, depressed: *Rumex;* ill humor and inability to work, irritable impatience: *Aloes;* indolence, with lassitude and ill humor: *Iodium;* would rather rest, lazy and out of temper: *Spongia;* want of activity, indifference: *Bellad.;* indifferent and indolent: *Argent.;* irritable, moody and disinclined to work: *Magn. mur.*

Heaviness. Of mind and body: *Phosphor.;* heavy body, inactive mind: *Phosph. ac.*

Stupor, heaviness and sleepiness: *Sanguin.;* heavy feeling of body, with drunkenness: *Stramon.;* whole body heavy, cannot express his thoughts: *Nux mosch.;* ill humor, after eating: *Graphit.*

Stiffness. Stiffness of body, senses leave him: *Camphor.;* rigidity and insensibility: *Nux mosch.;* stiffness and difficult comprehension: *Chin. sulph.*

From irritability, with children: *Pulsat.;* stiff body; limbs can be bent: *Veratr.*

Loss of Control. Hypochondriac, despondent, with helplessness: *Anac.* No confidence to make voluntary motions: *Angust.*

Restlessness and unsteadiness, does not know exactly what he wants, what he is to do or leave undone: *Natr. carb.*

Muscles do not obey the will: *Gelsem.;* unable to act upon her limbs: *Spongia;* as if not obeying the will: *Aster.*

Muscles refuse to obey the will when the attention is turned away: *Helleb.* Want of bodily feeling, with maniacal gestures: *Ant. crud.*

Staggering, Tottering, Reeling. Staggering: *Ant. crud., Borax;* with anxiety: *Nux mosch.;* with fear of falling: *Nux vom.*

Staggering walk, with delirium: *Stramon., Vip. torv.;* tottering walk, thinking only on one idea, he suddenly comes to consciousness: *Nux mosch.;* tottering walk, with stupor: *Stramon.;* tottering walk, if not very attentive: *Helleb.;* reeling about, staggering; drunkenness: *Stramon.*

Falling. Inclination to fall, with anguish: *Nitr. ac.*

Vertigo when sitting, cannot rise for fear of falling: *Kali carb.*

Falling in a fainting fit, with fear of death: *Moschus;* sudden falling, in mania: *Stramon.;* dazed and dull; falling: *Psorin.*

Tendency to fall powerless, stupefaction: *Alum.;* falling down, talks wildly: *Thuya;* disposed to fall, thinks he talks wrong: *Nitr. ac.*

From the chair, with insensibility: *Nux mosch.;* to the ground, senses leave him: *Camphor.;* after running about: *Veratr.*

Lameness, Mental Conditions and Concomitants. As if lamed, after a fright: *Stannum;* apprehensive: *Natr. mur.;* after vexation: *Sepia.*

Lamed on one side, after vexation: *Staphis.;* lamed feeling, with ill humor: *Conium.;* after every emotion: *Calc. phosph.*

Paralysis, with listlessness: *Nux mosch.;* with fear of being damned: *Conium.*

In occiput lame, cannot comprehend, weakminded: *Calc. ostr.;* as if paralyzed mentally and physically: *Phosphor.*

Senses torpid, with great mental depression: *Arnic.;* semi-lateral paralysis, with mania: *Hyosc.;* inability to move, loss of consciousness: *Amygd.;* sad, motionless, speechless: *Pet. tetr.*

A robust forest ranger, æt. 50, fell down in a fit in which he retained consciousness, six months ago. Limbs give way, particularly the right; when sitting he can lean neither forward nor backward without losing his balance. The arms are weak, speech difficult, mind dull; disposed to weep; urine and feces pass involuntarily; occasional attacks of dyspnœa. *Arnic., Aloes, Nux vom.* and counter-irritants were of no avail. After *Secale* in grain doses, three times daily, in three days the patient could retain his urine, and in sixteen days his health was fully restored.—A. H. Z., 52, 112.

SLEEP.

Gaping and Yawning. Frequent yawning without sleepiness, with cheerful mood: *Chamom.*

Yawns and is low-spirited, with chilliness: *Turpeth.;* yawning and anxiety: *Plumbum.*

Gaping, with hiccough and apprehensions: *Crot. tigl.;* and weariness after toothache, but could not fall asleep, fearing pain might return: *Rhus tox.*

Yawning, with ill humor: *Cinch. off., Gratiol., Zincum:* very sleepy, yawns all day, with ill humor: *Ol. anim.;* yawning and stretching, morose, peevish: *Selen.*

Children cry because they want to gape and cannot succeed: *Lycop.*

Yawning, no desire to speak when others talk: *Cinnab.*

Frequent yawning, with lassitude and aversion to mental occupation: *Magn. mur.*

Yawning, with idleness: *Cannab., Chinin.;* no desire to work, with constant gaping: *Mezer.;* with sleepy weariness, while walking: *Rhus tox.*

SLEEPINESS.

Feelings. Exhilaration of all the faculties, followed by a strong desire to sleep: *Ziz. aur.;* with activity: *Euphras.*

Somnolency after the least excitement, and after the least exertion of mind: *Nux mosch.*

After dinner much laziness and yawning, which disappears the moment he begins to work: *Natr. carb.*

Music makes sleepy: *Stannum.*

Many ideas keep him awake: *Agar.*

Drowsy, but cannot sleep; talkative, but losing the thread: *Laches.*

Painful. Dreary news makes him sleepy: *Ignat.;* cannot keep sleep off, with sadness: *Platin., Plumbum.*

Feels sick all over, with sadness and sleepiness: *Ol. anim.*

Drowsy and sad, all day long: *Paull. pin.*

Drowsiness, with hopeless despair: *Ant. tart.;* gloomy feeling: *Calc. phosph.*

Sleepy and melancholic: *Cepa;* and depressed: *Eup. purp.*

Sleepiness, with palpitation from apprehensions: *Aurum;* evening, early, with a peculiar anxiety as if he would be disturbed: *Agar.;* sleepy, with anxiety: *Arsen., Aurum, Borax, Caustic., Ledum, Nux vom., Rhus tox.;* anxiety and nausea: *Ledum.*

Disturbed by anxiety and restless dreams: *Arsen.*

Anxiety and drowsiness, with fever: *Asaf.;* heaviness all over: *Magn. carb.*

Drowsy weariness, with anxiety; could fall asleep while walking, followed by colic and heat, with thirst: *Rhus tox.*

Drowsy, with great anxiety, increasing till 11 P.M.: *Borax.*

Wants to lie down, anxiety, restlessness and sadness: *Rhus tox.*

MIND AND DISPOSITION.

Disposition to sleep, and uneasiness to despair: *Vip. torv.;* sleepiness after grief: *Phosph. ac.*

Indifferent Feelings: *Aloes, Corn. circ., Digit.;* quiet manner: *Carb. an.;* listless, inclined to doze: *Rhus rad.*

Indifferent and taciturn, with great drowsiness: *Tilia.*

Feelings and Conations Combined. Drowsiness, with changeable mood: *Nux mosch.;* dispirited: *Ant. tart., Ran. scel.;* fretful: *Canthar., Spongia;* irritability: *Ant. crud., Asar., Calc. ostr., Thuya;* ill humor: *Lycop., Sepia, Spongia;* and tired, most in the feet: *Acon.;* depression: *Argent., Eup. purp.*

Irritable and sad: *Calend.;* no ambition: *Mephit.;* has to lie down, but cannot sleep: *Borax;* depression of mind, tired body in moving while getting up: *Amm. gum.*

Feels unable to do his usual work, and contrary to his habits he falls asleep over it: *Ignat.*

Lassitude, disinclination to work: *Lauroc.*

Irritable, lazy, tearful and ill-humored: *Canthar.*

Sluggishness, weak and indisposed to work: *Magn. sulph.;* with lassitude and weariness: *Bryon.*

It is an effort to speak, cannot read, dullness, goes to sleep while sitting: *Mercur.;* taciturn, fretful, drags feet along: *Borax.*

Ill humor: ||*Asar.,* ❙*Calc. ostr.,* ❙*Carb. an.,* ||*Carb. veg.,* ||*Conium.,* ||*Magn. mur.,* ||*Platin.,* ||*Spongia;* and morose: *Calend., Platin.;* sleepy at 7 A.M.: *Calad.;* after the cheerful mood of the first days follows ill humor and drowsiness: *Clemat.*

Morose and peevish: *Selen.;* everything is disagreeable: *Spongia;* dissatisfied with the world: *Rhus rad.*

After supper, with stretching and impatience: *Nitr. ac.*

Idlers become dull and heavy: *Cepa.*

Actions. Drowsiness, with whining: *Canthar.;* weeping: *Platin.*

Ill-humored and sleepy, whining mood, with headache: *Lachnanth.*

Sad and moody, sits by herself without speaking; drowsiness, weeps when spoken to: *Platin.*

Drowsiness and complaining: *Opium.*

Aversions. Sleepy and indisposed to all kind of work: *Anac.;* not disposed to work: *Ran. scel.;* disinclined to business: *Triost. perf.;* disinclined to intellectual occupation: *Cinch. off.*

After eating, drowsy and averse to labor: *Anac.*

Disposed to do nothing: *Natr. mur.;* will not open eyes or mouth: *Ignat.;* drowsy and monosyllabic: *Aurum.*

Gets sleepy early in the evening, moody silence: *Kali carb.*

Idleness: *Calc. ostr., Carb. an., Carb. veg., Cinch. off., Clemat., Colchic., Crocus, Crotal., Magn. sulph., Nux mosch., Verbasc.*

Exaltations. With mental restlessness: *Hyosc.*

Almost unconquerable desire to sleep, changing to restlessness: *Arsen.*

From fright, with red face: *Opium.*

Starting as if frightened, palpitation: *Mercur.*

Production. Drowsy, but cannot sleep, with difficult comprehension: *Sol. mam.;* absentminded and drowsy: *Sumbul.*

Mental dullness: *Nuc. v. c.;* want of thinking power: *Hyosc.;* falls asleep as thinking becomes difficult: *Mercur.;* want of thought: *Natr. mur.;* sinking into absence of thought: *Nux vom.*

Drowsiness when at work, does not know what he is reading: *Bismuth.*

After dinner drowsy and dull, cannot do mental work: *Ferrum.*

Unable and indisposed to do mental work, better when lying down and dozing; worse when getting up and moving about: *Phosphor.*

Drowsiness and indisposition to mental labor: *Coloc.;* drowsy and weak-minded: *Chamom.;* dullness: *Nitrum, Nux mosch.*

Dullness and drowsiness in forenoon, getting worse after dinner: *Carb. an.*

Joyless and obtuse, sleepy, but cannot sleep: *Chamom.;* stupidity: *Opium;* sluggish and dull: *Digit.;* and weakness in head: *Stannum;* dreaminess and weakness of head: *Squilla;* drowsy and awake, as if dreaming: *Bellad.*

Insensibility following drowsiness, with constant muttering: *Ailanth.*

Muttering and smiling, with sleepiness: *Atrop.;* on falling asleep delirious: *Spongia;* alternately delirious and drowsy: *Nux mosch.*

Reproduction. Sleepy and tired in the evening, forgetful: *Formic.*

Drowsy and forgetful: *Guarœa;* sleepy, yet cannot sleep; distraction: *Bellad.;* drowsiness, as if sensation ceased: *Arg. nitr., Stannum;* inclination to fall asleep, with vanishing of thoughts: *Nux mosch.*

Drowsy and stupid: *Hyosc., Natr. mur., Nitrum, Nux mosch.*

Cannot read, cannot work, falls asleep while sitting: *Mercur.*

BEFORE SLEEP.

Sad. Cannot fall asleep until 2 A.M.; sadness: *Cuprum;* has to weep: *Hydroph.*

Very sad after going to bed; thoughts of death, with weeping: *Stramon.*

Anxiety. Until lying down in the evening, depression and anxiety: *Graphit.;* in bed, in the evening: *Sepia;* has to open her night-dress: *Baryt.*

Anxiety and restlessness: *Phosphor.;* cannot lie still: *Amm. carb.;* as if going to die: *Phosphor.*

Fear of being disturbed: *Agar.;* anxiety, has to get up: *Carb. an.*

Drowsiness, with anxiety, increasing until 11 P.M.: *Bovist.*

After lying down and going to bed: ❙*Arsen., Nux vom.,* ❙❙*Sulphur.*

Anxiety, with crowding of thoughts, has to get up: *Pulsat.;* anxiety, as if apoplexy would set in: *Pulsat.*

Anxious and restless, painful starting of the legs, has to move them up and down for several hours, two succeeding evenings, 10 P.M.: *Hepar s. c.*

Anxious feeling in the head, as if he would lose his reason: *Natr. mur.*

Restlessness and anxiety, has to draw the limbs up and stretch them out again: *Nux vom.*

Attack of fear, can scarcely lie still: *Carb. veg.*

Anxiousness, followed by sweat after midnight: *Nux vom.*

Before falling asleep, fearfulness: *Calad.;* before midnight: *Sarsap.;* early in bed: *Natr. carb.*

Anxious thoughts which come and go, mistakes objects in the room, fears the dark: *Calc. ostr.*

Anxious feeling as if his whole body had become monstrously large and heavy: *Natr. carb.*

Oppressing orgasm frightens: *Sepia.*

Anxiousness and palpitation: *Calc. ostr.;* stiffness and numbness of whole body, with anxiety: *Silic.*

Anxiety on going to sleep: *Calc. ostr., Hepar s. c., Lycop.;* dreams, with increase of catamenia: *Natr. mur.*

Starting, with illusion as if there was a light in the room, springs out of bed: *Ambra;* starts, like from a fright, feels it in her teeth: *Mercur.*

Anxiety Preventing Sleep. Anxiety about trifles: *Lauroc.*

Great anxiety after lying down, preventing sleep: *Sulphur.*

Anxious, feels too warm in bed: *Magn. carb.;* heat preventing her from sleeping before midnight: **Arsen.*

Tosses about, with anxious hot feeling: *Bryon.*

Anxious hot feeling prevents sleep: *Pulsat.;* has to uncover often: *Magn. carb.*

Cannot get to sleep before midnight on account of anxious heat: *Arsen., Graphit.;* has to uncover; when falling asleep vivid dreams: *Natr. mur.*

Fear: *Mercur., Rhus tox.;* fearfulness: *Kali carb.;* fearful when alone, most in evenings in bed: *Kali carb.*

Fear, with shuddering and weeping: *Carb. an.*

Anxiety and fearfulness, easily startled, from 4 P.M. until bed-time; objects appear larger when seen in half-light: *Berber.*

Fears to lose her reason on account of tearing and stitching in heart: *Magn. carb.;* fears apoplexy: *Coffea.*

Fear to go to sleep: *Natr. mur.;* painless pulsation in the head, with fear to go to sleep: *Nux mosch.*

Fear of death; afraid to lie down: *Laches.*

Could not fall asleep for fear the toothache might return: *Rhus tox.;* fears he will suffocate if closing the eyes: *Carb. an.*

Starts at every trifle; is apprehensive of great trouble: *Rhus tox.*

Before sleep difficult comprehension: *Bol. sat.*

Before going to sleep gloomy: *Thuya;* ill-humored: *Kali carb.;* restlessness: *Hura.*

Heat and restlessness, with pulsations in the head: *Arsen.;* tosses about in bed: *Magn. mur.;* before midnight: *Sarsap.*

Restless before falling asleep; when getting awake restlessness returns: *Phosphor.*

Great irritability in the evening, with unrefreshing sleep, broken by disagreeable dreams: *Lil. tigr.*

EXALTATIONS AND DELIRIUM BEFORE SLEEP.

Agar.
Alum.
Arg. nitr.
Atrop.
Bellad.
Bryon.
|| Calc. ostr.
Camphor.
Carb. an.
Caustic.
Cinch. off.
Coccul.
Fluor. ac.
Gelsem.
Graphit.
Gratiol.
Guaiac.
Helleb.
Hepar s. c.
Ignat.
Kali carb.
Ledum.
Lycop.
Mar. ver.
Mercur.
Natr. mur.
Nux vom.
Phosphor.
Phosph. ac.
Plumbum.
Psorin.
Pulsat.
Sabad.
Sepia.
Silic.
Spigel.
Spongia.
Staphis.
|| Sulphur.
Viol. tric.
Zincum.

Cannot get to sleep, as tired as she is, on account of many ideas: *Agar.*

Goes to bed sleepy, but cannot sleep on account of thoughts: *Fluor. ac.*

In the evening, after lying down, involuntary recollections: *Ignat.*; thoughts of an absent friend: *Plumbum.*

After lying down at night, unpleasant ideas: *Caustic., Graphit., Kali carb.*

Is awaked when falling asleep by startling fancies: *Cinch. off.*

Could not fall asleep before midnight on account of a fixed idea: *Graphit., Pulsat.*

Thoughts of the day's work keep him awake: *Coccul.*; crowding of thoughts prevents sleep: *Silic.*

Very much excited before going to sleep: *Psorin.*

Excitability, cannot get to sleep: *Gratiol.*; excitement, as after tea, does not sleep well: *Hyper.*

Mental excitement in the evening prevents sleep: *Calc. ostr., Mar. ver.; Zincum.*

Falls asleep late on account of many ideas: *Viol. od.*

Cannot get to sleep, one idea gives place to another, each lasting but a short time: *Cinch. off.*; thoughts cross each other and prevent sleep: *Nux vom.*

Rush of thoughts, keeps awake until midnight: *Hepar s. c.*

Profuse ideas make it difficult to fall asleep: *Sulphur;* before midnight: *Calc. ostr., Spigel.*; before midnight, full of various ideas: *Staphis.*

Thoughts are many and prevent sound sleep; gets up tired: *Cinch. off.*

Many thoughts of a disagreeable or pleasant kind prevent sleep: *Sulphur.*

Sleepless from a rush of ideas: *Pulsat., Sepia, Sulphur.*

After lying down, lively imagination; a hundred fleeting forms pass before his eyes: *Helleb.*; falling asleep, exalted imaginations: *Arg. nitr.*

Ludicrous visions in half slumber, loud laughing: *Sulphur.*

Falls asleep late on account of many images of the fancy: *Alum.*

When falling asleep and closing the eyes, visions and disposition to make verses, which appears ridiculous when awake: *Natr. mur.*

Starts, cannot get to sleep, has visions when closing the eyes: *Ledum.*

Restless wakefulness, horrible visions, sees queer faces: *Calc. ostr.*; sees horrible faces: *Carb. an.*; horrible images keep awake: *Mercur.*; frightful visions: *Lycop.*; horrible visions of strange masks when closing the eyes: *Sulphur;* frightening visions: *Atrop.*; shutting eyes she screams, is delirious: *Bryon.*

Delirious talk on falling asleep: *Gelsem.*

Delirium: |*Bellad.*, |*Bryon.*, || *Calc. ostr.*, | *Camphor.*, | *Caustic.*, | *Guaiac.*, | *Ignat.*, | *Mercur.*, | *Phosphor.*, | *Phosph. ac.*, | *Sulphur;* if he wants to fall asleep, horrible illusions disturb him: *Cinch. off.*

Cannot fall asleep, so many ideas and plans take hold of him, one crowds the other: *Cinch. off.*

Anxious ideas, mistakes one thing for another; fears the dark, desires bright light; better after passing wind: *Calc. ostr.*

MODEL CURE.

A hysterical lady was often very much disturbed by frightening visions shortly before going to sleep. Counter-irritants and leeches had been prescribed without effect. For three weeks she attended no evening companies, ceased drinking coffee and tea, and gave up her cold baths with no better success. She took *Atrop.* Since that time she has been undisturbed.—C. CASPAR.

SLEEPLESSNESS, WITH EXALTATION.

| Agar.
| Aloes.
|| Ambra.
| Arg. nitr.
|| Arsen.
| Borax.
| Bryon.
| Calc. ostr.
| Carb. an.
| Caustic.
| Cinch. off.
| Clemat.
|| Coca.
| Coccul.
| Coffea.
|| Colchic.
| Coloc.
| Gelsem.
|| Graphit.
|| Hepar s. c.
| Hydroph.
| Hyosc.
| Iodium.
|| Kali carb.
| Laches.
| Lauroc.
|| Lycop.
| Mercur.
| Myr. cerif.
| Nitrum.
| Nux vom.
|| Opium.
| Plant. maj.
| Platin.
|| Psorin.
| Pulsat.
|| Rhus tox.
| Sabad.
| Secale.
| Sepia.
|| Silic.
| Sol. tub. ægr.
| Staphis.
| Sulphur.
| Sumbul.
| Therid.
|| Thuya.
| Veratr.
| Viol. tric.

After mental exertion he cannot get to sleep until midnight: *Kali carb.*

Inclination to study, with liveliness until after midnight: *Gelsem.*

Long awake in the evening and much disposed for mental labor: *Therid.*; sleepless; memory stronger: *Opium.*

Continues mental work until late at night, with great ease: *Laches.*

Towards morning involuntary activity of mind which prevents sleep: *Arsen.*

Sleepless after midnight, thoughts keep him awake as sleepy as he is: *Cinch. off.*

All night in a pleasurable state: *Opium;* with cheerfulness: *Secal.*

Sleepless, with serenity: *Secal.*

Excited, merry, little sleep and vivid dreams: *Clemat.*

Restless sleep, excited, cannot get to sleep before 2 o'clock: *Carb. an.*

Keeps awake long and is lively in the evening: *Laches.*

Contented, happy mood: *Aloes.*

Exhilaration of the nervous system in the evening, with sleeplessness: *Myr. cerif.*

Sleepless, with good humor: *Opium;* after pleasant excitement with inclination to work, wakeful and brisk feeling: *Coca, Hydroph., Lauroc., Veratr.*

Excitement prevents sleep: *Coffea.*

Cannot sleep in the night, after talkativeness: *Ambra.*

Nightly nervous excitement: *Arg. nitr.*

Sleeplessness from nervous excitation, with restlessness: *Sulphur, Sumbul.*

No sleep, full of ideas: *Coffea;* sleepless from intrusion of ideas: *Calc. ostr., Coloc., Lycop., Nitrum, Thuya.*

SLEEPLESSNESS, WITH EXALTATION.

Sleepless from a rush of ideas: *Calc. ostr.*, *Laches.*, *Pulsat.*, *Sepia*, *Sol. tub. œgr.*; after midnight: *Hepar s. c.*; crowded thoughts: *Bryon.*, *Coca.*

Sleepless all night from unpleasant ideas, one after the other: *Cinch. off.*

No sleep till midnight from constant intrusion of a melody or the like: *Pulsat.*

From exaltation: *Opium*: ecstasy: *Hyosc.*

After waking in the night, rush of thoughts: *Kali carb.*

Sleep prevented by one idea: *Baryt.*, *Coffea*, *Graphit.*, *Platin.*, *Petrol.*

Cannot sleep; sees nothing but cyphers: *Phosph. ac.*

Vexatious ideas preventing sleep: *Sulphur.*

Sleepless all night from unpleasant ideas: *Cinchon.*, *Opium*; tormenting ideas: *Graphit.*; inward uneasiness, could not fall asleep: *Paris.*

Sleeplessness, with homesickness: *Capsic.*; sadness: *Carb. an.*, *Rhus tox.*, *Sulphur.*

Insatiable thirst and tossing about: *Arsen.*

Great melancholy, with restlessness: *Act. rac.*

|| Acon.
| Act. rac.
| Agar.
 Ambra.
 Arnica.
| Arsen.
| Baryt.
| Bellad.
| Bryon.
|| Carb. an.
| Carb. veg.
| Caustic.
| Chamom.
| Chin. sulph.
| Cinch. off.
|| Coccul.
| Coffea.
| Conium.
| Cuprum.
| Graphit.
| Hepar.
| Hyosc.
|| Jatroph.
| Kali carb.
 Kali hydr.
| Lauroc.
|| Magn. carb.
 Magn. mur.
 Mercur.
 Merc. subl.
| Natr. carb.
| Natr. mur.
| Nitr. ac.
|| Plant. maj.
 Ran. scel.
 Rhus tox.
|| Sepia.
|| Silic.
| Sulphur.
| Thuya.
| Veratr.

Sleeplessness, with Anxiety. About trifles: *Lauroc.*; distressing: *Kali hydr.*; as if he had committed a crime: *Thuya*; anguish: *Carb. an.*, *Rhus tox.*, *Sulphur*; very restless and uncomfortable: *Mercur.*; drawing pains in all the limbs: *Bellad.*; trembling: *Thuya*; warm feeling: *Arnic.*, *Magn. mur.*; heat, cannot fall asleep before midnight: || *Arsen.*; in the evening: *Carb. an.*, *Lauroc.*, *Natr. carb.*; at night, with constriction: *Jatroph.*; lasting an hour: *Sulphur.*

Apprehensive and sleepless, pregnant women: *Act. rac.*

Sleepless in child-bed; as if she would die: *Conium.*

Cannot sleep half the night on account of apprehensions: *Graphit.*, *Rhus tox.*

Imagines he had something very important to do; keeps from sleep: *Bellad.*

Fear, Grief, Vexation. Fear of suffocating when closing the eyes: *Carb. an.*

Wakeful at night, with grief: *Coca*; vexatiousness: *Calc. ostr.*; as if he had committed a crime: *Thuya.*

Loss of mental energy, with sleeplessness: *Corn. cir.*

Faint-hearted, no courage: *Pulsat.*; timorous: *Rhus tox.*

Depressed and discouraged: *Rhus rad.*; despondent: *Nux vom.*; ill-humored: *Chamom.*; irritable, peevish, fretful: *Calc. ostr.*; complaining, whining and ill humor: *Chamom.*, and praying: *Stramon.*

With crying and twisting about of sucklings: *Senna.*

Silent brooding; melancholy: *Stramon.*

Sleep Disturbed by Restlessness: || *Arsen.*, *Bryon.*, *Carb. an.*, *Cinch. off.*, *Graphit.*, || *Iodium*, *Mercur.*, *Plant. maj.*, || *Pulsat.*, || *Rhus tox.*, *Sulphur*; and whimpering: *Arsen*

Hypochondric restlessness and despondency: *Graphit.*

Restlessness and heat: *Carb. an.;* tossing about in bed, with sadness and great thirst: *Arsen.*

Restlessness and anxiety, has to get out of bed; crowding of thoughts: *Bryon.;* nightly restlessness, cannot stay in bed: *Rhus tox.;* goes from place to place; cannot sleep at night; seems like a crazy person: *Iodium.*

Restlessness all night long: *Mercur.*

Great mental anxiety, pacing backward and forward in the room; then throwing himself on the bed, and from one side to the other in the greatest mental agitation; sleep with the most horrible and frightful dreams, which awaken him: *Plant. maj.*

Day and night furious, with cries: *Hyosc.;* sings and trills: *Veratr.*

No sleep until 2 A.M.; delirium: *Veratr.*

Imaginations: *Ledum;* great depression, with delusions, with persistent sleeplessness and dread of impending destruction of all near her: *Kali brom.*

Transient sleep in mania: *Colchic.;* sleepless in mania: *Hyosc., Stramon.*

Sleepless day and night, with mania; *Cuprum;* and red face: *Cicut.*

Puerperal mania, with complete sleeplessness: *Ver. vir.*

Ridiculous dreams, with restlessness all night: *Myg. las.*

Disagreeable dreams cause sudden wakefulness: *Scut. lat.*

Sleeplessness, with weeping mood, ill humor and general lassitude: *Chamom.*

Restless and fearful, cannot sleep, with cold legs: *Thuya.*

Anxiety as if he had committed a crime, easily startled, trembling, cannot sleep: *Thuya.*

Sleepless from exaltation, with heat: *Lauroc., Veratr.*

Anxious sweat preventing sleep: *Bryon.*

Sleepless before midnight, anxious heat: ||*Arsen., Kali carb., Pulsat., Veratr.;* until after: *Gelsem.;* after midnight: *Cinch. off., Colchic., Hepar;* until 2 A.M.: *Carb. an.;* from 1 A.M. to 3 A.M.: *Hepar;* from 3 A.M. until morning, with anxiety: *Arsen., Rhus tox.*

General uneasiness in the night: *Cyclam.*

Toothache is bearable during the day but drives to destruction in bed at night; better from keeping quiet: *Clemat.*

Tossing about in bed all night, with dullness in head: *Dulcam.*

MODEL CURES.

Mania; he thinks he is lying in his sepulchre; confessing, praying, wants to be killed by slaying; laughs as if tickled; wants to be kissed; accuses his wife as faithless; scolding, beating in a rage, will not be taken hold of by his attendants, takes them for dogs, and barks at them; talking in the Jewish jargon, this he never did before; supposes his house to be surrounded by carts, Jews and geese, offending him, driving him into a rage; pale, eats nothing, does not sleep, while the muscles of his face are in a constant twitching motion. Case of long standing. *Stramon.*[9], cured in a few days.—SCHELLHAMMER.

Pressure at stomach, nausea, eructations, rumbling in abdomen, sensation as of a round ball going to and fro under the ribs, with various sounds; fluid food aggravates it, tight clothing or bandage around the abdomen relieves; *sleeplessness;* amelioration from lying quiet; during three weeks. *Cuprum.*—LEMBKE.

SLUMBER.

Conscious in sleep, hears everything, but cannot rouse himself: *Opium.*

As if in slumber; is vexed at having to open his eyes to see or his lips to speak: *Ignat.*

Slumber, with difficult comprehension: *Stannum.*

Rattling breathing in slumber, starts in fright and looks wildly about: *Bellad.*

Remembers forgotten things in slumber: *Calad.*

Starts from half slumber, with anxiousness, sadness and oppression: *Strontian.*

Half sleeping, half waking condition; she hears others talk of things which frighten her, although she knows she is dreaming; can rouse herself only with difficulty: *Kali carb.*

Attack of anxiety in the night, as if she must die: *Amm. carb.*

After vexation falls asleep, with twitching of arms and hands, and staring eyes: *Conium.*

Tosses about anxiously; lies as if unconscious and groans: *Bryon.*

Restless sleep disturbed by vivid dreams, which he cannot remember; after midnight half wakeful condition: *Spigel.*

Half slumber, with strange ideas, as if the mind was active: *Sabad.;* sleep is made up of flighty dreams: *Silic.*

Delirious talk, with anxiousness before midnight; with open eyes: *Sulphur.*

Nightmare in half slumber, with great fear: *Silic.*

At night heat and great excitement; during the day a difficulty to attend to mental work: *Arg. nitr.*

Confused talk at night: *Digit.;* in the evening: *Bellad.*

Flightiness. Dreaminess at night: *Cahinc;* flightiness: *Therid.;* nightly fancies: *Laches.*

Disturbed sleep at night, tosses about, wakes up flighty, thinks he is in different places: *Lycop.*

Flighty dreams: *Graphit.;* with stupor as in fever: *Baryt.*

Half waking, half dreaming; finds himself in different places, everything appears real yet he knows he is in bed: *Psorin.*

Happy ecstasies all night, elevated contemplation, memory stronger: *Opium.*

Delirium especially at night, with ecstasy: *Acon.*

Coma. Coma and melancholy: *Plumbum;* delirious: ‖*Acon.,* ׀*Ant. crud.,* ׀׀*Arnic.,* ‖*Bryon.,* ׀*Camphor.,* ׀׀*Coloc.,* ‖*Pulsat.,* ׀*Secal.;* stupid: *Hyosc.*

Stupefied slumber, with flightiness; is often on the water; when about to fall in, starts and awakes: *Nitrum.*

After sound sleep, dreams which exert the mind: *Alum.*

Eyes Shut. Imagines awful things during the night: *Calc. ostr.*

When closing the eyes, sees fanciful visions and faces: *Arg. nitr.*

When lying awake at night with closed eyes, she sees ghosts and animals in a bright light approaching from afar and then slowly retreating: *Thuya.*

Seeing spirits: *Spigel., Thuya;* in dreams: *Hippom., Sarsap.*

Night Walking. Gets up and walks, for a long time does not know where he is: *Silic.;* gets up in her dream, walks to the door as if intending to go out: *Bryon.;* walks about the room: *Natr. mur.*

Flighty talk, with heat; children move around in bed with closed eyes, without speaking: *Rheum.*

Gets out of bed from an anxious dream, thinking there is a fire, dresses, and talks out of the window; is frightened when told there is nothing going on: *Sulphur.*

Gets up unconsciously: *Bryon., Natr. mur., Petrol., Phosphor., Silic.*

Flightiness in sleep, gets out of bed: *Silic.*

Gets up and walks from room to room, with closed eyes: *Alum.*

Getting up in the night and walking up and down in deep thought: *Bellad.*

Goes about furiously with closed eyes, breaks everything in the room, goes back to sleep and is unconscious of what happened after waking: *Phosphor.*

Unbearable anxiety, springs out of bed and seeks to take his life, but is afraid of the open window or the knife: *Cinch. off.*

Fearful anxiety, great inward woe as if the soul would separate from the body, at night: *Thuya.*

Strikes her hands together above her head, in the night: *Bellad.;* and sings: *Veratr.*

MODEL CURES.

Nightly attacks of anxiety; afraid of the cholera, gets cramps in the calves from fear; nausea, heavy feeling in abdomen, rolling in umbilical region; another time thinks there are robbers in the house and wants to jump out of the window; often thinks the visions are real; weary of life, looks at everything from the dark side. Symptoms last through the morning and get better during the day. The least noise disturbs sleep. Vertigo. *Laches.*—C. Hg.

A boy, æt. 4, light complexioned, blue eyed, sandy haired. For more than two years was disturbed every night with the most horrid nightmares. The child would always awake once, and sometimes three or four times, nightly, with fearful fright, uttering *sudden, startling and piercing cries,* and vow there was some *dreadful beast* under his bed or in the room, and not until the gas was lit and the room thoroughly searched, would he be appeased so as to be induced to go to sleep again. Disposition of the boy is naturally good, but has been rendered nervous, peevish and fretful, in consequence of these sudden and repeated frights. *Chamom.*[200], two doses, put to flight the above symptoms most effectually. Von Tagen.

Miss C., æt. 20, during morning, headache, pain in lumbar region, arms, legs and left side of throat. After 3 p.m., chilly feeling in the lumbar region, extending up as far as between the shoulder-blades, cold hands and feet, fingernails blue, general coldness. After from one to three hours, fever, flushed face, suffused eyes, lachrymation, running at nose; constant thirst; desire for cold and acid drinks; hands and feet cold; loss of appetite; *restless sleep with frightful dreams*: *Eup. purp.*—Von Tagen.

SLEEP AND ANXIETY.

Alum.
Al. p. s.
Ant. crud.
Arsen.
Ars. hydr.
Aurip.
Aurum.
Bellad.
Calc. ostr.
Carb. an.
Carb. veg.
Caustic.
Chamom.
Cinch. off.
Coccul.
Conium.
Cuprum.
Cyclam.
Digit.
Dulcam.
Ferrum.
Graphit.
Jatroph.
Ignat.
Kali carb.
Laches.
Lauroc.
Lithium.
Lycop.
Magn. carb.
Magn. mur.
Mangan.
Mercur.
Merc. subl.
Natr. carb.
Natr. mur.
Nitr. ac.
Nux vom.
Oleander.
Petrol.
Phosphor.
Pulsat.
Rhus tox.
Sepia.
Silic.
Spongia.
Squilla.
Stramon.
Sulphur.
Veratr.
Zincum.

Anxiety all night: *Nitr. ac., Sepia, Veratr.*
Anxious heat in the evening from 5 to 6 and in the morning from 4 to 5: *Sepia.*
With suicidal inclination at 8 P. M. and 2 A. M.: *Cinch. off.*
In the evening, after lying down and after midnight: *Arsen.;* after going to bed, till near midnight: *Veratr.;* in the evening and night intense anxiety: *Carb. an.;* and apprehension: *Mercur.*
As if going to die, before but more after midnight: *Rhus tox.*
Before midnight, awakening from sleep with a start: *Mercur.*
Anxiety as if he had to die: *Oleand., Rhus tox.*
The greatest anxiety before midnight, thinks he will die: *Ars. hydr.;* anxiety and heat before midnight: *Magn. mur.*
Awakes with anxiety about midnight: *Sepia.*
About midnight gets half awake with anxious torturing restlessness, lasting until near morning: *Mangan.*
After Midnight: *Alum., Ant. crud.,* **Arsen.,** *Cinch. off., Dulcam., Lycop., Mangan.,* **Nux vom.,** *Rhus tox.;* at 2 A.M.: *Cinch. off.*
Inclined to self-destruction: *Cinch. off., Nux vom.*
In half slumber great anxiety, with thoughts of death: *Conium.*
Anxiety and apprehension worse after midnight: *Nux vom.*
Anxiety and fear of the future: *Dulcam.*
With wind colic: *Aurum;* pain in stomach till 1 o'clock: *Kali carb.;* palpitation: *Nux vom.*
Increased anxiety after midnight: *Aurip.;* anxious heat, with inclination to uncover: *Arsen.*
Wakes after midnight, with anxiety and nausea: *Squilla.*
At 2 A.M. with mental inquietude, everything troubles his mind: *Graphit.;* wakes near 2 o'clock with cardiac anxiety, cannot go to sleep again: *Kali carb.*
Anxiety about 3 A.M.: *Arsen., Rhus tox.;* anxious palpitation: *Arsen.*
Anxiety from 3 to 5 A.M.: *Ant. crud.;* anxious heat from 4 to 5 A.M. and from 5 to 6 P.M.: *Sepia.*

Nightly Anxiety, with other Mental Symptoms. Anxious and homesick: *Mercur.;* dejected: *Carb. an.*
Anxiety, as if she had done wrong: *Ferrum.;* as if he had taken some one's life: *Phosphor.;* anxious heat, driving to distraction: *Petrol.*
Anguish all night: *Veratr., Zincum;* anxious and restless: *Lith. carb.*
Cannot sleep for anxiety and foreboding: *Rhus tox.*
With weeping and indistinct talking: *Caustic.*
Child is restless and anxious, cries much, reaches for this thing and that, without taking anything: *Kali carb.*

Anxiety, starting and loud crying: *Bellad.*
Anxious sleep in mania: *Stramon.*

Anxiety and Bodily C.C. Head. Buzzing, with drawing motions in belly: *Veratr.;* heat: *Nitr. ac.;* congestion, with rising of hair: *Carb. veg.*

Eyes. Rapid dilatation and contraction of pupils: *Chamom.*

A pressing pain under the right eye drives her out of bed, with anxiety: *Arsen.*

Oversensitiveness of hearing, the slightest noise reverberates in the ear: *Carb. veg.*

In his sleep he thinks he hears some one approaching the bed, which awakes him, with anxiety: *Carb. veg.*

Face. Neuralgia, with fearful anxiety, driving out of bed: *Magn. carb.*

Anxiety, with spasmodic drawing in jaws: *Sepia;* heat in the left cheek with toothache: *Oleand.*

Throat. Feeling of anxious soreness in the œsophagus, particularly at night: *Spongia, Zincum;* gagging: *Kali carb.;* vomituritio: *Cyclam., Oleand.*

Gastric. When lying on the right side, oppression and anxiety, has to sit up: *Kali carb.;* belching relieves: *Kali carb.*

Stomach. Violent, constrictive pain going into the chest, with anxiety: *Kali carb.;* anxious pressure in the epigastrium: *Sulphur.*

Abdomen. With incarcerated wind: *Aurum, Sulphur;* drawing motions in the abdomen: *Veratr.;* anxious, restless feeling in abdomen: *Nitr. ac.*

Colic at night, with agony, anxiety and oppression: *Al. p. s.*

Bladder. Anxious feeling from constant urging to urinate: *Natr. mur.;* frequent urination: *Oleand.*

Chest. Dyspnœa: *Kali carb.*

Dry cough, causing vomiting and anxious sweat, has to get up: *Silic.*

Anxiety and constriction of chest: *Jatroph.*

Spasmodic drawing in chest: *Sepia;* pain into chest from stomach: *Kali carb.*

Ebullition, with fear of apoplexy, has to get up: *Natr. carb.*

Anxiety, with ebullition: *Mercur.;* has to sit up: *Carb. an.*

Precordial anxiety: *Lycop.;* palpitation, with anxiety at 3 A.M.: *Arsen.;* anxious palpitation, feels as if she had done wrong, cannot stay in bed: *Nitr. ac.*

Wakes from an anxious dream, with palpitation and anxiety: *Silic.*

Frightful dream, after which anxiety and inability to go to sleep: *Caustic.*

Limbs. Stitches in axilla: *Kali carb.;* heat in hands: *Nitr. ac.*

Positions. Anxiety when lying on the right side; has to sit up until the wind is belched up: *Kali carb.*

Restless. Tossing about: *Arsen., Ferrum, Mangan., Merc. subl., Phosphor.;* children: *Sulphur;* running about: *Bellad.*

Spasms. Of limbs: *Alum.;* starting: *Bellad.;* when falling asleep: *Alum.;* trembling: *Calc. ostr.;* twitches and spasmodic drawing in thighs: *Sepia.*

Wakes with anxious heat and spasmodic feeling in whole body: *Sulphur.*

Sleep. Great restlessness and anxiety at night: *Phosphor.;* cannot sleep: *Caustic.;* awakes with anxious restlessness: *Nitr. ac.*

Anxiety, keeps awake two or three hours every night: *Natr. mur.*

Half wakeful, anxious condition: *Conium.*

Wakes frequently, as if from anxiety, and thinks it must be time to get up: *Digit.;* anxiousness in bed: *Lauroc.*

Sitting up relieves faceache; pain in jaw, driving out of bed: *Magn. carb.*

The toothache is relieved after getting out of bed, and returns when getting in again: *Oleand.*

Attacks of anxiety, driving out of bed: *Arsen., Graphit., Rhus tox.*

Great anxiety when in bed; none when out of it: *Chamom.*

Anxiety, with fear of getting crazy: *Calc. carb.*

Dreams. That she is on a sinking raft, awakes with anxious feeling: *Alum.;* restless sleep from many dreams, with anxiety: *Laches.*

Nightmare, feels as if her body was constricted, wanted to call but could not, could not open the eyes or move a limb: *Natr. mur.*

Anxious and flighty; is frightened in her dream, and wakes with anxiety and trembling: *Calc. carb.*

Restless sleep, with anxious frightening dreams, from which it takes some time to recover: *Chin. off.*

Sleep full of dreams; unrefreshing sleep after attack of anxiety: *Cuprum.*

Cold and Heat. With chill about midnight: *Sepia.*

Throws the covers off in sleep: *Nux vom.*

After midnight anxious heat, with inclination to uncover: *Arsen.*

Heat mounts to the face, with precordial anxiety: *Nux vom.*

Heat in left cheek: *Oleand.*

Cannot rest in one place on account of anxious heat: *Merc. subl.*

Restless sleep, tossing about, hot and anxious, with twitching: *Alum.*

Great anxiety, with general heat; spasmodic feeling: *Sulphur.*

Anxious heat, worse in hands and feet: *Ignat.;* heat and itching: *Petrol.*

Heat before sweat, with thirst; before midnight: *Magn. mur.;* short sweat: *Kali carb.*

Attacks. Frequent attacks from 1 o'clock till morning: *Kali carb.*

Night attacks, with restlessness: ∎*Arsen.,* ∎*Chamom., Cyclam.,* ∎*Ignat., Pulsat.*

Touch. Lies hard, as if on stones, has to turn continually: *Magn. carb.*

Skin. Feeling as if a hand was stroking her body, with formication when moving in bed: *Carb. veg.;* itching and heat: *Petrol.*

MODEL CURE.

Cardiac anxiety, fearfulness, frightful dreams; religious melancholy from pangs of conscience after a misdeed; weeping, praying; great lassitude, emaciation and sweat in the morning; painful menstruation: *Aurum.*—SEIDEL.

OTHER MENTAL COMPLAINTS AT NIGHT.

|| Aloes.
|| Arg. nitr.
Arsen.
Bellad.
| Berber.
|| Calc. ostr.
| Carb. an.
Carb. sulph.
Cinnab.
|| Coca.
| Coffea.
Graphit.
| Hyper.
| Laches.
Lauroc.
|| Lycop.
| Mezer.
| Moschus.
Opium.
|| Sepia.
Therid.
|| Zincum.

Excitability. Disturbing sleep: *Lycop.*
With heat and fullness in head: *Arg. nitr.;* and heat and redness of the face: *Aloes;* lasting till after midnight: *Mar. ver.;* with restlessness: *Carb sulph.*

Exalted imagination: *Arg. nitr., Therid.;* and good humor: *Opium.*

Wakeful at night; crowding of thoughts: *Cinnab., Coca, Graphit.;* great talkativeness, waking or sleeping: *Arsen., Bellad.*

Writes with facility in evening and all night: *Laches.*

Merriness: *Alum., Bellad., Caustic., Crocus, Hyosc., Kreosot., Lycop., Opium, Phosph. ac., Sepia, Silic., Stramon., Sulphur., Veratr.*

Cheerfulness in bed: *Hepar.;* sings and trills quite gaily: *Veratr.*

Sad. After midnight sad ideas: *Rhus tox.;* sad, then merry dreams: *Mancin.*

Hypochondria: *Alum., Calc. ostr., Laches., Magn. sulph., Arnic., Natr. mur.*

Apprehension: *Arnic., Calc. ostr., Dulcam., Laches., Rhus tox.*

Feels as if he was going out of his mind at night: *Eup. perf.*

Fear. *Crotal., Ipec., Phosphor., Rhus tox., Stannum.*

Fear of damnation: *Pulsat.;* of spectres: *Carb. veg.;* of thieves: *Ignat.;* of having been poisoned: *Ars. met.;* of cholera: *Laches.*

Fearfulness. Timidity: *Caustic., Rhus tox.;* in bed: *Kali carb.;* ceases after belching: *Stramon.;* afraid of being alone: *Tabac.;* fears every motion of the head on account of unbearable pains: *Bovist.*

After midnight, fear: *Ignat.;* timid at night: *Caustic.*

Sorrow. Sad thoughts all night, and weeping all day: *Caustic.*

Sleeps till 2 o'clock A.M.; inconsolable: *Veratr.*

Full of care and trouble: *Dulcam.;* in the night, and apprehension about his disease: *Ars. hydr.;* despondent: *Carb. an., Graphit.*

Ill Humor: *Anac., Borax, Chamom., China, Lycop., Rhus tox., Sabad.*

Vexation: *Castor., Graphit., Lycop., Rhus tox.*

Irritability: *Lil. tigr., Spongia.*

After a slight vexation she weeps all night: *Natr. mur.*

The slightest noise in the house vexes him: *Cinnab.*

Complaining and scolding: *Veratr.*

Singing in sleep: *Crocus.*

Loud laughing after midnight: *Silic.*

Weeping. In sleep (comp. p. 196): | *Caustic.,* || *Carb. an.,* || *Chamom.,* | *Conium,* || *Kali carb., Lycop.,* || *Natr. mur.,* | *Nux vom.,* | *Pulsat., Rhus tox., Thuya;* incessant: *Camphor.;* tearfulness: *Baryt.*

Nursing children refuse the breast, weep, start from sleep, and grow pale and wilted: *Borax.*

OTHER MENTAL COMPLAINTS AT NIGHT.

Cannot get into a comfortable position, which makes him weep: *Lycop.*
The cough causes weeping and restlessness: *Sulphur.*
Weeps in sleep, and sobs when getting awake: *Carb. an.*
Children weep and toss about in sleep: *Kali carb.*
Weeps all night; laughs during the day: *Stramon.*
Weeping in dreams: *Carb. an., Natr. mur.,* ||*Pulsat., Silic.;* weeping wakens: *Ignat., Nux vom., Sulphur;* three hours after midnight: ▮*Arsen., Bryon.*
Moaning after falling asleep: *Alum.;* in sleep: *Bellad.*
Whimpering: *Apis,* ||*Arsen., Aurum, Chamom., Cinch. off., Ipec., Laches., Lycop., Mercur., Natr. mur., Opium, Rheum, Veratr.;* 3 P.M.: *Bryon.;* with motion of limbs: *Hyosc.*
Low weeping: *Phosphor.;* loud: *Phosph. ac.*
Growling: *Lycop.;* and howling: *Chamom.;* and praying: *Stramon.*
Crying (comp. p. 198), moaning and groaning: ||*Alum.;* and howling: *Silic.*
At 2 A.M. moaning on account of heat, wants to be more thinly covered: *Ignat.*
Terrible anxiety, would like to scream out loud from inward woe: *Thuya.*
Screams out loud at 3 A.M., in anxious dreams: *Bryon.*
Starts often in sleep and screams out: *Caustic.*
Nightly spasm of the abdominal muscles, with loud screaming: *Lycop.*
Anxious screaming in sleep, with children: *Borax.*
Screaming and tossing about in sleep: *Borax.*
Tired of life at night: *Ant. crud., Nux vom.;* terrified at night: *Ascar.*
Hastiness: *Laches.*
Restlessness. Mental inquietude: *Argent., Arsen., Digit., Graphit., Iodium, Kali carb., Laches., Mercur., Spongia, Sulphur.*
Before midnight mind and body restless: *Sarsap.;* restless, with anxious constriction in stomach: *Natr. mur.*
Nervous motions in paroxysms every night: *Arg. nitr.*
Restlessness, can lie on neither side: *Staphis.;* tosses from one side to the other: *Spigel.;* cannot get into a comfortable position: *Carb. an.*
Throws herself anxiously about in bed: *Camphor.*
Something prompts him to get out of bed: *Rhus. tox.*
Restlessness driving out of bed, disposition to shoot himself: *Ant. crud.*
Wants to go from one bed to another: *Arsen.*
Gets in and out of bed, finds rest nowhere: *Mercur.*
Cannot stay in bed: *Acon.*
Tosses about in bed, with a burning feeling and anxious dreams: *Rhus tox.*
Starts from sleep, with an involuntary jerk of the left leg: *Zincum;* with trembling of the limbs: *Petrol.*
Starts as if frightened, makes many motions and talks in sleep: *Acon.*
Restless tossing: *Sulphur;* of children, with crying: *Kali carb.*
Dreams. Restless, with many dreams: *Ambra, Cicut.;* merry dreams: *Digit.*

Troubled and confused dreams, with restless sleep: *Menisp. can.*
Dreams full of danger and trouble, with unquiet sleep: *Rumex.*
Smells sulphur and spunk; the illusion continues after awaking: *Anac.*
Starts and screams; dreams he is quarreling with a beggar: *Magn. carb.*
Unpleasant ideas at night: *Cinch. off.;* after midnight: *Rhus tox.*
Cannot get rid of one idea at night: *Acon., Coffea, Graphit., Ignat., Petrol., Psorin.;* intruding ideas: *Aloes, Coloc., Graphit., Psorin.*

Delirium. Great restlessness and flighty talk: *Digit.*
Delirium during sleep: *Cactus;* in evening: *Valer.;* in bed: *Kali carb.*
Alternately sleeping and delirious for several hours: *Nux mosch.*
On shutting the eyes: *Calc. ostr.;* after closing the eyes objects appear, which are now too thick now too thin, changing as rapidly as the pulse beats: *Camphor.*
All kinds of images: *Graphit.;* when closing the eyes feels as if he had lost his reason: *Opium.*
Fanciful images: *Sepia, Spongia.*

With Talking. Flighty talk: *Aurum, Bryon., Cannab.;* restless sleep, with delirious talk: *Phytol.*
When waking and sitting up in bed confused talk: *Chamom.;* asks confused questions: *Aurum.*
Delirium about his business; worse at night, after 3 A.M.: *Bryon.*
Delirious and restless all night, with talk about his business: *Mygal.*
Converses with spirits all night: *Stramon.;* delirium and fear of ghosts: *Acon.;* fancies some one came in at the door: *Conium;* runs about searching for thieves: *Arsen.*
After midnight more restless; raving in the morning: *Bellad.*
Nocturnal delirium: *Bellad.;* violent: *Plumbum;* swearing and making a noise: *Veratr.*
Delirium, with increase of pain: *Dulcam.;* pain makes delirious: *Veratr.*

Intellect. Madness, rage: *Bellad., Cicut., Digit., Phosph. ac., Veratr.*
Mania at night: *Bellad., Stramon.;* loss of senses: *Bellad.*
Coma, weakminded: *Plumbum.*
Snoring, loss of consciousness: *Stramon.*
When falling in a slumber, absence of mind and stupidity: *Stannum.*
Difficult comprehension at night: *Arnic., Bol. sat., Cinch. off.,* ǁ *Platin., Staphis.;* at 11 o'clock: *Mercur.*
Got up confused after midnight: *Stramon.*
Mental dullness at night: *Kali carb., Ran. scel.*
Feeling of weakness and difficulty of connecting ideas at night: *Mur. ac.*
Anxiety in epigastrium, mental confusion, stupid slumber: *Stramon.*

MODEL CURE.

An old lady had a vision every night since six weeks, in which many persons, all strangers, came into her room and to her bedside, causing her such fear that she had to leave the bed: *Stramon.*—BECKER.

ON AWAKENING OR BEING WOKE.

NOTE.—Being woke by certain sensations or other symptoms ought to have been separated from getting awake and suffering the one or other complaint, but it has thus far not always been done.

|| Acon.
   Agar.
|| Alum.
   Amm. carb.
|| Arg. nitr.
|| Arnica.
   Arsen.
   Ars. hydr.
|| Aurum.
.| Bellad.
   Berber.
|| Borax.
|| Bryon.
   Calc. ostr.
   Cannab.
   Capsic.
   Carb. an.
   Carb. veg.
   Castor.
|i Caustic.
   Chamom.
   Chelid.
   Chin. sulph.
   Cina.
   Cinch. off.
   Clemat.
   Coca.
   Coccul.
   Colchic.
   Conium.
   Cuprum.
   Cyclam.
   Digit.
   Dulcam.
   Graphit.
   Guaiac.
   Hepar s. c.
   Hyosc.
|| Ignat.
   Janiph.
| Kali carb.
   Kali hydr.
| Laches.
   Lact. vir.
   Lepid.
| Lycop.
   Magn. mur.
   Magn. sulph.
   Mercur.
|| Mezer.
   Mur. ac.
   Myrist.
   Natr. carb.
|| Natr. mur.
   Nitr. ac.
   Nitrum.
   Nuc. v. c.
   Nux vom.
|| Opium.
   Ox. ac.
   Paris.
|| Petrol.
   Phelland.
   Phosphor.
   Phosph. ac.

Feelings. Gets wide awake before midnight and cannot go to sleep again: *Mur. ac.*

Awakes with a pleasant face: *Ignat.*; with pleasant ideas: *Nitr. ac.*

Cannot get to sleep again after being woke by sweat at 4 A.M.: *Petrol.*

On getting awake, gloomy: *Nuc. v. c.*

Awakes about midnight, with great thirst and sorrowful ideas: *Platin.*

Sad: *Lepid.*; wakes from dreams with sad ideas: *Sulphur*; depressed: *Cyclam.*; low spirited: *Kali carb.*; out of spirits: *Nitr. ac.*; hypochondriac humor: *Alum., Lycop.*; after 2: *Nux vom.* Wakes suddenly from anxious dreams, with gloomy thoughts: *Platin.*

Apprehensive mood on getting awake: *Ars. hydr.*

Getting awake at 1 A.M. with gloomy, apprehensive thoughts *Phosph. ac.*

Fear and Fearfulness: *Alum., Amm. carb., Bellad.,* I *Coccul., Conium, Hepar s. c., Ignat., Laches., Lycop., Magn. sulph., Natr. carb., Natr. mur., Nitr. ac., Phosph. ac., Pulsat.,* I*Silic.,* I*Sulphur, Zincum.*

After waking, great fearfulness: *Amm. carb.*; fearful ideas *Conium*; tormenting dreams, leaving a fear of death: *Alum.*; fear of damnation: *Magn. sulph., Pulsat.*; fear of spectres: *Coccul.*; of thieves: *Ignat., Natr. mur.*; as if somebody entered his door: *Conium*; fear of thunder-storms: *Hepar s. c., Laches., Natr. carb., Nitr. ac.*

Getting awake at 2 A.M. with trembling and fear, which makes her start up in bed: *Ratanh.*

Awakes at midnight with fear, thinks there are robbers in the room: *Natr. mur.*

Apprehension. As if something would happen: *Lycop., Nux vom., Pulsat.*

On getting awake lassitude, irritability, anxious restlessness and apprehension of evil: *Clemat.*

Anxiety. Awakes with anxiety: *Agar., Alum., Arg. nitr., Arsen., Carl. an., Caustic., Digit., Lycop., Natr. mur., Nitr. ac., Nux vom., Phosph. ac., Pulsat., Sepia, Silic., Sol. nigr., Zincum.*

Awakes at midnight: *Arg. nitr.*; after: *Ignat., Lycop., Phosph. ac.*; at 2 A.M.: *Natr. mur.*; at 3 o'clock: *Arsen., Silic.*; with a chill: *Sepia.*

MIND AND DISPOSITION.

Phytol.
|| Platin.
Plumbum.
Psorin.
Pulsat.
Ratanh.
Rhus tox.
|| Sambuc.
|| Sepia.
Silic.
Sol. nigr.
Spongia.
Stannum.
Stramon.
|| Sulphur.
Sulph. ac.
|| Veratr.
Zincum.

Awakes frequently: *Agar.*, *Digit.*, *Nitr. ac.*, *Zincum;* early: *Nux vom.;* as if it was time to get up: *Digit.*
Wakes frequently in the night, as if woke by fear: *Lycop.*
Is woke by anxiety, which keeps her awake long: *Conium.*
Sleep is interrupted by anxiety and heat: *Veratr.*
A strange feeling of heat in the head wakes him, and is followed by anxiety: *Arnic.*
Cramp-like pain in the mouth after being woke by anxiety: *Sepia.*
Melancholy: *Carb. an.;* is bowed down with it: *Alum.;* continuing: *Pulsat.;* fear as from an evil conscience: *Magn. sulph.;* as if he had committed a crime: *Pulsat.*

Feels a heavy lump in scrobiculum, causing desire to vomit: *Arg. nitr.*

Incarcerated wind, better from walking up and down the room: *Silic.*

Awakes at midnight, with an anxious feeling of a heavy lump in the stomach, causing nausea: *Arg. nitr.*

Awakes with anxiety and nausea, coming from abdomen into stomach, followed by diarrhœa: *Phelland.*

Awakes with nausea and inclination to vomit about midnight: *Bellad.*

Is woke by painful pressure in abdomen: *Mezer.*

Is woke in the night by great anxiety, and a cramp-like pain in the chest and abdomen: *Sepia.*

Crampy sensation rising from chest into throat, wakes with anxiety: *Veratr.*

Wakes with anxiety at 1 A.M., as if suffocating with stoppage of nose: *Amm. carb.;* anxious awakening after midnight, heavy breathing: *Calc. ostr.*

When awaking, dyspnœa and anxiety: *Nitr. ac.;* anxiety, oppression and sweat: *Alum.*

Short breath, as if he would suffocate: *Sambuc.*

Attack of anxiety on waking after midnight, cannot get her breath: *Lycop.*

Anxiety and oppression of chest wake at midnight: *Ignat.*

Starts up from sleep before midnight, cannot get his breath, calls anxiously for help: *Hepar s. c.*

Is awakened several times in the night with constriction of chest and anxiety, has to sit straight up: *Lact. vir.*

Starts up from sleep with anxiety, dyspnœa and trembling: *Sambuc.*

Infants awake at night with anguish; they are able to inhale but not to exhale: *Sambuc.*

Suffocating jerks waken every few minutes from sleep in hydrothorax: |*Lact. vir.;* starts, running from below up, as soon as he falls asleep; with cerebrospinal meningitis after a sunstroke in the nape of the neck: |*Bellad.*

Violent palpitation when lying on the back, awakens at midnight with anxiety, has to sit up: *Nitrum.*

Is awakened towards 4 and 5 A.M. with cardiac anxiety, better when getting up: *Alum.*

Restlessness; after sleeping a short time is awakened by anxiety, has to sit up; head drops from one side to the other: *Caustic.*

Awakens as if frightened; trembling and violent palpitation: *Mangan., Mercur.*

Awakes with anxious trembling: *Caustic., Sambuc.;* anxious heat: *Natr. mur., Nux vom., Sepia, Sulphur.*

Frequent starting from sleep, followed by anxious feeling and sweat: *Clemat.*

After waking indifference to life and disgust for the business of the day: *Phytol.;* when awaking tired of life: *Lycop., Natr. carb.*

Feelings and Conations. After getting awake, discontented with his lot: *Plumbum;* dissatisfied: *Nuc. v. c.;* no courage: *Graphit., Pulsat.*

Bad humor: *Cyclam., Janiph.;* every night after midnight: *Phosphor.*

Dispirited, irritable: *Petrol.;* angry thoughts: *Kali carb.*

Peevish: *Carb. an., Chamom., Sulph. ac.;* irritable: *Platin.*

Vexatious: *Bellad., Carb. an., Castor., Caustic., Chamom., Petrol., Rhus tox., Sulph. ac.;* and suspicious: *Laches.*

Vexes herself about unpleasant events which have happened long ago: | | *Lycop.*

When disturbed in sleep, angry: *Cuprum.*

Conations; Actions. Frequent waking, with moaning and groaning: *Amm. carb.;* pitiful weeping, moaning and sobbing, tossing about: *Cina;* very pettish: | | *Bellad.;* weeping a long while: *Pulsat.;* could not stop his tears for a long while: *Phosphor.*

Weeping wakens: *Cina;* before midnight: *Alum.;* towards morning: *Kali hydr.*

Awakes at 11 o'clock as if with a fright and weeps aloud: *Mercur.*

Awakes with a feeling as if the limbs were being stretched and screams about headache: *Rhus tox.*

Nightmare when lying on the back; awakes screaming: *Guaiac.;* awakes with screams: *Hyosc.*

Awakes after midnight with attacks of anxiety and loud screaming, cannot stop it: *Chin. sulph.*

Awakes about midnight with screaming and convulsions: *Laches.*

Exaltations. Restlessness wakes from sleep: *Amm. carb.;* at 2 A.M. and drives out of bed: *Magn. mur.*

Restlessness and feeling of hunger awake him: *Natr. mur.*

Nightly cough and great restlessness: *Sulphur.*

Restlessness on waking from sleep: *Bellad.;* a long time on awakening in the morning: *Bellad.;* with sadness when waking: *Carb. an.;* in the morning in bed, with ill humor: *Pulsat.;* after a night of anxiety: *Spongia;* on awaking from a dream could not stop his tears for fifteen minutes or more, in the morning: *Phosphor.*

When awaking, fright: *Spongia;* about trifles: *Laches.;* waking as if from fright: *Aurum;* after a frightful dream the spectres haunt him for awhile: *Sulphur;* fear after sad dreams: *Lepid., Pulsat.;* with starting: *Ox. ac.;* with fright as if falling from a height or into the water: *Digit.;* dreams of robbers; wakes in affright and believes the dream true: *Veratr.*

Intellect. Awakes from vivid dreams at 2 A.M. and cannot compose himself to sleep again: *Mezer.*

After getting awake he cannot sleep again on account of thoughts: *Kali carb.*

Gets awake at 1 A.M. and is kept awake by crowding of thoughts until four: *Borax;* gets awake at 2 A.M. and cannot sleep again on account of a rush of thoughts: *Silic.;* thinks he is in a strange place when getting awake: *Paris;* is confused, cannot recollect where she is nor what time it is: *Platin.;* thinks he is turned round in bed: *Calcar.*

When awaking does not recognize persons present: *Chamom.;* difficult waking and difficult comprehension: *Berber.;* after waking deranged: *Opium.*

When awaking cannot get rid of one idea: *Acon., Bryon., Ignat., Platin., Psorin., Silic.*

Wakes up as if frightened and confused, does not know where he is: *Pulsat.*

When roused from sleep difficulty of collecting thoughts: *Coca.*

After dreams difficult comprehension: *Arnic., Bellad., Capsic., Coccul., Cinchon., Silic.*

Waking visions: *Acon.;* delirium: *Aurum, Carb. veg., Colchic., Dulcam., Mercur., Natr. mur., Paris.*

After waking gets up suddenly and talks nonsense before she is aware of it: *Ignat.*

Starting in sleep; after waking as if drunk and half crazy: *Opium;* rage: *Bellad.*

Stupefaction: *Chelid., Natr. carb., Phosphor.*

When awaking, weak memory: *Stannum.*

After awaking, awkward: *Stramon.*

MODEL CURES.

Child six months old. Screaming; fever and hot head; all worse at night; starts in sleep as if frightened; pale in the evening; light green colored, slimy discharges from bowels, the light colored part appeared to be undigested milk; discharges more frequent during afternoon and evening. While talking with the mother, the child being asleep upon her arm, she bent forward to pick something from the floor, the child immediately threw up its hands. Upon questioning her, she said the child appeared to be afraid of falling, and she "didn't see how a child so young should know anything about falling." About a month previous the child's mouth had been sore, but had been cured as the mother supposed; *Borax*[lm] (F.), next morning the child was well.—H. N. MARTIN.

An infant, nine months old, has been affected with a species of laryngismus, attacking it at longer or shorter intervals since its birth; the laryngeal spasms have now become quite frequent, appearing several times in the day and night; it *awakes from sleep with suffocation;* is able to inspire but not to expire, becomes livid in the face, gasps in great anguish, and very slowly recovers its breath: *Sambuc.*[2c]; the child never had an attack subsequently.—C. WESSELHŒFT.

WHEN AWAKING IN THE MORNING.

Waking Early in Bed. Gets awake early, is bright and cheerful and disposed for mental work: *Aloes.*

Could not sleep after 3 A.M. for anxiety: *Rhus tox., Veratr.;* restlessness: *Zincum.*

Palpitation, with anxiety: *Phosphor.*

Anxious feeling in the abdomen: *Sulph. ac.*

Anxiety, as if sweat would break out: *Phosphor.*

Ill humor, pushes the pillows around, throws the covers off, does not want to see anyone: *Arsen.*

Cutting bellyache, screams, tosses about and gets beside himself: *Acon.*

Disinclined to get up, irritable and tired: *Thuya.*

Tired of life: *Lycop.;* confused, does not know whether he has slept: *Carb. an.;* absentminded: *Natr. carb., Phosphor.;* weak memory: *Stannum.*

Pleasurable Feelings and Exaltations. Very lively: *Nux mosch.;* good humored: *Hepar;* cheerful: *Clemat.*

All things appear new to him, even his friends, as though he had never seen them: *Stramon.*

Greater flow of thoughts: *Hura;* disposition for mental labor: *Aloes;* brain is more excited: *Aloes.*

Unpleasant Feelings. Is not refreshed by slumber: *Bellad.*

Dullness in head, as if not slept enough, uncheerful: *Kali carb.;* dull, uncomfortable feeling: *Phosphor.*

Few hours after waking lassitude and discomfort, would rather have slept: *Sepia.*

Sadness: *Alum., Carb. an., Phosphor., Sepia;* melancholy: *Ignat.;* grief: *Alum.;* dejected: *Arsen., Kali carb., Nitr. ac.;* looks cross and gloomy, very sad, unhappy, distressed, as if weighed down by sorrow: *Alum.;* lazy, sleepy and depressed: *Amm. gum.;* unpleasant ideas: *Sulphur.*

Feels extremely sad, unhappy and distressed in mind: *Laches.*

Hypochondric mood: *Alum., Lycop.;* fear: *Gelsem.;* and starting: *Ox. ac.;* on awaking in the dark, anxiety: *Natr. mur.;* for a moment after waking he is full of fear: *Nitr. ac.;* afraid to leave the room after waking, that an accident might befall him: *Psorin.;* wakes with fear of death on account of imagined pains in sleep: *Alum.*

On rising from bed apprehension: *Arg. nitr., Nux vom.*

Melancholy and anxious on getting awake: *Carb. an.*

When awaking in the morning from a deep sleep, anxious idea that she would now have to die: *Lycop.*

Anxiety: *Alum., Caustic., Cinch. off., Coccul., Graphit., Magn. carb., Magn. mur.;* and restlessness: *Lycop.;* apprehension: *Rhus tox.*

Trembling anxiety: *Carb. veg.*

Anxious imaginings: *Cinch. off.;* fear as from a bad conscience: *Magn. sulph.*

Anxious, fearful and desponding after a dream: *Pulsat.*

Irritable and anxious, as if something had happened in his dream to make him weep: *Platin.*
Anxiety drives him out of bed: *Anac., Chin. sulph.*
Anxiety and lassitude: *Magn. carb.*
Awakes with a shrinking look, fear: *Stramon.*
Weariness of life: *Lycop., Natr. carb.*
Sense of entire indifference to life and disgust for the business of the day on waking early in the morning: *Phytol.*
No ambition, as if no will; wavering: *Natr. carb.;* faint-hearted: *Pulsat.*
Ill humor: *Argent., Arsen., Bellad., Bryon., Conium, Janiph., Kali carb., Lycop., Mezer., Magn. mur., Natr. sulph., Nitr. ac., Nux vom., Petrol., Phosph. ac., Platin., Plumbum, Pulsat., Rhus tox., Sulph. ac., Thuya.*
Morose, disposed to bite: *Bellad.;* fretful: *Bellad., Bovist., Carb. an., Kali carb., Sulphur;* moody: *Cyclam.;* discontented: *Plumbum, Pulsat.;* dejected: *Hepar;* does not want to speak: *Hepar;* discontented look: *Ignat.;* irritable look: *Magn. carb.*
Children wake with ill humor: *Arsen., Kali carb., Laches.,* **Lycop.**
After getting up in the morning, until breakfast, out of humor: *Natr. sulph.*
Discontented and moody: *Nuc. v. c.;* dissatisfied with his destiny: *Plumbum.*
Irritability: *Canthar., Carb. an., Castor., Cyclam., Kali carb. Petrol., Sulph. ac.*
After getting out of bed irritable and apprehensive: *Arg. nitr.;* peevish: *Bovist., Carb. an., Chlorof., Gambog.;* impatient, throws things from him: *Dulcam.;* irritable, violent: *Graphit.,* **Sulph. ac.**
Children or grown people are irritable when getting awake, scream, strike about them and do not wish to be spoken to: **Lycop.** C. G. Raue. Similar: *Kali carb.*
Weeping: *Amm. mur., Borax, Carb. an., Prun. spin., Pulsat*
Ill-humored, weeps when looked at: *Ant. tart.*
After getting up from bed slow thinking: *Stramon.*
Laziness: *Hyper., Natr. mur.;* and lassitude: *Digit., Natr. carb.*
After rising in the morning moody, does not want to speak: *Coccul., Hepar.;* lazy and sleepy: *Verbasc.*
Joyless, taciturn, is averse to everything: *Magn. mur.*
Cannot bear contradiction: *Chamom.*
As if drunk: *Graphit.*
Rush of ideas; is scarcely conscious: *Nux vom.*
Difficult comprehension: *Aesc. hipp., Arnic., Berber., Carb. an., Cannab., Capsic.,* **Cinch. off.,** *Ignat., Kali carb., Mercur., Nitrum, Platin., Pulsat., Rheum, Staphis., Silic., Sol. mam., Thuya.*
Dazed feeling: *Arsen., Calcar.;* dullness: *Capsic.;* cannot comprehend the least thing: *Anac.*
Sees the vision of a burning house: *Hepar.*
Illusion on first waking, sees persons who are not there: *Sulphur.*
Delirium: *Ambra, Dulcam., Helleb., Hepar, Natr. mur.*
Full of fancies: *Conium.*

After sleep rage, mania: *Cicut.*
When awaking thinks it is much later: *Aloes.*
After getting up from bed weak memory: *Stramon.;* want of memory, forgetful: *Stannum.;* vertigo or loss of thoughts: *Stramon.*
Headache, which disappears when thinking of the pain: *Cicut.*
Stupor: *Chelid., Natr. carb.*
On sitting up in bed senses forsake her: *Natr. mur.*

AFTER LOSS OF SLEEP.

|| Ambra.
| Bryon.
|| Cinch. off.
|| Coccul.
| Colchic.
| Cuprum.
|| Ipec.
 Natr. mur.
| Nitr. ac.
|| Nux vom.
 Opium.
|| Phosph. ac.
|| Pulsat.
| Ruta.
| Sabin.
| Selen.
 Sepia.
| Sulphur.

Sufferings from loss of sleep night after night; effects of long continued strain on the mind by nursing, requiring mental and bodily attention; consequences of grief for loss or threatened loss of that which is most dear: *Nitr. ac.*

Sleeplessness from long continued nursing: *Coccul.,* |*Sulphur.*

The slightest loss of sleep tells on him: *Coccul.*

Feels very weak after passing a restless night, looks worn and sad: *Natr. mur.*

She is affected by getting up half an hour earlier than usual: *Kreosot.*

ANECDOTE.—While waiting towards evening at the office of Dr. Hlbg, there came running in the wife of a neighbor, a cabinet-maker, who years ago had been a prover of the *Nux moschata.* She wanted the doctor to go with her at once, for she said: "my husband fell down while working and lies on the floor in convulsions, the children screaming." She came near screaming herself, when she heard the doctor was out. But here is a doctor! said Mrs. Hlbg. Having become a foreigner in the fatherland, and knowing the personal hatred of Dr. Tr., who that same day had been seen walking intimately over the bridge with the Coroner, a Dr. S——r, a man so fond of persecuting others, that he had a Rabbi arraigned for murder, because a little boy died after circumcision, this and the possibility of the cabinet-maker dying in convulsions and thus getting me into trouble, kept me from going with the woman; but I put the following questions:—"What ailments has your husband been liable to?" "None, he was always well, never had a spasm in his life." "What has happened to-day, before he fell?" "Nothing at all!" "What did he say, what were his last words?" Sobbing, she answered: "after hurrying from the supper table to his bench, he said I must finish this coffin to-day and I want to go to bed as soon as I can!" "He lost sleep last night," she said, "he had to keep the watch in a house of mourning." Immediately a dose of *Coccul.* was ordered. As soon as Dr. Hlbg came home, he hastened there, and found the man in bed asleep. His wife had with much difficulty poured the powder, dissolved in water, into his mouth. The convulsions ceased soon after; he became conscious, asked "what is the matter?" and went to bed. He was well next day and nearly a year after he had not had another fit. Compare Hahnemann's Materia Medica, Vol. I., p. 184, sympts. 440 and 454.—C. HG.

MIND AND DISPOSITION.

AFTER SLEEP.

NOTE.—Sleep, soon after the first dose of a well-chosen medicine often warrants the improvement of the sick.—Feeling refreshed by sleep, particularly the mind, is a sure sign of the beginning of healing.—Hence, we ought never to forget asking the patient: "How do you feel when first wakening from sleep?" Or the mother: "How is the child when waking up by its own accord?"

Being better after sleep is mostly an indication to leave the patient without any more medicine. In rare cases only it indicates the remedy.

Better and worse after sleep. Both according to B. R., with some additions; the marks after the name signify aggravation after sleep; those before, amelioration; the cypher signifies that nothing has been observed.

Better after Sleep. Heaviness in abdomen as from a load, with anxiety: *Amm. mur.*

General aversion and irritability: *Capsic.*

Sudden blindness, with anxious sweat and bright light before the eyes: *Calc. ostr.*

Forgetfulness better after siesta: *Gymnoc.*

Getting out of bed, suicidal inclination: *Ant. crud.*

Worse after Sleep. Ill humor: *Anac., Bellad., Caustic., Chamom.;* quiet manner: *Anac.;* rage: *Bellad.;* irritability: *Caustic.*

On rising from bed, morose: *Caustic.;* getting up moody: *Hepar;* morose: *Magn. mur., Nitr. ac.*

After rising from bed, anxiety: *Magn. carb.*

Worse after Sleeping too long: *Acon., Anac., Arnic., Arsen., Camphor., Carb. veg., Caustic., Chamom., Conium, Euphras., Ferrum, Hepar, Kali carb., Laches., Lycop., Opium, Stramon., Sulphur;* on being disturbed after a long sleep, gets angry: *Cuprum.*

Worse after the Siesta. Mental depression and all other symptoms: *Bryon.*

Irritability and vexation: *South pole of Magnet;* with anger and weak feeling in the feet: *Clemat.*

Weak, lazy, irritable and thirsty: *Borax.*

Indifferent: *Mur. ac.;* and depressed, knees falter: *Rhodod.*

Depressed in mind from a laming stiffness in all the limbs: *Cinch. off.*

Irritability and vertigo: *Clemat.*

Ill humor, easily exasperated: *Caustic.*

Dullness in head: *Carb. veg.;* unfit for mental work: *Graphit.;* difficult comprehension: *Stannum.;* want of memory: *Conium.*

Better after siesta; inability to think: *Gymnoc.*

During sleep in the day time, whining and crying: *Anac., Canthar.*

TIMES OF DAY.

NOTE.—The times of the day as a modality have the highest value among our characteristics, but like precious pearls, they call for many and very deep divings.

As every symptom of the prover has to appear at a certain time of day, it is always very uncertain if this time has anything to do with it, in most cases it may be accidental; many coincidents and corroborations by practice have to be collected and compared, before we may suppose and then acknowledge that it is more than accidental, and finally regard it as characteristic. It should never be forgotten to observe what *kind* of symptoms appear at given times of the day. What we find in B. R., p. 299, is thus nearly useless. H. Gross' remissions are somewhat better than B.'s aggravations. (Comparative Materia Medica, *Aurum* and *Platin*.)

The hours of sleep, breakfast and other meals, the whole manner of living has generally more influence than the position of the sun.

MORNING.

Aloes.
|| Alum.
|| Ambra.
Amm. carb.
Amm. mur.
Amphis.
Anac.
August.
Argent.
Arsen.
Aster.
Berber.
| Borax.
| Bovist.
Bryon.
Calad.
| Calc. ostr.
|| Canthar.
|| Carb. an.
Carb. veg.
| Castor.
Caustic.
Cepa.
Chelid.
|| Chlorum.
Cinch. off.
Cinnab.
| Coccul.
Colchic.
|| Conium.
|| Cotyl.
Cyclam.
Dulcam.
| Fluor. ac.
Gambog.
Gelsem.
|| Graphit.
Guaiac.
Helleb.
|| Hepar s. c.
|| Hippom.
Hura.
Hydroph.
Hyosc.
Ignat.
| Kali carb.
Kalmia.
|| Kreosot.
|| Laches.
Lactuc.

Pleasurable Feelings. Mind symptoms better: *Graphit.;* cheerfulness: *Conium, Graphit., Hepar, Platin., Psorin., Spigel.*

A peculiar but agreeable sense of cheerfulness: *Cinnab.*

Merriness: *Bovist., Colchic.;* moodiness: *Hepar s. c.;* everything in nature wears a smiling aspect: *Fluor. ac.*

Painful Feelings. Homesick; feels as if forsaken: *Carb. an.;* dark mood: *Sulph. ac.*

Sadness: *Alum., Carb. an., Kreosot.,* ||*Laches., Mancin., Nitr. ac., Nuc. v. c., Petiv., Petrol., Phosphor., Platin.*

Dejection: *Calc. ostr., Petrol., Platin., Sepia, Sulphur.*

Low-spirited: *Kali carb., Platin., Sepia;* unhappy: *Tarax.*

Heavy spirits and melancholy: *Carb. an., Phosphor., Sepia.*

Apprehension: *Lycop.,* |*Magn. sulph., Mur. ac., Nux vom., Pulsat.*

Thinks he will lose his senses: *Mercur.*

Fear of an epileptic attack: *Alum.*

Anxiety about a trifling indisposition: *Coccul.*

Full of care about domestic affairs: *Pulsat.*

Anxiety: *Caustic.;* as if he had to expect something very important: *Canthar.;* as from an evil conscience: *Magn. sulph.;* after a meal: *Conium;* in doors: *Magn. mur.;* with fainty weakness every other morning: *Nitr. ac.;* better in the morning: *Carb. an., Castor., Rhus tox.;* anguish: *Alum., Nux vom., Pulsat., Veratr.;* awe: *Nux vom.;* with nausea: *Calc. ostr.*

Sits brooding, fears not to be saved: *Psorin.*

Cannot think of his affairs without grieving: *Pulsat.*

Ennui, is absorbed in himself: *Natr. carb.*

Inconsolable grief: *Phosphor.;* better in morning: *Graphit.*

Neutral Feelings. Indifference: *Magn. mur.;* and dullness: *Mancin.*

Uninterested, quiet: *Coccul., Hepar s. c., Petrol.;* apathy: *Cepa.*

Lauroc.
Lycop.
ǀ Magn. mur.
ǀǀ Magn. sulph.
ǀ Mancin.
ǀ Mangan.
Mercur.
Mezer.
Mur. ac.
ǀǀ Natr. carb.
ǀǀ Natr. sulph.
ǀǀ Nitr. ac.
ǀ Nitrum.
Nuc. v. c.
ǀ Nux vom.
Ox. ac.
Pedic.
ǀǀ Petiv.
ǀ Petrol.
ǀǀ Phosphor.
Phosph. ac.
ǀ Platin.
Plumbum.
Prun. spin.
ǀǀ Psorin.
ǀ Pulsat.
Ran. scel.
Rhus rad.
ǀǀ Rhus tox.
Sabad.
Sabin.
Sarsap.
ǀǀ Sepia.
Silic,
Spigel.
ǀ Spongia.
Squilla.
ǀ Staphis.
ǀ Stramon.
ǀ Sulphur.
ǀ Sulph. ac.
Tarax.
ǀ Thuya.
Veratr.
Zincum.

Feelings and Conations. Out of humor: *Amm. carb., Cyclam.,* ǀǀ *Kreosot., Magn. mur., Natr. sulph., Nitr. ac., Sabad., Sarsap., Thuya;* and inclined to weep: ǀǀ *Hippom., Sulphur.*

Indisposed to business and talk: *Tarax.;* and feels as if beaten: *Hydroph.;* until after breakfast: *Natr. sulph.*

Children are ill-humored, and cry for things, which, after getting, they petulantly throw away; worse early in the morning: *Staphis.*

Discontented: *Plumbum, Pulsat.*

Discouraged: *Hippom., Platin., Sepia, Sulphur;* and lazy: *Platin.;* and inclined to weep: *Sulphur.*

Does not wont to get up and dress: *Rhus tox.*

With gaping and belching: *Mangan.*

Morose: ǀǀ *Amm. mur., Conium, Hepar s. c., Hippom., Magn. mur., Mangan., Natr. sulph., Nitr. ac., Phosphor., Sulphur, Zincum.*

Wrinkled forehead: *Mangan., Zincum.* -

Lachrymose: *Hippom., Sulphur.*

Disposed to criticize, utters reproaches: *Rhus rad.*

Inclined to get angry: ǀǀ *Petrol.;* impatient: *Dulcam.;* disgusted: *Magn. mur.;* vexed: *Petrol.;* fretful: *Amm. carb., Amm. mur., Calad., Calc. ostr., Carb. an., Natr. sulph., Petrol., Sepia, Staphis.*

Does not wish to talk nor to be spoken to: *Natr. sulph.;* and is sleepy: *Calad.;* peevish: *Amm. carb., Bovist.,* ǀ *Calc. ostr., Canthar., Carb. an., Castor.,* ǀǀ *Chlorum, Kali carb., Mangan.,* ǀ *Petrol., Sepia, Staphis., Sulph. ac.,* ǀǀ *Thuya;* all things he takes in his hands he wants to throw from him: *Staphis.*

Irritable and excitable: *Calc. ostr., Canthar., Cinch. off., Conium, Kalmia, Natr. carb., Natr. sulph.,* ǀ *Nux vom., Spongia;* and depressed after a little work: *Calc. ostr.*

Very passionate and disposed to violent anger: *Calc. ostr., Graphit., Gambog.,* ǀǀ *Petrol.,* ǀǀ *Psorin.;* constant thoughts of dying: *Psorin.*

Actions. Inclined to be active: *Aloes;* hastiness: *Ignat.*

Inclination to laugh: *Graphit., Hura;* to weep: *Amm. carb., Borax; Carb. an., Hippom., Kreosot.,* ǀǀ *Petiv., Phosphor., Platin., Prun. spin., Pulsat., Spongia;* also in the evening: *Sulphur.*

Discontented: *Pulsat.;* groaning: *Bellad.;* inconsolable: *Phosphor.;* fears a misfortune and is very melancholy: *Magn. sulph.;* very much displeased, fretful and inclined to weep, morning and evening: *Sulphur;* slow in thinking: *Nitrum, Ox. ac.*

Aversions. Indisposed to think: *Nitrum, Nux vom.;* to work: *Angust., Tarax.;* to conversation: *Tarax.;* laziness: *Amm. carb., Amm. mur., Canthar., Chelid., Coccul., Lactuc.,* ǀǀ *Natr. carb., Nux vom., Platin., Ran. scel., Rhus tox., Squilla.*

Disgusted with all headwork: *Ran. scel., Squilla.*

Says very little during a walk: *Sabin.;* not disposed to speak: *Sabin.;* does not want to speak nor be spoken to: *Natr. sulph.;* disinclined to answer: *Magn. mur.;* talks very little, shuts his eyes: *Petrol., Silic., Thuya.*

Exaltations. Exalted imaginations: *Conium;* exalted spirits: *Laches.;* overactive, too busy, without strength: *Hyosc.*

Disposition to work: *Aloes.*
Oversensitive in the morning: *Calc. ostr., Graphit.*
Early in the day sensitive, better in afternoon: *Natr. sulph.*
Mental restlessness: *Dulcam., Hyosc*

Depressions. Indisposition: *Cepa;* mental relaxation: *Canthar.;* mental and bodily relaxation: *Laches., Phosphor.*

Sadness and lassitude, better from walking about: *Amphis.*
Anxiety, weak and faint feeling: *Arsen.*
After getting out of bed vertigo and loss of thoughts: *Stramon.*

Intellect. Head confused when getting up: *Pedic.*

Difficult comprehension: *Aster., Berber., Carb. an., Lauroc., Mezer., Thuya;* difficult thinking: *Ox. ac.*

Uncheerfulness, inability to think, with dull headache: *Gelsem.*

Early in the morning felt as if going out of her mind, elevated, careless state, lasting five minutes, followed by a sensation as of blood trickling down the left arm, from the shoulder to the finger-joints: *Cotyl.*

Abstracted; ennui: *Natr. carb.*
Deficiency of clearness in ideas: *Borax.*
Mental dullness: *Berber., Canthar., Carb. veg., Graphit., Phosphor.;* and indifference: *Mancin.;* dull and gloomy: *Sulph. ac.*
Hardly able to answer questions: *Ox. ac.;* unable to think: *Anac., Gelsem.*
Aversion to thinking, not to reading or memorizing: *Nux vom.;* aversion to mental occupation: *Ran. scel.*
Full of fantasies: *Conium, Mercur.*
Delirious: *Ambra, Bryon., Conium, Dulcam., Helleb., Hepar s. c., Mercur., Natr. carb.*

A momentary stitch in the region of the heart, as if in the pleura; frequent spasmodic contraction of the muscles of the heart, worse when lying on the back; he has an idea that he will have a stroke of apoplexy, which causes him no anxiety: *Argent.*

Stares before him thoughtlessly: *Guaiac.*
Absentminded: *Guaiac., Natr. carb., Phosphor., Phosph. ac.*
Absence of thought if alone: *Phosph. ac.*
Slow thinking: *Stramon.;* stupid: *Graphit.;* want of mind: *Nux vom.;* awkward in talking: *Ignat.;* forgetful and dizzy: *Silic.*
Revived memory: ||*Fluor. ac.;* memory useless: |*Anac.*

On Rising or After It. Anxiety, weariness and trembling: *Arg. nitr.*
Uncomfortable: *Ignat., Nitr. ac.*
Sadness and tired feeling: *Carb. an.;* peevish for an hour: *Bovist.;* and disposed to anger: *Gambog.;* dejected and irritable after the least exertion: *Calc. ostr.;* depressing stiffness in limbs: *Cinch. off.*

284 MIND AND DISPOSITION.

Oppression, with trembling of heart: *Spigel.*
Anxiety, with heat: *Carb. an., Petrol.;* irritable and apprehensive: *Arg. nitr., Magn. sulph.;* fretful: *Canthar., Magn. mur.;* vexed: *Nitr. ac.;* morose: *Canthar., Nitr. ac., Magn. mur.;* fear lasting after a dream: *Pulsat.*
Mind and body relaxed, weary: *Amm. carb., Laches., Phosph. ac.;* and indisposed to work: *Lact. vir.*
Disposed to weep: *Amm. carb.;* throng of ideas: *Nux vom.;* stupidity: *Magn. mur.*

FORENOON.

Aethus.
Aloes.
II Alum.
II Amm. carb.
II Amm. mur.
II Anac.
I Ant. crud.
Apis.
Argent.
Arg. nitr.
Arsen.
Baryt.
Bellad.
Bismuth.
II Borax.
Calad.
II Calc. ostr.
I Cannab.
Canthar.
Carb. an.
II Carb. veg.
II Caustic.
Chamom.
Cinnab.
II Clemat.
Colchic.
Conium.
I Graphit.
Gratiol.
II Hippom.
Hura.
Hydroph.
Kali carb.
Laches.
.I Lycop.
I Magn. carb.
Magn. mur.
Mezer.
Mur. ac.
I Natr. carb.
II Natr. mur.
I Natr. sulph.
II Niccol.
Nitrum.
II Nux mosch.
Ox. ac.
Platin.
Plumbum.
Phelland.
II Phosphor.
Psorin.
Ran. bulb.
Ran. scel.

Pleasurable Feelings and Exaltation. Unusual well feeling: *Plumbum;* good-humored, conversational: *Caustic.;* cheerful and merry: *Borax;* cheerful and lively: *Aethus.. Natr. sulph.;* gay, merry: *Graphit., Phosphor.;* lively and talkative: *Caustic.;* lively comprehension: *Ox. ac.*
Disposition for work; hastiness: *Aloes.*
Bright humor: *Caustic., Colchic., Natr. mur., Phosphor., Tinct. acr., Zincum;* in a reconciling mood: *Aloes.*
Voluptuous fancies: *Hippom.*
Laughing: *Graphit.;* cheerful and happy: II *Clemat.*

Unpleasant Feelings. Uncomfortable and dreary: *Phelland., Phosphor.*
Gloomy: *Arg. nitr.;* and sad: *Phelland., Sarsap.*
Sad: *Amm. carb., Ant. crud., Cannab., Graphit.;* and morose: *Phelland.*
Sad ideas and longing for death: *Apis;* dejected, with apprehension and cold feeling: *Amm. carb.;* doleful and sorrowful; the sound of bells makes him weep: *Ant. crud.;* dejected: *Amm. carb., Cannab.;* and unhappy: *Alum.;* melancholic: *Thuya;* hypochondric: II *Anac., Hippom., Nux mosch.*
Anxiety: *Alum., Canthar., Natr. mur., Sarsap., Sulphur;* anguish: *Lycop.*
Apprehensive and lachrymose: *Niccol.;* and feeling cold: *Amm. carb.*
Anxiety and melancholy, vexed about trifles, no desire for mental occupation: *Clemat.*
Sick headache, with nausea and anxiety: *Calc. ostr.*
Anxiety, with contraction in the rectum: *Calcar.;* constriction of chest, with anxious breathing: *Nitrum.*
Cardiac anxiety: *Bellad.;* anxiety, with palpitation: *Mezer.;* sudden anxiety and palpitation: *Natr. mur.*
Constrictive, tensive feeling all over, with anxiety: *Baryt.*
Anxiety and trembling sensation all over: *Platin.*
Inward fear and trembling: *Lycop.*

Rumex.
Sabad.
ǁSarsap.
Seneg.
ǀSepia.
Serpent.
Silic.
Sulphur.
ǀSulph. ac.
Tinct. acr.
Thuya.
Zincum.

Anxious heat: *Calcar.*
Disinclined for any work, with ennui: *Alum.;* indifference: *Alum., Sarsap.*

Feelings and Conations. Discomfort: *Serpent.;* disgust: *Sarsap.*
Ill humor: *Amm. carb., Argent.,* (excited in the afternoon) *Caustic., Gratiol., Magn. carb.;* and grumbling: *Caustic.;* nothing is good enough: *Hippom.*

Morose: ǁǀ*Amm. carb., Caustic., Colchic., Tinct. acr.;* at 7 o'clock: *Calad.;* sometimes with headache: *Amm. carb.*

Peevish: *Amm. carb., Amm. mur., Carb. veg.,* ǁǀ*Phosphor., Ran. bulb., Seneg.;* weary and tired: *Gratiol., Magn. mur.*

Fretfulness: *Carb. an., Phosphor., Ran. bulb., Seneg.;* and serious face, better at noon: *Aethus.;* with headache: *Serpent.;* heat in head: *Aethus.*

Vexed: *Caustic., Gratiol., Natr. carb., Phosphor.;* vexing ideas: *Ran. bulb.;* after a vexation, prostration, palpitation and trembling: *Lycop.*

Irritable: *Cinnab.;* better after dinner: *Amm. mur.;* and impetuous: ǁǀ*Carb. veg.;* disposed to quarrel: *Ran. bulb.;* vehement: *Natr. carb.;* and angry: *Silic.*

Actions. Disposed to weep: *Ant. crud.;* with ill humor: *Sarsap.*
Sighs a great deal; laughs at trifles, but in the evening is disposed to grieve and weep: *Graphit.*

Desires. Depressed and joyless, wishes to be alone: *Alum.;* longing for death: *Apis.*

Aversions. Introverted: *Phosphor.*
Aversion to everything: *Calad., Sarsap.*
Taciturn: *Hippom., Natr. mur.;* till noon: *Aethus.*
Sluggish: *Natr. mur.;* with stretching: *Magn. carb., Mur. ac.;* and sleepiness: *Magn. carb.,* ǁǀ*Sarsap.;* dull and stupid: *Laches., Psorin.*
No desire to work: *Alum.*

Restlessness: *Anac., Calad., Hydroph., Phosphor., Silic.,* oversensitiveness: *Amm. mur.;* as after vexation: *Natr. carb.*

Intellect. Not inclined to think: *Rumex;* difficult comprehension: *Arsen.;* unable to think: *Sepia;* dullness is increased by serious thoughts: *Sulphur;* dull and weak in the head: *Arsen.;* when reading does not know what he reads: *Bismuth.;* dull and disinclined to work: *Psorin.;* dull and stupid: *Sarsap.;* fullness: *Sulph. ac.;* absent: *Phosphor., Silic.;* forgetful: *Calad.;* awkward: *Anac.*

NOON.

Towards noon less moroseness and grief: *Aethus.*
Sadness: *Zincum;* anxiety and weakness, with headache: *Chin. sulph.;* cardiac anxiety: *Bellad.;* palpitation renewed by thinking of it, with anxiety: *Baryt.;* great anxiety with palpitation, has to lie down: *Mezer.*

Low-spirited: *Canthar.;* low spirits at noon, in the evening hilarity: *Zincum.*

Irritable: *Amm. mur., Natr. mur., Rumex;* fretful: *Kali carb., Mar. ver.;* peevish and cross; every little thing worries him: *Kali carb.;* irritable, peevish and frightened: *Zincum;* oversensitive: *Zincum;* nervous excitement, impatience: *Hura;* restless mind: *Hydroph.*

Lassitude; weary and drowsy; goes to sleep while talking or standing; inability to think: *Magn. carb.*

Sluggish, disinclined to move: *Aloes.*

It gives him too much trouble to think; stupid: *Ars. met.*

Dull and weak headed: *Arsen.*

Absentminded: *Moschus;* from 11 A.M. till 4 P.M.: *Nitrum.*

Headache and stupefaction: *Aethus.;* stupefied: *Zincum;* stupid and weak in head: *Arsen., Conium.*

ALL DAY.

Cheerful: *Anac., Magn. mur., Mur. ac.;* gay and merry: *Aurum, Caustic.:* bright: *Sarsap.*

Oversensitive: *Carb. veg.;* sad: *Droser., Phelland., Sulphur.*

Anxious: *Ant. crud., Bellad., Caustic., Lauroc., Mercur., Natr. carb., Nitr. ac., Phytol., Platin., Ruta, Sulph. ac., Zincum.*

Repeated attacks of anxiety: *Chamom.*

Terrible anxiety in the head, confused vision, walks his room wringing his hands and lamenting, from 5 A.M. to 5 P.M.: *Psorin.*

Cardiac anxiety in a light degree, with irritability: *Platin.*

Anxiety; hasty and restless; cannot keep the limbs still, wants to stretch them: *Natr. carb.*

Restlessness in all the limbs, a sort of crawling, with anxiousness: *Ambra.*

Restlessness, with constriction of chest: *Ambra.*

Restlessness: *Ambra, Natr. carb., Sulphur;* anguish: *Magn. carb., Graphit., Mercur., Natr. carb., Pulsat., Stannum;* dolefulness: *Bovist.;* grief: *Staphis.*

Day and night inconsolable: *Carb. an.*

Indifference: *Anac., Digit., Mercur., Veratr.*

Music, of which he is fond, does not please him: *Carb. veg.*

Timidity: *Carb. an., Natr. mur., Verbasc.;* melancholy and depressed, with anxious timidity: *Natr. mur.*

Discontented: *Arsen., Ledum;* out of humor for days: *Dulcam., Petrol., Sepia, Zincum;* dejected: *Ant. crud., Natr. mur.;* low-spirited: *Stannum;* hypochondric: *Agn. cast.*

Ill-humored: *Ant. crud., Bismuth., Ipec., Magn. carb., Phelland., Pulsat., Sarsap., Sulph. ac., Viol. tric.;* fretful: *Anac., Calc. ac., Carb. veg., Caustic., Cyclam., Mercur., Natr. carb., Platin., Ruta, Stannum, Staphis., Sulphur, Verbasc.;* morose: *Mercur.;* vexed: *Carb. veg.;* vexing ideas: *Sulphur.*

Irritable all day long, at war with himself, apprehensive and dissatisfied, not disposed for mental labor: *Caustic.;* impetuous: *Nitr. ac.*

Pain in head so violent, has to weep aloud: *Phosphor.;* whining all day, better in the evening: *Zincum;* whining day after day: *Natr. mur.*

Weeping all day: *Bryon., Lycop.;* for weeks: *Alum., Mezer.*

Whining and lamenting on account of terrible pains in the knees: *Canthar.*

Head is dull, as after turning round in a circle: *Calc. ostr.*

Great dullness and depression, with pains in the limbs: *Gelsem.*

Palpitation when sitting and fixing the attention on anything: *Natr. carb.*

AFTERNOON.

Feelings. Feels better in the afternoon: *Amm. mur., Anac., Argent., Cannab., Magn. carb., Natr. sulph., Ox. ac., Phosphor., Plumbum.*

Better humor, more inclined to work: *Anac.*

Mental depression in forenoon, cheerfulness in afternoon: *Argent., Cannab., Magn. carb.*

More decided than in the forenoon, playful and mirthful: *Ox. ac.*

More lively in the afternoon: *Phosphor.*

Good humored: *Anac., Sarsap.;* cheerful: *Argent., Calc. ac.,* I *Cannab., Clemat., Lauroc., Magn. carb., Ol. anim., Sarsap.,* I I *Thuya.*

Cheerful and more interested: *Lauroc.;* greater mobility: *Ol. anim.;* can work better: *Aloes;* very active, lost in his work: *Plumbum;* more inclined to work: *Sarsap.*

Very cheerful towards evening, inclined to dance and sing: *Natr. mur.*

Merry: *Staphis.;* exalted: *Argent.*

Great liveliness and activity of mind, but cannot keep his thoughts fixed on one thing on account of an inward restless feeling, such as one feels when having great expectations: *Angust.*

Very bright and active: *Ox. ac.*

Cheerful in forenoon, dull in afternoon: *Natr. mur.*

Sadness: *Aethus., Carb. an., Conium, Digit., Ignat., Ol. anim., Phosphor., Ruta, Zincum.*

Great melancholy: *Phosphor.;* in latter part of P.M. and evening: *Calc. sulph.;* out of spirits: *Conium;* weary of life: *Ruta;* dejected: *Cannab., Mangan., Ol. anim.;* weary and depressed: *Sulphur;* depression of spirits: *Alum., Rhus rad.*

Weary, anxious and sad: *Carb. an.*

Fearful, melancholy, does not know what ails her: *Niccol.*

Hypochondric mood: *Coccul., Graphit., Zincum.*

Apprehensions: *Amm. carb., Carb. veg., Magn. carb., Natr. carb., Nux vom., Tabac.*

Great apprehension and anxiety from noon to 3 P.M.: *Aster.;* at 5 P.M.: *Nux vom.;* fear of damnation: *Carb. veg.*

Anxiety, with fear of the future, at 6 P.M.: *Digit.*

Restlessness and anxiety, with feeling as if something was going to happen: *Tabac.;* anxiety as if going to die, with heat: *Ruta.*

Anxious apprehension of an accident, with sensation as if diarrhœa would set in: *Crot. tigl.*

Anxiety: *Calc. ostr., Carb. veg., Magn. carb., Magn. mur.,* I I *Natr. carb.,* I I *Nitrum, Phelland., Phosphor., Pulsat., Tabac., Zincum.*

Fearfulness, no confidence in himself, hypochondric: *Canthar.*

Every afternoon between five and six great anxiety, as if she had done a crime: *Amm. carb.*

Restlessness and anxiety every afternoon, feels as if he had done a great crime, ends in weeping, even on the street: *Carb. veg.*

Fearfulness and anxiety relieved by weeping: *Tabac.*

Fearfulness, no ambition, with vice-like headache: *Magn. carb.*

Anxiousness after nausea and headache in the forenoon: *Calc. ostr.*

Anxiousness, with sick headache: *Nitr. ac.*

Anxiety, with constant sighing: *Tabac.*

Cardiac anxiety: *Rhus tox.;* precordial anxiety: *Canthar.*

Anxiousness, with constriction of chest: *Sulphur.*

Anxiety, with insupportable feeling of distress in the breast, increasing to tears and screams, daily from 4 to 5 P.M.: *Thuya.*

Weakness and fearfulness, does not know what to do with herself: *Amm. carb.*

Every afternoon restlessness and anxiety: *Carb. veg.;* runs hither and thither, tries to sleep but cannot: *Lamium.*

Great worriment, has to lie down: *Phosph. ac.*

Anxiety and trembling: *Carb. veg.;* of hands: *Pulsat.*

Anxiety from twelve to three: *Aster.;* at four: *Tabac.;* four to five: *Thuya;* four to six: I I *Carb. veg.;* five: *Nux vom.;* six: *Digit.;* five to six: *Amm. carb.*

While walking heat in face, with anxiety: *Strontian.*

Anxious and weak, with sweat on epigastrium: *Nitrum.*

Constriction and oppression, with anxiousness: *Sulphur.*

Anxiousness, with flushes of heat and sweat: *Plumbum.*

Fear: *Digit., Sulphur.*

Anguish: *Amm. carb., Nux vom., Phosph. ac., Rhus tox.*

Indifferent Feelings. Tired of life: *Mur. ac.;* ennui; quiet manner: *Plumbum;* seeks company: *Zincum;* introverted, quiet mood: *Helleb.;* with a discomfort in the whole body, four afternoons in succession: *Mangan.*

Afternoon clouded forehead: *Zincum.*

Quiet mood: *Anac., Mangan.;* loss of the usual cheerfulness: *Ignat.;* no ambition: *Gratiol.*

Indifference from three to six: *Conium.*

Feelings and Conations. Long deliberation after every question: *Gratiol.*

Scrupulous conscientiousness and anxiety, which take away her peace of mind from 4 to 8 P.M.: I *Lycop.*

AFTERNOON.

Faint-hearted: *Carb. an., Ran. bulb.;* discouraged: *Conium;* fearful: *Amm. carb.*

Ill humor: *Aethus., Aloes, Alum., Anac., Bovist., Cannab., Conium, Ignat., Iodium, Mangan., Magn. carb., Mur. ac., Nitr. ac., Ox. ac., Plumbum, Sarsap.;* from noon till evening: *Iodium;* after half-past one till evening: *Alum.;* afternoon and evening: *Ox. ac.*

Ill humor and indifference every afternoon from three to six; feels as if a heavy guilt weighed him down: *Conium.*

Morose: *Aethus., Borax, Cannab., Magn. sulph., Mangan., Pulsat., Sarsap., Zincum;* at 4 P.M.: *Borax;* four days in succession: I I *Mangan.;* will not speak: *Magn. sulph.*

Morose and quarrelsome until 4 P.M.: *Hydroph.*

Irritable and quarrelsome from noon to 2 P.M.: *Aster.;* quarrelsome humor without getting angry: *Dulcam.*

Criticises others: *Dulcam.*

4 P.M. crossness, bursts into tears: *Pulsat.*

Very irritable, is disgusted with everything, inclined to quarrel and make an uproar: *Alum.*

Hypochondric mood after irritability in the forenoon: *Graphit.*

Irritability of temper: *Colchic., Graphit.;* with headache: *Lil. tigr.*

Nervousness, especially afternoon and evening: *Platin.;* nervous and impatient about half-past one: *Hura;* very impatient: *Nitr. ac.*

Fretful and indisposed after dullness all forenoon: *Sarsap.*

Peevishness after dinner, abating towards evening: *Natr. carb.*

Reproachful and peevish after 4 P.M., several days: *Borax.*

Peevish, fretful and sullen: *Alum., Borax, Bovist., Cannab., Canthar., Cinnab.,* I *Colchic., Kali carb., Lauroc., Mangan., Mur. ac.,* I I *Natr. carb., Sarsap., Zincum;* with pressing headache in forehead: *Kali carb.;* painful quivering on a small spot: *Bovist.;* jerking and heaviness from 2 P.M., increasing till evening: *Magn. carb.;* after dinner: *Natr. carb.;* 1 P.M.: *Alum.;* 2 P.M.: *Lauroc.;* 4 P.M.: *Borax;* several days in succession: *Borax, Mangan.*

Suspicious: *Nux vom.*

After a vexation, headache increasing from 1 P.M., until it passes off in bed: *Magn. carb.*

Actions. Impetuous: *Caustic.*

Crossness and weeping at 4 P.M.: *Pulsat.*

Oppression and sighing at 5 P.M.: *Hura.*

Groaning and moaning: *Cina.*

Morose, vexed with himself, scolds and abuses: *Aloes.*

Desires. Pensive, anxious longing, weak and sentimental: *Castor.*

Quiet thoughts of death, with weakness: *Zincum.*

Aversions. Close and introverted: *Helleb., Plumbum;* fribbling, lazy: *Borax;* displeased with everything: *Gratiol., Natr. mur., Zincum;* disinclined to mental work: *Nux vom.*

Heavy and drowsy, cannot accomplish anything that requires attention: *Lepid.*

Out of humor, would rather not talk: *Magn. sulph.*
Lassitude, weariness and aversion to labor, indisposed to talk: *Sulphur.*
Indisposed to speak: *Viol. tric.*
Disposed to do nothing: *Natr. mur.*
Sluggish and weary, yawning: *Chelid.*
It is hard for him to stick to his work: *Aster.*
Disgust for work: *Bufo.*
No ambition, dissatisfied with all kinds of work: *Plumbum.*

Exaltations. Mental excitement: *Aloes, Angust.*
Strange excitement of the fancy, loves to dwell on adventurous occurrences of his past life: *Argent.*
Crowding of thoughts; waking dreams: *Angust.*
Bright humor: *Phosphor., Plumbum;* from 3 o'clock till evening: *Zincum;* flow of ideas at 5 P.M.: *Sol. tub. œgr.;* exalted imagination from five to seven: *Staphis.*
He does not know whether that which dwells in his imagination has really happened or whether it is the recollection of a dream: *Staphis.*
Restlessness of mind: *Angust., Carb. veg., Hyosc., Ruta, Tabac.*
Restlessness driving from place to place: *Staphis.*

Depression. Loss of liveliness: *Ignat.*

Intellect. Difficult comprehension: *Arg. nitr., Conium, Gratiol.;* intellectual labor difficult: *Rhus rad.;* weak mind: *Mur. ac.;* can scarcely think: *Sepia.*
Confused and absentminded, forgets things: *Cepa.*
Cannot read, write or think: *Silic.*
Dullness and inability to think: *Sepia.*
Mental dullness: *Anac., Graphit., Helleb., Lauroc., Natr. mur., Sepia, Silic.;* does not want to speak: *Viol. tric.*
Sudden loss of consciousness: *Ol. anim.*
Stupid from 11 A.M. to 6 P.M.: *Arsen.;* from 3 A.M. to 4 P.M.: *Calc. ac.;* stupid and absent from 3 to 7 P.M.: *Natr. mur.;* attacks of stupefaction: *Zincum.*
Quick acting memory: *Anac., Angust.*
Forgetfulness: *Cepa*; weak memory: *Lauroc.;* says words he does not want to say during a chill: *Chamom.;* forgets things or gets them mixed up: *Cepa.*
Puttering, does not accomplish anything: *Borax*
Absentminded: *Gratiol., Mangan., Plumbum.*
Slight emotions cause palpitation: *Phosphor.*

Better in the Afternoon. The sensitiveness of the early day: *Natr. sulph.;* the disgust: *Sarsap.*

EVENING.

Better in the Evening. Anxiousness: *Magn. carb., Sulph. ac., Zincum.*
Trembling anxiety and fear as if something would happen: *Magn. carb.*
Pectoral anxiety; anxiety and tearfulness: *Zincum.*
Ill humor of the day: *Amm. carb., Bismuth., Calc. ac., Calc. ostr., Magn. carb., Niccol, Viol. tric.*
Taciturnity: *Clemat.;* weak mind and memory: *Bufo.*
Better in the Evening than during the Day. Better after eating: *Amm. carb.;* more able to do mental labor than during the day: *Cicut., Pulsat.*
During the day depressed mood, merry in evening: *Sulphur;* sadness of day gets better: *Castor.;* whining all day, better in the evening: *Zincum.*

Pleasurable Feelings and Exaltations. Religious thoughts; hopefulness: *Hyper.*
Mental excitement: *Anac., Carb. veg., Cinch. off., Laches., Phosphor., Zincum.*
Excitement like that after tea: *Hyper.*
Feeling as if the mind was brighter and more active: *Valer.;* more inclined to study: *Cicut.;* disposed to intellectual occupation: *Pulsat.;* and talkative, keeps awake longer: *Therid.*
Good humor: *Pulsat.;* spirits best about 6 P.M.: *Calc. sulph.*
Happy humor: I*Aloes;* towards evening joyous, lively imagination: *Cyclam.;* bright humor: *Chelid., Zincum.*
Writes with great ease and power without getting sleepy: *Laches.*
Stimulated fancy; copious flow of ideas from 9 to 10 o'clock: *Anac.*
Towards evening excited humor: *Zincum.*
Feels unusually well and strong: *Cina.*
Great cheerfulness and mental activity: *Nuc. v. c.;* uncommon liveliness: *Valer.;* lively and talkative: *Laches.*
Cheerfulness: *Bismuth., Cistus, Clemat., Graphit., Laches., Natr. carb., Natr. mur., Platin., Verbasc., Viol. tric., Zincum.*
Merriness: *Alum., Aster., Bellad., Castor., Cuprum, Ferrum, Natr. mur., Phelland., Zincum;* great gaiety: *Bufo, Pedic.;* immoderately gay: *Castor., Phelland.*
Feels gayer and stronger: *Sarsap.*
In the evening merry; depressed by day: *Sulphur.*
Gay, merry: *Calc. ostr., Magn. carb.*
Exaltation: *Cinch. off., Mar. ver.;* exalted imagination: *Cyclam., Phosphor.;* from nine to ten: *Anac.*
Hot face after animated conversation: *Fluor. ac.*

Care and Sorrow: *Arsen., Digit., Graphit., Kali carb.;* towards evening gloomy: *Amm. carb.;* sad: *Murex;* doleful: *Ignat., Nitr. ac.;* homesick: *Hippom.*
In the dusk, sadness: *Ignat.;* same hour: *Phosphor.;* and confusion of ideas: II*Murex;* later: *Ant. crud., Baryt., Bovist., Ferrum,* II*Kali carb., Phosphor., Platin., Ran. scel.,* II*Sepia;* after lying down: *Stramon.;* in bed: *Arsen., Graphit., Sulphur.*

With apprehension: *Arsen.;* as if forsaken: *Baryt.;* life-weary: ||*Kali chlor., Ruta;* fretful: *Ant. crud.;* melancholic: *Ran. scel.;* has to shed tears without cause: *Kali carb.;* prostration: *Bovist., Laches.*

Melancholic: *Arsen., Lycop., Nitr. ac., Ruta, Seneg.;* woeful: *Ignat.;* low-spirited: *Lycop., Ran. scel.;* weeping: *Platin.;* depressed: *Kreosot., Ran. scel., Rhus rad.;* dejected: *Alum., Carb. an., Graphit., Magn. carb., Kali carb., Ruta,* ||*Sepia, Spigel., Sulphur;* despairing: *Ant. tart.; Kreosot.*

Such inner weakness, that he fears he will have to give up his practice, while riding in his carriage: *Osmium.*

Hypochondric mood: *Hydroph., Kreosot., Nux vom., Phosphor.;* in bed: *Pulsat.*

Apprehension. Afternoon, till evening: *Natr. carb.;* towards evening: *Tabac.;* at twilight: *Rhus tox.;* early: *Carb. an.*

In evening: *Alum., Anac., Baryt., Carb. an., Digit., Hepar, Hippom., Kali carb.;* as if something would happen: *Kali hydr., Magn. mur., Natr. mur., Nux vom., Pæon., Zincum;* for an hour: *Rhus tox.;* after being cheerful during the day: *Anac.*

As if something would happen: *Alum., Tabac.*

As if forsaken: *Baryt.;* with ennui: *Magn. mur.;* as if going to die: *Phosphor..*

As if lamed by a fright; dark foreboding, afraid something will happen: *Natr. mur.*

Apprehension and inconsolable weeping: *Veratr.*

In bed: *Arsen., Graphit.;* gloomy forebodings; fears his friends may have met with an accident: *Arsen.*

MODEL CURES.

Periodic melancholy with a woman, æt. 65. The attacks come only at dusk, before the lamps are lighted and in the night: *Arsen.*—HAYNEL.

Towards evening anxiety and apprehension about his family, which he left behind while going on a short journey; the anxiety increases until he becomes inconsolable: *Petrol.*—HAYNEL.

A woman, æt. 50, became weakminded, childish, and laughed without cause. She had two paralytic attacks, each at 8 o'clock in the morning. She lay quietly on her back with closed eyes. Delirious talk always *worse in the evening*. Wants to get away, throws things out of the window, laughs much. At 3 A.M. violent spasms, which return every half hour. Wants to scream but cannot; gurgling sound in the throat; foams at the mouth; opistholonos; strikes with one arm, with the other she only grasps; pale face, unconsciousness: *Stramon.*[30]—HARTLAUB.

Very restless in the evening in bed; converses with spirits who approach his bed, lays hold of a sword and strikes about him to drive the fiend who is after him from the room. Red face, glistening eyes, great thirst, distended abdomen and great sexual excitement: *Stramon.*—TRINKS.

Acon.
‖ Ambra.
Anac.
‖ Arsen.
‖ Bellad.
Borax.
Calc. ostr.
I Carb. an.
Carb. veg.
Caustic.
Cinch. off.
‖ Digit.
Droser.
Graphit.
Guarœa.
Hepar s. c.
Hippom.
Hyper.
Kali carb.
Kali hydr.
Lauroc.
Ledum.
Lycop.
Magn. carb.
Magn. mur.
‖ Mezer.
Mur. ac.
Natr. carb.
Natr. mur.
Nitr. ac.
Nitrum.
Pæon.
Petrol.
‖ Phosphor
Pulsat.
Ran. bulb.
Rhus tox.
Ruta.
Sepia.
I Stannum.
‖ Sulphur.
Tabac.
Veratr.

Anxiousness. After brightness all day: *Anac.;* afternoon, till evening: *Nitrum.*

Anxiousness, shuddering and awe as soon as the evening approaches: I *Calc. ostr.*

Towards evening: *Borax, Natr. mur., Sepia;* several days: *Tabac.;* with dry heat in the face: *Acon.;* in twilight: *Calc. ostr., Rhus tox.;* at 6 P.M.: *Digit.;* from 7 to 8 P.M.: *ɔser.;* at 8 P.M.: *Mur. ac.;* increasing for several hours: *Carb. ι ʃ.*

Most violent attacks: *Mezer.*

After lying down: *Carb. veg., Graphit., Nux vom.;* in bed: *Magn. carb., Sulphur;* at 11 P.M.: *Borax, Ruta.*

And dejection: *Carb. an.;* indifference and irresolution: *Guarœa;* pusillanimity: *Ran. bulb.;* weeping relieves: *Digit.;* suicidal disposition: *Hepar;* does not know where to turn: *Veratr.;* oversensitive: ‖*Ran. bulb.;* anxious ideas attack him: *Kali carb.;* confusion of ideas: *Guarœa.*

Head. Feels as if drunk. *Nux vom.;* weakness: *Natr. mur.;* heat: *Carb. veg.,* ‖*Ruta;* sweat: *Mur. ac.*

Disturbed sight: *Natr. mur.;* confusion before eyes: *Lycop.;* all things appear to get narrower and smaller: *Carb. veg.*

Face. Dry heat: *Acon., Carb. veg., Graphit.*

Tongue stiff, boring in a tooth: *Natr. mur.*

Stomach. Grasping sensation: *Petrol.;* belching: *Carb. veg.*

Abdomen. Painful expansion, has to open clothing: *Mezer.;* fullness to bursting: *Mur. ac.*

Before menses: *Nitr. ac.*

Breathing. Short and oppressed: *Caustic., Nux vom.;* short, has to breathe quickly, until with one deep inhalation it passes off: *Stannum;* constriction of chest: *Stannum;* with restlessness: ‖*Arsen.*

Heart. As if it was squeezed: *Cactus, Carb. veg.;* rising up, followed by nausea and trembling: *Nux vom.;* beating in region of heart: *Graphit.;* palpitation, with short breath: ‖ *Caustic.;* with weeping and coldness: *Mezer.*

Limbs. Tingling in arm, hand and points of fingers; rising up in throat: *Natr. mur.;* arms fall down as if paralyzed: *Mur. ac.;* leg asleep, joints as if dead: *Natr. mur.*

All the limbs prostrated, can hardly walk across the room: *Mezer.*

Trembling of limbs and whole body: *Mezer., Nux vom.*

Positions. Has to lay the head on the table: *Nux vom.;* cannot sit, has to walk about: *Nitr. ac.*

Cannot lie on the left side; beating, which moves the bed-cover, turning over relieves: *Graphit.*

Feverish restlessness: *Ruta;* prevents sleep: *Carb. an., Lauroc., Natr. carb.*

Coldness of whole body: *Mezer.;* chilliness and shuddering, with gaping. *Mezer.;* at full moon: *Sulphur.*

Dry heat: *Hyper.;* hot hands: *Carb. veg.;* sweat runs down the face: *Mur. ac.;* on forehead: *Carb. veg.*

<small>Arnica.
Bryon.
Calc. ostr.
Carb. an.
Carb. veg.
II Caustic.
Digit.
Droser.
Guaræa.
Kali carb.
Laches.
II Lycop.
Magn. carb.
Mercur.
II Phosphor.
Phytol.
I Pulsat.
Ran. bulb.
I Rhus tox.
II Sarsap.
Valer.</small>

Fear. The fearfulness of the afternoon lasts through the evening: *Amm. carb.*

Towards evening fear of becoming delirious: *Bryon.;* in twilight: *Calc. ostr.*

Fear of the future, with sadness and weeping: *Digit.*

Full of fear inspiring ideas: *Caustic.*

And horrible visions drive out of bed: *Carb. veg.*

As if a horrible face peered from every corner: *Phosphor.*

Fear of horrible visions, which force themselves on her imagination: *Lycop.;* fear takes hold of him on trying to open a door in the dark, which opens with difficulty: *Lycop.*

Fearfulness in the dark, afraid he may be hurt: *Valer.*

Afraid of staying by herself, fear of ghosts: *Ran. bulb.*

Afraid of ghosts: *Pulsat.*

Fear of losing reason, with excitement: *Guaræa.*

Fearfulness and shuddering: *Phosphor.*

Towards evening alarmed as if going to die: *Phytol.;* timid and fearful: *Caustic., Phosphor., Valer.;* terrified: *Phosphor.;* frightened and sensitive: *Crocus, Laches.;* fear of being harmed: *Arnic., Valer.;* fearful and starting: *Mercur.*

Fear in bed: *Calc. ostr., Kali carb., Magn. carb., Mercur.*

Anguish: *Bellad., Carb. veg., Graphit., Hura, Phosphor., Pulsat., Rhus tox., Sulphur, Veratr.;* anguish from 4 to 6 P.M.: *Carb. veg.;* and suicidal disposition: *Hepar s. c.;* better in evening: *Amm. carb., Magn. carb.*

Very uncomfortable: *Sulphur;* depressed: *Graphit., IIKreosot.;* cast down about his broken health: *Calc. ostr.;* despair of ever getting well: *Kreosot.*

Sad thoughts of the future rise up before him, feels quite forsaken: *Baryt.*

Ill humor, with backache worse in the evening: *Aloes.*

Inconsolable, lamenting and weeping: *Veratr.;* vexation and despair, doubts arise on subjects of the truth of which he is thoroughly convinced: *Argent.*

Life weary: *Aurum, Droser., Hepar, Kali chlor., Rhus tox., Ruta, Spigel.;* ennui: *Magn. mur.;* quiet humor: *Amm. mur.;* introverted: *Ignat.;* tranquillity: *Mancin.;* indolence: *Rhus rad.;* indifference: I*Aloes,* II*Digit., Kali chlor., Lycop.*

Feelings and Conations. Irresolute: *Baryt.;* discouraged: *Ran. bulb.;* and morose: *Sulphur, Sulph. ac.;* timid: *Ant. tart.;* full of timorous ideas: *Caustic.;* vascillating mood: *Crocus.*

A woman, æt. 28, became melancholy after suppressed itch; emaciated, pale earthy complexion, weakness of limbs. Flushes of heat and palpitation prevent sleep, sleep comes towards morning, would like to stay in bed until midday. Aversion to work, indifference, weeping; seeks solitude, despairs of recovery, she is irritable and forgetful: *Psorin.*—F. J. BRENFLECK, near Heidelberg. Hygea, v. 6, p. 131.

EVENING.

Aloes.
‖ Amm. mur.
‖ Ant. crud.
‖ Baryt.
‖ Bovist.
‖ Calc. ostr.
‖ Cinch. off.
‖ Conium.
Fluor. ac.
‖ Ignat.
Indigo.
‖ Kali carb.
Kalmia.
‖ Magn. carb.
‖ Magn. mur.
‖ Mur. ac.
Ox. ac.
‖ Pulsat.
Rhus tox.
‖ Spigel.
‖ Sulphur.
Verbasc.
‖ Zincum.

Ill humor. Better in the evening: *Bismuth.*, *Magn. carb.*, *Sarsap.*, *Zincum.*

Towards evening: *Kalmia*, *Bovist.;* at sunset: *Pulsat.;* about 7 o'clock: *Magn. carb.;* from 8 o'clock till falling asleep, with headache: *Magn. carb.;* in bed: *Cinch. off.*, *Kali carb.*, *Rhus tox.*

Morose: ‖ *Magn. carb.;* and sad: *Magn. mur.;* and passionate: *Psorin.;* and easily offended: *Pulsat.;* and peevish: *Zincum;* and taciturn: *Zincum;* everything worries him, every noise is unpleasant: *Kali carb.*

Discontented. Sees everything in the worst light: *Fluor. ac.*

Dissatisfied with the present: *Hippom.;* with everything, nothing suits him: *Ignat.;* everything is repugnant: *Magn. carb.*

Taciturn. Sleepy and uninterested: *Conium;* and morose, easily offended: *Pulsat.;* takes no interest, feels uneasy and does not know what he wants: *Sulphur.*

Out of humor, with backache: *Aloes.*

Irascibility, would like to fight: *Niccol.*

Quarrelsome and vexatious: *Silic.*

Irritable: *Kalmia*, *Zincum;* and sensitive: *Calc. ostr.*

Irritable in the evening, with disagreeable dreams at night and unrefreshing sleep: *Lil. tigr.*

Irritability of temper, with headache coming on when waking; increasing, very severe at noon, passing from forehead and temples to protuberance of occiput; dull, pressing, heavy, continuing through afternoon, evening and night: *Lil. tigr.*

In the evening insane jealousy: *Laches.*

Aloes.
Amm. carb.
Ant. crud.
Ant. tart.
‖ Calc. ostr.
Canthar.
Crocus.
Kali carb.
‖ Magn. carb.
Magn. mur.
‖ Mur. ac.
Natr. carb.
Natr. mur.
Nux jugl.
‖ Psorin.
Pulsat.
Silic.

Fretful and Peevish. Better in evening: *Magn. carb.*, *Verbasc.*

Towards evening peevish and discontented: *Nux jugl.;* after sunset cross, takes everything in bad part: *Pulsat.;* at 7 P. M.: *Magn. carb.*

Out of humor without a cause: *Calcar.;* easily vexed, cannot brook opposition: *Natr. mur.*

Torturing irritability, making his own and others lives a misery: *Psorin.*

Ill-humored and irritable, with backache: *Aloes;* fretful; fatigued, especially the feet: *Ant. crud.*

Sad and peevish: *Ant. crud.*

Sleepy and irritable: *Calc. ostr.*

Towards evening out of sorts and irritable: *Bovist.;* vehement: *Natr. mur.*

Easily vexed, readily angered: *Natr. mur.;* impetuous, angry and impatient, cannot bear opposition: *Niccol.*

Peevish, irascible and abusive: *Amm. carb.*

Extremely irritable and angry, with general heat: *Hippom.*

Irritable, vexed and vehement: *Psorin.*
Violent and hot-headed: *Caine.*
Less and less cheerful, in the evening quite out of humor: *Mur. ac.*
Feels best in the morning, is anxious and depressed in the evening: *Carb. an.*
Cheerful mood in the morning, depressed in the evening: *Graphit.*
Irritable and moody in the evening, cheerful through the day: *Magn. mur.*
Actions. Laughter alternating with weeping: *Aurum.*
Unusual inclination to laughter in the evening: *Cuprum, Natr. mur.*
Great desire to laugh, cannot get done laughing over things which are not ludicrous: *Iodium.*
Exuberant spirits, inclined to sing and whistle: *Bellad.*
Talkative: *Calc. ac., Laches., Sulphur, Viol. tric.*
Talking delirium from 4 P. M., all night: *Hepar s. c.*
Wide awake and talkative: *Laches.*

Amm. carb.
Amm. mur.
Aurum.
Calc. ostr.
Carb. an.
Clemat.
Digit.
Graphit.
Kali carb.
Kali chlor.
Kali hydr.
Lact. vir.
Lycop.
Mezer.
Natr. mur.
Platin.
Stramon.
Sulphur.
Thuya.
Veratr.

Weeping. Tendency to weep: *Amm. carb., Calc. ostr., Graphit., Kali hydr., Natr. mur., Platin., Sulphur;* and gloominess: *Platin.;* and sadness: *Kali carb.;* and grief: *Graphit.*
Imagined trouble makes her unhappy, runs about the room crying and screaming, or sits weeping in a corner, refusing to be comforted: *Veratr.*
Sheds tears from a feeling of moral weakness: *Clemat.*
Anxiousness, weeping mood, apprehension of evil: *Kali hydr.*
Gloomy, almost inclined to weep: *Amm. carb.*
Irritable and ill-humored in the morning, disposed to weep at night: *Sulphur.*
Violent fit of spasmodic weeping: *Thuya.*
Laughing alternating with crying: *Aurum.*

Disposed to weep; in the morning she laughs about trifles: *Graphit.*
Scolding. Irritable, angry and scolding: *Amm. carb.*
Screams from a tearing pain in right mastoid: *Canthar.;* from a shooting in region of heart: *Rhus tox.;* pain on outside of foot: *Hepar s. c.*
Desires and Aversions. Desire for solitude: *Rhus tox.*
Anxiety, with desire to drown himself: *Droser.*
In twilight anxiety, with inclination to commit suicide: *Rhus tox.*
Terrible anxiety and despair, inclined to take his life: *Hepar;* aversion to talk: *Ignat., Amm. mur.*
Sits wrapt in thought, averse to speaking: *Amm. mur.*
Sadness, with aversion to conversation; confusion of ideas: *Mur. purp.;* does not answer: *Pulsat.;* indisposed to speak: *Viol. tric.*
Disposed to criticise: *Rhus rad.*
Indisposed for everything: *Sulphur;* sluggishness: *Carb. veg., Magn. mur., Mur. ac., Pulsat., Ran. scel.;* not inclined to work: *Spiggur.*
Lazy, drowsy and uninterested: *Carb. veg.*
Forgetful, absentminded; melancholy; fear of dying, thinks himself above others; colicky pains in umbilical region, worse in the evening: *Platin.*—HERMEL.

EVENING.

Alum.
| Amm. carb.
Argent.
Arsen.
Calc. ostr.
Carb. an.
|| Carb. veg.
|| Caustic.
Natr. carb.
Nitr. ac.
Rhus tox.
Ruta.
Veratr.

Restlessness. Contented mood but restless, has to go from place to place; desire for company: *Argent.*

Restless during mental occupation; *f. i.*, reading: *Natr. carb.*

Mental inquietude in bed: *Amm. carb.*; has to change position constantly: *Rhus tox.*; cannot keep the legs still: *Calc. ostr.*

Unbearable restlessness in the limbs: *Caustic.*

Terrified feeling, shudders and weeps: *Carb. an.*; spirits affected: *Platin.*

Depressed and easily frightened: *Sepia.*

Mental exhaustion: *Turpeth.*

Intellect. Evening and night full of plans, projects and schemes: *Cinch. off.*

Unpleasant ideas: *Caustic.*

All sorts of ideas, mostly from the past, crowd upon her and prevent sleep: *Sulphur.*

Waking dreams, gets confused and imagines himself away from home: *Acon.*

In the evening, in bed, vexing ideas: *Sulphur;* one fixed idea: *Baryt., Phosph. ac.;* fixed ideas of music: *Ignat.*

When alone feeling as if he had to turn round and would then see an apparition: *Bromum.*

Has no control over his thoughts: *Natr. mur.*

Difficult comprehension at 6 o'clock: *Capsic., Kali carb., Pulsat., Sepia;* intellectual labor difficult: *Rhus rad.*

Thinking and speaking are difficult towards evening: *Ignat.;* difficult thinking: *Armor.;* inability to think: *Silic.*

Cannot study: *Gymnocl.*

Thoughtlessness: *Sepia;* attacks of insensibility: *Calc. ostr.*

Pressure in the forehead and temples as if on the surface of the brain, not interfering with thinking: *Phosph. ac.*

Absentminded, buried in thought: *Amm. mur.*

When riding out, inward mental weakness: *Osmium.*

Want of mind: *Carb. an., Lycop., Natr. mur.*

Easily affected: *Platin.*

Mental dullness, inability to think: *Amm. carb., Ignat., Natr. mur.;* indifference: *Digit.;* head feels dull and stupid: *Dulcam., Kali carb.*

Dullness when standing or walking, relieved by lying down: *Gratiol.*

Dazed feeling in head, with irritability: *Mercur.*

Stupefaction: *Acon., Coloc., Lycop.;* in the evening, in the warm room, with chilliness: *Pulsat.*

Vertigo, with insensibility: *Thea;* attacks of stupefaction: *Zincum.*

Heaviness of spirits: *Lycop.*

Forgetfulness: *Millef.;* weak memory: *Ars. hydr., Bufo;* imagination and memory weakened: *Anac.*

Incoherent conversation: *Bellad.*

Familiar places appear strange: *Rhus rad.*
At 9 o'clock imagines she will have a goitre: *Zincum.*
Delirium: *Bryon., Laches., Lycop., Sulphur;* insatiable thirst, with burning heat and delirium; talking from 4 P.M. all night: *Hepar s. c.*
Mania: *Mercur.;* from 8 P.M. to 2 A.M.: *Cinch. off.;* rage: *Crocus.*
Angry and quarrelsome: *Niccol.*
Converses with spirits; strikes about him with a sword to drive the devil away: *Stramon.*
Clumsiness: *Agar.;* does not succeed with any work: *Mur. ac.;* awkward in talking: *Lycop.*
Mind symptoms get worse in the evening, with heat in the face: *Hippom.;* evening in bed: *Borax.*

WARMTH.

Sunlight. Lessens the imagination of being larger: *Platin.;* increases the restlessness: *Kadm. sulph.;* the dullness in head: *Nux vom.;* (in the cold moonlight sentimental mood: *Ant. crud.*).

Heat. Lessens the pain over the whole chest, with strange imaginations: *Amyl. nitr.*

If he gets agreeably warm, everything appears brighter to him: *Phosphor.*
With warmth of body the good humor increases: *Mar. ver.*
Indifference to the heat and cold of the weather: *Fluor. ac.;* in mania: *Mercur.*

Warmth. Of bed; makes mind easier: I *Caustic.,* II *Magn. carb.;* improves anxiety: *Graphit.*

Warm cloths applied lessens violent pain in belly and anxiety: *Phosphor.*

Desire for Open Air. Weakness with anxiety, relieved by breathing out-door air: *Calcar.*

Restlessness in lower limbs when in a close room, desire for open air: *Aster.*
Dull and irritable, desire to go into the open air: *Anac.*
Anxious feeling in the region of the sternum, as if he could not stay in the room, desire for open air and activity: *Anac.*
Has to leave the room and go into the air: *Lauroc.*
Is impelled to seek the open air: *Sulphur.*
Dizziness and dullness in the head at dinner, has to seek the open air: *Magn. mur.*
Runs out of the house after a domestic quarrel: *Mercur.*
Flies from the house into the open fields: *Bellad.*
Wants to jump out of the window to get into the air: *Kali hydr.*

Covering. Chilliness returns when uncovering, even during the hot stage: *Arg. nitr.*

Cannot bear to be uncovered in spite of the heat: *Cinch. off.*
Restlessness in the limbs, especially in the bends of the arms, cannot bear to be covered: *Aster.*

Toothache with anxiety, better when getting out of bed: *Oleand.*
Anxiety in the evening, has to open her night dress: *Baryt.*
Has to uncover herself in the night, but feels cold and cannot stand it: *Magn. carb.;* heat and chill, with inclination to uncover: *Opium.*
Cannot bear uncovering during the sweat, from the agony of toothache: *Clemat.*
Hot hands and feet, but cannot bear to have them uncovered: *Ignat.*

Taking Cold. After a foot-bath anxiety and sleeplessness for hours: *Natr. carb.*
After taking cold very irritable: *Calc. ostr.;* mania: *Bellad.*

Better in Open Air: *Aloes, Bryon., Calc. ostr., Coffea, Lauroc., Magn. mur.,* ❙*Platin.,* ❙❙*Pulsat.*
Cheerful in the open air: *Angust.;* happy and laughing; ecstasy: *Platin.*
Inability to persevere: *Asaf.;* unsteadiness: *Graphit.;* vexing ideas: *Coffea.*
Anxiety lessens: *Gratiol., Lauroc., Magn. mur., Rhus. tox.*
Better in sunshine: *Platin.;* and heat: *Gratiol.;* oppression: *Lauroc.;* being angry about himself: *Aloes.*
Forsaken mood: *Rhus tox.;* ill humor: ❙*Coffea;* fretfulness: *Aloes, Calc. ostr.; Platin., Pulsat.,* ❙❙*Stannum.*
Lachrymose humor, gloominess: *Platin.*
Inconsolability, howling: *Coffea;* moroseness: *Calc. ostr., Stannum.*
Delusion of fancy, imagining to be too large: *Platin.*
Inability to attend to a lecture: *Cinnab., Graphit.;* overirritability: *Sabin.;* difficult thinking: *Menyanth.;* dull and indisposed to work: *Cinch. off., Sulphur;* will not speak: *Calc. ac.;* anxious feeling in head: *Lauroc.*

Better when Walking in the Open Air. Contented, cheerful: *Angust., Fluor. ac.*
Feels better: ❙❙*Aloes, Asar.,* ❙❙*Graphit., Ignat., Mar. ver.,* ❙*Pulsat., Rhus tox., Stannum.*
Ill humor, better from walking in the open air but no inclination to do so: *Aloes.*
Drowsy and irritable, with headache; better when walking in open air: *Asar.*
Irritability and discomfort after eating: *Borax.*
Absence of mind: *Graphit.*
Dullness in head as after having been drunk: *Dulcam.*
When going into the open air everything appears ludicrous: *Nux mosch.*
When walking in open air feels unusually well: *Plumbum.*
On coming in the room after a walk cheerful: *Phosph. ac.*
Vascillating mood: *Asaf.*

Better Out-doors, Worse In-Doors. Anxiety worse in-doors: *Bryon., Magn. mur.*
Has to leave the room, it appears dreary, with anxiety: *Valer.*
Heat and restlessness in-doors: *Lycop.;* and anxiety: *Spongia.*
Melancholy, ill humor and anxiety, worse in-doors: *Rhus tox.*

Irritability and indisposition to talk on coming into the house: *Calc. ostr.*
Goes in the open air to weep: *Hura;* <in-doors, >out-doors: *Platin.*
Stupefaction >out-doors, <in-doors: *Bellad.;* and vertigo: *Mercur.*
Dull headache in the room, with difficult flow of ideas; better in the open air: *Menyanth.*

Worse in the Room. Anxiety: *Arsen., Bryon., Magn. mur.*
Gets fainty in a warm room: *Lil. tigr.*
Fear: *Valer.;* gloominess: *Platin.;* sadness: *Platin., Rhus tox.;* melancholy, as if left solitary: *Rhus tox.;* hypochondric mood: *Valer.;* irritable: *Anac.;* ill humor: *Anac., Ignat.*
Fretfulness, moroseness: *Calc. ac., Pulsat.*
Imagines to be larger in-doors: *Platin.;* did not know what she was doing: *Bryon.;* difficult thinking: *Menyanth.*
Awkwardness in-doors: *Bryon.*

Coming in the Room. On coming in the room from open air morose, indisposed to speak: *Calc. ac.*
Bellyache, with weeping mood: *Sulphur.*
Anxious feeling on entering the room, with nausea: *Alum.*
Headache and faceache, with great irritability: *Tongo.*
On returning from a walk irritable: *Pulsat.*

Better In-Doors: *Ant. crud., Ignat., Phosph. ac.;* sadness: *Phosph. ac.;* peevishness and ill humor: *Aethus.;* seeing persons larger: *Caustic.;* laughing at everything: *Nux mosch.*

Better In-doors, Worse Out-doors. Sadness and despondency: *Phosph. ac.*
Anxiousness out-doors, ill humor in the house: *Ignat.*
Irritability and ill humor: *Aethus.*
Cannot bear the slightest breeze, it makes him shrink and shudder like a person falling into cold water: *Psorin.*
Sensitive to the least breath of air, with anxiousness: *Graphit.*
Fear of taking cold: *Natr. carb., Sulphur.*
Great sensitiveness to cold, shrinking and shuddering, followed by heat, anxiety and apprehension: *Cyclam.*

Worse Out-doors. Ecstatic desire for an ideal woman: *Ant. crud.*
Indescribably happy, would like to embrace everybody and laugh at the saddest things: *Platin.*
Inclined to laugh at everything: *Nux mosch.*
Cheerfulness: *August., Mar. ver., Plumbum.*
All objects appear new, as after a long sickness: *Helleb.*
Feels anxious and sick on going in the open air: *Spigel.*
Apprehension: *Anac., Hepar, Nux vom.;* despondency: *Phosph. ac.*
Tired of life: *Mur. ac.;* hypochondric mood: *Conium, Petrol.;* indifference: *Mur. ac.;* indifference when in company: *Platin.*
Ill humor: *Aethus., Amm. carb., Arnic., Borax, Calc. ostr.,* **|** *Conium, Mur. ac., Nux vom., Pulsat., Sabad.;* with heavy pressure in occiput: *Kali carb.;* fretfulness: *Acon., Mur. ac.;* irritability and drowsiness: *Rhus tox.*

Vertigo, persons appear larger: *Caustic.;* stupefying weakness of head: *Sulphur.*

In open air and sunshine dullness in head: *Nux vom.*

Attacks of vertigo worse from thinking: *Silic.*

Worse from a draft of air; restlessness, with headache: *Kadm. sulph.*

Chilliness, cannot get warm; sadness: *Ol. anim.*

Worse when Walking Out-doors or after it. Uncomfortable feeling and flushes of heat: *Caustic.*

Sad, has to weep: *Calc. ostr.;* sad and unusually tired: *Nux vom.*

After getting tired, dreary and sad: *Kali carb.*.

Sad: *Ant. crud., Coffea, Conium, Cuprum, Phosph. ac., Sepia, Sulphur;* and grave: *Phosph. ac.;* and gloomy: *Sepia;* becomes sad suddenly: *Sulphur;* with fainting weakness: *Sepia.*

When walking, apprehension about the heart: *Cina;* about his family: *Hepar;* when driving, apprehension of distant evil: *Laches.*

Anguish: *Bellad., Canthar., Cina, Platin., Tabac.*

Suicidal inclination: *Bellad.*

Anxiety: *Anac., Arg. nitr., Bellad., Cina, Hepar s. c., Ignat., Platin.;* sudden faint-feeling and inability to act with her will on her limbs; *Spongia;* with gloomy, melancholy thoughts: *Tabac.;* lachrymose and weary of life: *Bellad.;* with bellyache: *Mezer.;* with palpitation: ‖*Nux vom., Platin.;* tired feeling around heart and chest: *Spongia;* tired in the thighs: *Spigel.;* trembling in the knees: *Hepar s. c.;* as if the clothes pressed him and were too tight: *Argent.*

Suspicious that some one is following him: *Anac.*

Anxious; unable to use his limbs but conscious: *Spongia;* with sweat and fear of dying after bellyache: *Mezer.;* loses his senses, has to lie down; looseness of bowels: *Ledum.*

Quiet manner: *Arnic., Borax, Calc. ostr., Phosph. ac., Sabin.;* indifference: *Conium;* wavering mind: *Asaf.;* despondency: *Phosph. ac.*

Laziness, indisposition to think or speak: *Arnic.*

Difficult comprehension: *Hepar s. c.*

Lassitude and vexation: *Amm. carb., Borax;* with headache: *Kali carb.;* vexing ideas: *Sulphur.*

Everything grieves her: *Mur. ac.;* weeping: *Bellad., Coffea.*

Inclination to scream, with pain in the back: *Calc. ostr.*

Disposition to bend the body forward in walking, to hurry and sing, but all in a dragging forced manner: *Mezer.*

During a walk not disposed to speak: *Sabin.;* or think: *Arnic.*

Sluggishness: *Coccul.;* dullness and headache: *Conium.*

Erroneous suppositions: *Anac., Bromum, Baryt.*

Inclination to pull people's noses in the street: *Mercur.*

Does not know where he is: ‖*Glonoin.*

Loss of consciousness: *Canthar.;* attacks of unconsciousness: *Hepar;* as if reason were going: *Acon.;* vertigo, as if senses would leave her: *Thea;* stupefaction, weakness and gloomy ideas: *Sulphur;* distracted: *Platin.*

SEASONS.

Winter, Spring, Summer, Fall, according to B. R., with many additions.

	W.	Spr.	S.	F.
Acon.	I			
Agar.	I			
Ambra.		I		
Amm. carb.	I			
Ant. crud.				I
Argent.	I			
Arsen.	II			
Aurum.	II	II		II
Baryt.	II		I	
Bellad.	II	I	I	
Bovist.	I			
Bryon.	I	II	I	I
Calc. ostr.	II	I		
Camphor.	I			
Capsic.	II			
Carb. an.	I			
Carb. veg.	II	I	I	
Caustic.	I			II
Chamom.	II		I	
Cicut.	I			
Cina.	I			
Cinch. off.				I
Cinnab.			I	
Coccul.	II			
Colchic.	I			II
Conium.	II			
Dulcam.	I	I	I	
Ferrum.	I			
Graphit.			II	
Helleb.	I			
Hepar.	I			
Hyosc.	II			
Ignat.	II			
Ipec.	II			
Kali carb.	I			
Laches.		II		II
Lycop.	II	I	II	
Magn. carb.	I			
Mangan.	II			
Mercur.	II	I		II
Merc. subl.				II
Mezer.	I			
Natr. carb.	I		II	
Natr. mur.	,I	II	I	
Nux mosch.	I			
Nux vom.	II	I	I	I
Petrol.	I			
Phosphor.	II		II	
Phosph. ac.				II
Pulsat.	I	II	I	
Rhodod.	II			
Rhus tox.	II	II		II
Ruta.				
Sabad.	I			
Sarsap.		II	II	
Secale.	I			
Selen.			II	
Sepia.	I	II		
Silic.	I	II	I	
Spigel.	I			
Spongia.	I			
Stramon.				I
Strontian.	I			
Sulphur.	II	II		
Thuya.		I		
Veratr.	I	II		II

In the height of summer and in the depth of winter, more than in the seasons between: *Baryt.*, *Bellad.*, *Bryon.*, *Carb. veg.*, *Chamom.*, **I I***Fluor. ac.*, *Lycop.*, *Natr. carb.*, *Nat. mur.*, *Nux vom.*, *Pulsat.;* most in the changeable seasons: *Laches.*, *Rhus tox.*, *Veratr.*

Better and Worse in Kind of Weather.

Irritable, thoughtful, dissatisfied in cloudy, cold, rainy weather: *Aloes.*

In cloudy weather very morose, out of humor: *Amm. carb.*

Would like to ride out even in wet weather: *Psorin.;* great aversion to wet weather: *Elaps.*

Dreads the cold in hot weather and the heat in cold: *Sulphur.*

Worse before Thunder-Storms:
Petrol., *Phosphor.*, *Psorin.*, **I I** *Rhodod.*, *Sepia*; during: **I I** *Bryon.*, I *Caustic.*, **I** *Gelsem.*, **I I** *Laches.*, **I I** *Natr. carb.*, **I I** *Natr. mur.*, **I I** *Nitr. ac.*, **I I** *Petrol.*, **I** *Phosphor.*, I *Psorin.*, **I** *Rhodod.*, **I** *Sepia*, **I** *Silic.*

Gets faint if a storm is near: *Petrol.*, *Silic.*

Affected by the atmosphere of a storm: *Psorin.*

The sultry air oppresses him, but when it begins to thunder and lighten he brightens up: *Sepia.*

Uneasy, restless and anxious: *Phosphor.*

During a thunder-storm more anxious than before: *Nitr. ac.*

Less fear of a thunder-storm: *Natr. carb.*

Great fear during a thunder-storm at night; anxious sweat drives her out of bed: *Natr. mur.*

A nervous young lady, uneasy already before a thunder-storm, set up a terrific scream after a heavy thunder-bolt, and continued it without cessation in spite of the consoling efforts of the alarmed family, until they had time to run for the doctor. One dose of *Gelsem.* high quieted her very soon. Since then she has kept well by resorting at the return of the least fear to the same remedy.—A. LIPPE.

NOTE.—Dr. Grauvogl's doctrines of the agreement and disagreement of the different kinds of weather with the oxygenoid, hydrogenoid and carbonitrogenoid constitutions will be left for the last volume of this work, as Grauvogl is engaged with a new edition.

CHILL, HEAT, SWEAT.

NOTE.—Among all the good practitioners our struggling school has been blessed with, Bönninghausen is one who had more cases of *intermittent fever* to treat than the majority of others practicing in so-called febrile districts. His position in society kept him above all harassing cares. Two days in each week he stayed at home, to enter in his repertory every symptom which according to his latest experience had been overcome. Forty years of his life he followed this same plan. His experience with intermittents he has laid down condensed in a small volume, "Bönninghausen's Homœopathic Therapia of Intermittent and other Fevers," translated by Dr. A. Korndœrfer. With such a key true homœopathists can be successful in overcoming our Western and Eastern fevers, although they may *differ each year*.

In the "Analytical Therapeutics" the mind symptoms have been arranged comparatively, so that every one can see at a glance how the different stages differ. The three columns relate to chill, heat and sweat. If there are only two it means heat and sweat.

It was a very tedious and tiresome work, but it will enable everyone to see what relation certain drugs have to the different stages of fever. We learn to observe the symptoms of the mind better than before, are more successful and sometimes find that the most objective characteristics correspond with the symptoms of the mind.

Bönninghausen was induced by a so-called "moonshine" symptom to give *Taraxacum*; his cure led Raue to the discovery of the "mapped tongue," a most significant symptom, reducing our choice in most important cases to a few drugs only. Bringing a plant from a rich family, one of the old famous class of "Amara," within the neighborhood of acrid minerals, we consider a very important acquisition, not only for the practitioner but also for such who attempt to build up a science out of the facts of our Materia Medica.

Pleasant Feelings. During the heat thoughts clearer and brighter: *Thuya.*

Agreeable warmth, cheerfulness and greater mobility of body: *Phelland.*

Clemat.	‖	‖	Chill: ❙*Cannab.*, ❙*Nux mosch.*, ❙*Phosphor.*, ‖❙*Pulsat.*, *Rhus tox.*, ❙*Veratr.*
Coffea.	❙	‖	❙
Crocus.	❙		‖
Natr. carb.	❙	❙	Heat: ❙*Acon.*
Opium.	‖	‖	‖
Platin.	‖	‖	Sweat: ❙*Apis*, ‖❙*Arsen.*, ❙*Bellad.*
Sarsap.	‖	❙	‖ Excited and cheerful during the sweat: *Clemat.*

Unpleasant Feelings. Flushes of heat and uncomfortable feeling after a walk: *Caustic.*

Lassitude and discomfort, with anxious heat and sweat: *Magn. carb.*

Chill when talking of unpleasant things: *Calc. carb.*, *Gelsem.*, *Mar. ver.*

When reading exciting news creeping chilliness: *Gelse.n.*

Chilliness from unpleasant news: *Sulphur.*

All complaints worse during chill: ‖❙*Calc. ostr.*, *Ci...i.*, *Ignat.*, ❙*Mar. ver.*

Violent febrile rigor after a surprise: *Mercur.*

Disposition to dwell on unpleasant subjects; shudders on seeing a cripple: *Benz. ac.*

Sweat after disagreeable news: *Calc. phosph.*

Acon.	‖	❙	❙ Oversensitiveness. Chill: ❙*Bryon.*, ❙*Capsic.*,
Aurum.	‖		‖❙*Cinch. off.*, ‖❙*Colchic.*, ‖❙*Hepar*, ❙*Natr. carb.*,
Chamom.	‖	‖	❙ ❙*Petrol.*, ‖❙*Phosphor.*, ‖❙*Veratr.*
Coffea.	‖	❙	‖
Conium.	❙		Heat: ‖❙*Bellad.*, ❙*Carb. veg.*, ❙*Lycop.*, ‖❙*Mar. ver.*,
Nux vom.	❙	‖	‖
Selen.	‖	‖	❙*Natr. mur.*, ❙*Nitr. ac.*, ❙❙*Pulsat.*, ‖❙*Valer.*
Sepia.	❙	‖	❙

Sweat: ❙*Baryt.*, ‖❙*Bellad.*, ‖❙*Cinch. off.*

Overexcitability, with inclination to sweat: *Sabin.*

Oversensitiveness of Hearing. In chill, heat and sweat: ❙❙*Capsic.*; in chill and sweat: ❙*Arnic.*; heat: ‖❙*Acon.*, ‖❙*Bellad.*, ❙*Calc. ac.*, ❙❙*Conium*, ❙*Ipec.*, ❙*Lycop.*, ‖❙*Nux vom.*

304 MIND AND DISPOSITION.

Sweat: **II** *Chamom.*, **I I** *Cinch. off.*, **I** *Coffea*, **I I** *Lycop.*, **I I** *Natr. carb.*, **II** *Nux vom.*, **I** *Sabad.*, **I** *Zincum.*

Acon.	II	II	I
Aurum.	I		II
Bellad.	II	II	II
Calc. ostr.	II	I	I
Chamom.	II	I	I
Graphit.		II	II
Ignat.	II	I	
Lycop.	II	I	II
Petrol.	I	I	I
Platin.	II	I	II
Pulsat.	II	II	I
Spongia.		II	II
Sulphur.	II	I	II
Veratr.	I		I

Tearful and Weeping Mood. Chill: *Arsen.*, *Cannab.*, *Carb. veg.*, *Conium*, *Hepar s. c.*, *Kali carb.*, *Mercur.*, *Natr. mur.*, *Selen.*, *Silic.*, *Viol. od.*
Heat: *Coffea*, *Spigel.*
Sweat: *Bryon.*, *Cinch. off.*, *Nux vom.*, *Rheum*, *Rhus tox.*, *Sepia.*
With chilliness: *Bellad.*, *Lycop.*, *Pulsat.*
With a cold chill in back: *Lil. tigr.*; rigor: *Arsen.*

Feels chilly all over, oppressed and disposed to weep: *Hura.*
Weeping mood, with chilliness: *Pulsat.*
Heat and chill, both inward, at the same time, with weeping mood: *Petrol.*
Fever and chill, with weeping mood: *Cannab.*
Heat of the whole body, with sweat in the face and weeping mood: *Carb. an.*
Chilliness, with mournful weeping, changing into howling: *Bellad.*
Child screams and cries uninterruptedly and puts its fists in its mouth, with pale face and cold body: *Ipec.*

Bellad.		I	II
Chamom.		I	I
Rheum.		II	I
Acon.	II	II	I
Bellad.		I	I
Bryon.		II	I
Calc. ostr.	I		I
Coccul.	II	I	
Graphit.	I	I	II
Ignat.	II	II	II
Lycop.	I	II	
Natr. mur.	II	II	I
Nitr. ac.	II		I
Nux vom.	I		I
Platin.	II	I	
Pulsat.	I	II	II
Rhus tox.	II	I	I
Sepia.	I	II	
Staphis.	I	II	
Sulphur.	I		II

Whimpering and Whining. Heat: *Pulsat.*
Sweat: *Acon.*, *Bryon.*, *Camphor.*, *Mercur.*
Sadness. Chill: *Cannab.*, *Chamom.*, *Conium*, *Cyclam.*, *Kali chlor.*, *Laches.*, *Mercur.*, *Spigel.*, *Veratr.*
Heat: *Arsen.*, *Digit.*, *Natr. carb.*, *Nux mosch.*, *Phosphor.*, *Phosph. ac.*, *Silic.*, *Staphis.*, *Sulphur.*
With the sweat—homesick: *Mercur.*
Pensive mood, with chill: *Ant. crud.*
Feels a lack of vital warmth, with sadness: *Conium.*
Shuddering and chill in the afternoon, followed by heat and better humor: *Conium.*

Coldness after walking in the open air, could not get warm for a long while: *Ol. anim.*
Flushes of heat with ill humor, sadness and anxiousness: *Natr. carb.*
Sadness with sick feeling, sees things as they appear in a fever: *Digit.*

Apis.	I	I	I
Arsen.	I		II
Cinch. off.	II	II	I
Conium.	II	I	II
Hepar.	I		I
Rhus tox.	I		I
Sulphur.	II	II	I

Dejected, Depressed, Cast Down. Great mental depression, with chilliness: *Helleb.*
Low-spirited, with chilliness: *Turpeth.*
Chilly, sluggish and depressed, has to lie down on the floor near the fire: *Laches.*

Cold feeling: *Amm. carb.*
Chill: *Cannab.*, *Laches.*, *Spigel.*
Depression of spirits, cold chills in back: *Lil. tigr.*
With heat alone: *Chamom.*, *Ignat.*, *Lycop.*, *Natr. carb.*, *Opium*, *Petrol.*, *Pulsat.*, *Stannum.*

Heat and sweat: |Acon., ||Bellad., ||Sepia.
Sweat alone: |Calc. ostr., |Nux vom., ||Sabin., ||Spigel., ||Thuya.

Arsen.	||	||	
Calc. ostr.				
Conium.			||	
Ignat.				||
Lycop.					||
Natr. mur.				
Selen.	||		||
Sepia.	||	||	

Melancholy. Chill: ||Helleb., |Phosphor., ||Platin.
Heat: |Graphit., |Nux mosch., |Phosph. ac.
Sweat: |Aurum.
Chilly as if deluged with cold water and melancholy: Veratr.
Hopeless, disposed to give up, with chilliness: Ant. tart.
Hypochondria. Hypochondric mood, with chill: Arsen., Conium, Pulsat.
In febrile state: Calc. ostr., Petrol.
Hypochondria in the evening, with heat: Hippom.
Ill humor, inclined to melancholy, with a feverish condition: Petrol.

Alum.
Amm. carb.
Arg. nitr.
Arsen.
Carb. an.
Cyclam.
Droser.
Graphit.

Apprehension. Cold feeling: Amm. carb.; coldness: Arsen.; crawling: Carb. an.; chilliness: Arg. nitr.; shuddering: Droser., Natr. mur.; chilly: Arsen., Cyclam.; forenoon: Amm. carb.; evening: Carb. an.
Apprehension of evil, with chilliness and shuddering on single parts: Cyclam.
Anxiety and flushes of heat as if he would receive bad news, chilliness: Droser.
Her nerves are so badly affected she fears she will go crazy; is always chilly: Arg. nitr.
As if something had occurred, with external heat and anxiety: Alum.
Internal heat, with apprehensiveness: Phosph. ac.
Cold sweat on forehead, with apprehension and trembling: Sepia.

Acon.
Arsen.
Bryon.
Nux vom.
Phosphor.
Platin.
Pulsat.
Rhus tox.
Veratr.

Fear of Death. During heat alone: Calc. ostr., ||Coccul., |Ipec., |Moschus, |Nitr. ac., ||Ruta; sweat alone: |Nitrum.
Sudden attacks of heat, with fear of dying: Calc. ostr.; hot all over with anxiety, as if about to die: Ruta.
Anguish. With inner chill: Lycop.; with coldness of body: Nitr. ac.; with attacks of flying heat: Arnic., Pulsat.
In hot stage, high fever: Stramon.; with heat and sweat at night: Natr. mur.
Agony and heat: Acon.
Fear. With chill: Calc. ostr., Carb. an.
Fear of heat during the chill, fear of chill during the heat: Sulphur.
Flying heat, with fear of ghosts: Pulsat.
During heat: Nux mosch., Spongia.
Fear of something under the bed when waking, with dry heat: Bellad.
Heat and sweat, with fear and terror: Spongia.
Cold sweat, frequently with fear and starting: . . . .

MIND AND DISPOSITION.

ANXIETY.

Acon.	‖	‖	‖
Apis.		‖	‖
Arnic.		‖	‖	‖
Arsen.	‖	‖	‖
Berber.			‖
Bovist.	‖	‖	‖
Calc. ostr.	‖	‖	‖
Capsic.	‖	‖	
Carb. veg.	‖	‖	‖
Chamom.	‖	‖	‖
Cinch. off.	‖	‖	‖
Coccul.	‖	‖	‖
Coffea.	‖	‖	‖
Conium.	‖	‖	
Digit.	‖		‖
Hepar.	‖	‖	‖
Ignat.	‖	‖	‖
Mercur.	‖	‖	‖
Natr. mur.	‖	‖	‖
Nux vom.	‖	‖	‖
Phosphor.	‖	‖	‖
Platin.	‖	‖	
Pulsat.	‖	‖	‖
Rheum.	‖	‖	‖
Rhus tox.	‖	‖	‖
Sulphur.	‖	‖	‖
Thuya.	‖	‖	‖
Veratr.	‖	‖	‖

Anxious Mood. Coldness not relieved by warmth: *Cuprum.*

Coldness of body: *Nitr. ac.;* inner heat and outer coldness of limbs: *Arsen.*

Inner chill, with restlessness and trembling anxiety: *Calc. ostr.*

Coldness of external parts: *Coloc.*

Before the chill: *Ars. hydr.*

With chill: ‖*Calad.,* ‖*Calend.,* ‖*Camphor.,* ‖*Cimex,* ‖*Lamium.*

With coldness: *Caustic.,* ‖*Cuprum, Jatroph.,* ‖*Mezer., Nitr. ac.;* shuddering: *Ol. anim.*

Heat. ‖*Ambra,* ‖*Amm. carb.,* ‖*Anac.,* ‖*Argent.,* ‖*Asaf.,* ‖*Carb. an.,* ‖*Cina,* ‖*Colchic., Crotal.,* ‖*Cyclam.,* ‖*Droser.,* ‖*Euphorb.,* ‖*Gratiol.,* ‖*Guarœa,* ‖*Hyosc.,* ‖*Ipec.,* ‖*Laches.,* ‖*Lauroc.,* ‖*Magn. mur.,* ‖*Niccol.,* ‖*Opium,* ‖*Paris,* ‖*Petrol.,* ‖*Rhodod.,* ‖*Ruta,* ‖*Sabin.,* ‖*Secal.,* ‖*Spigel., Valer.,* ‖*Viol. tric.,* ‖*Zincum.*

Sweat: ‖*Ambra, Amm. carb.,* ‖*Ant. crud., Benz. ac., Cannab.,* ‖*Caustic.,* ‖*Cicut., Cimex, Crocus, Fluor. ac.,* ‖*Kreosot.,* ‖*Mangan.,* ‖*Mezer.,* ‖*Nitrum,* ‖*Sabad.,* ‖*Selen.*

Cold sweat: *Ant. tart., Mur. ac., Sepia, Stramon.;* runs down all over the body: ‖*Arsen.*

Cold sweat covering the cold skin: *Cuprum;* after palpitation and constriction of chest: *Calc. ostr.*

Anxiousness, with sweat: *Benz. ac.,* ‖*Calc. ostr., Caustic., Cuprum;* anxiety drives out sweat: *Rhus tox.*

Anxiousness; during and after it sweat: *Nux vom., Phosphor.;* one hour after it: *Bellad.*

Alum.	‖	‖
Angust.		‖
Baryt.	‖	‖
Bellad.	‖	‖
Bryon.	‖	‖
Canthar.	‖	‖
Ferrum.	‖	‖
Graphit.	‖	‖
Lycop.	‖	‖
Magn. carb.	‖	‖
Merc. subl.	‖	‖
Mur. ac.	‖	‖
Natr. carb.	‖	‖
Nitr. ac.	‖	‖
Phosph. ac.	‖	‖
Plumbum.	‖	‖
Sepia.	‖	‖
Spongia.	‖	‖
Stannum.	‖	‖
Staphis.	‖	‖
Stramon.	‖	‖

Heat and Sweat. Hot sweat: *Angust.*

Is suddenly covered with hot sweat, with moaning and fear: *Laches.*

Anxious, short-lasting sweat over the whole body: *Arnic.*

Sweat, with agony: ‖*Acon.;* with anguish: *Calc. ostr., Graphit., Nux vom., Rhus tox., Sepia.*

Alternately. Coldness, with heat: *Bovist.*

Chill and heat: *Rheum;* with vertigo and nausea: *Veratr.*

Heat followed by rigor: *Droser.*

Inward chilliness: *Lycop.;* external and internal chill: *Arnic.;* crawls: *Natr. mur.;* crawling all over, no heat or thirst: *Droser.*

Coldness: *Jatroph.;* chill and crawling: *Arsen.*

Heat and Cold. Heat with anxiety, but feels cold to the touch: *Carb. veg.*

Hot and cold by turns, after anxiety: *Bellad.*

Hot head, cold hands and feet: *Sulphur.*

Inner heat: ❙❙*Phosph. ac.;* blood boiling: ❙❙*Anac., Carb. veg.,* ❙❙*Nux vom.*

Heat without thirst: *Capsic., Cinch. off., Phosph. ac., Rhus tox.*

Flushes of heat: *Angust., Platin., Sepia;* rapid flush: *Droser.;* rising: *Angust., Bellad., Opium, Phosphor.*

Flying heat: *Ambra, Arnic., Calc. ostr., Ignat., Platin.,* ❙❙*Pulsat.,* ❙*Sepia;* sudden: *Graphit., Spongia.*

Warmth: ❙❙*Anac., Arsen., Magn. carb., Spongia.*

Heat all over, externally: *Alum., Gratiol., Ruta.*

Dry heat: *Hyper., Stramon.*

Unbearable heat: ❙❙*Opium.*

Heat and Sweat. Anxious heat as if sweat would break out: *Ignat., Phosphor., Stannum;* sweat breaks out from the slightest motion: *Stannum;* anxious feeling of heat, with sweat: *Nux vom.*

Heat and sweat with restlessness, weak memory and sensitiveness to noise: *Capsic.*

Head. Fear of getting crazy, with chill and sensation as if beaten: *Calc. ostr.*

After headache external and internal chill, with anxiety: *Arnic.*

Heat of the whole body, cool hands, pressing headache and anxious moaning: *Pulsat.*

Pressing headache, with great anxiety and short-lasting sweat: *Arsen.*

Anxious heat mostly in head: *Magn. carb., Sulphur;* heat in hands and head: *Nitr. ac.*

Great heat in the head, with feverish restlessness and anxiety: *Ruta.*

Heat in head with anxiety driving out of bed and room: *Thuya.*

Anxiousness, with increased warmth in head and body: *Zincum.*

Head turns from side to side involuntarily; gets hot, has to seek the open air: *Caustic.*

Burning heat mounts to the head and spreads over the whole body, with restlessness and confused ideas: *Opium.*

Heat in the eyes, with backache and great anxiety: *Nitr. ac.*

Heat of outer ear, with chill: *Aurum.*

Face. Cold after the chill: *Droser., Pulsat.;* followed by crawling: *Pulsat.*

Outer and inner warmth in forehead, better in open air: *Lauroc.*

Heat most in face: *Droser.;* with palpitation: ❙*Acon.*

Towards evening dry heat in the face, with anxiety: *Acon.*

Increasing anxiety with heat in face, in evening: *Carb. veg.*

Great anxiety in the evening as if something had happened, with hot face and cold hands and feet: *Graphit.*

MIND AND DISPOSITION.

Anxiety with heat in the face and disposition to sweat, after stool: *Caustic.*
Anxious heat as if deluged with hot water; forehead cold: *Pulsat.*
Heat in left cheek with anxiety as if going to die during nightly toothache: *Oleand.*
Flushes of heat, mostly of hands and face, when sitting, with anxiety and sweat: *Calc. ostr.*
Inward heat caused by anxiousness, followed by sweat on the forehead: *Nux vom.*
Flushes of heat and anxiousness, with lassitude and mental dullness: *Alum.*

Red Face. Flushed cheeks, with hoarseness: *Hepar.*
Anxiousness in evening, with flushed face and flushes of heat: *Sepia.*
Sudden heat with anxiousness, red face and sweat: *Spongia.*

Face-sweat: *Natr. carb.;* with maniacal gestures: *Arsen.*
Sweat on forehead and chest: *Phosphor.*
Attacks of heat without red face but with anxiousness and bead-like sweat on the forehead: *Nux vom.*
Sweat only in face, rolling down in large drops: *Pulsat.*

Cold Sweat on Face: *Arsen., Bryon., Calc. phosph., Mur. ac., Natr. mur., Veratr.*
When lying insensible: *Bryon.;* with crawling over the back: *Natr. mur.*
Child is cold all over and screams: *Calc. phosph.*

Teeth. Toothache driving to despair, with anxious sweat; cannot bear to be uncovered: *Clemat.*

Mouth. Feverish state, with dryness of mouth and thirst; anxiety, restlessness and pain in the limbs: *Canthar.*

Throat. Rising up in pit of stomach, then in the throat: *Nux vom.*
Burning down into the stomach: *Euphorb.;* in back part of pharynx: *Arnic.*
Anxious, disagreeable heat, with sweat and dryness in the throat, in the morning in bed: *Sulphur.*
Flushes of heat as if deluged with hot water, red face, sweat, anxiousness and dryness in throat: *Sepia.*

Thirst. First shuddering, then heat causing anxiety followed by thirst for beer: *Nux vom.*
Violent thirst, with heat and increasing anxiety: *Platin.*
Anxious heat after breakfast: *Phosphor.*
After eating soup heat beginning in abdomen, with anxiousness and sweat in the region of stomach and chest: *Ol. anim.*
After beer soup heat and anxiousness: *Ferrum.*
Heat rising from below up, anxious sweat, nausea and great fear: *Bellad.*
Anxiety and nausea, with sweat: *Calc. ostr.*
Anxiety, cannot sit still, with sweat and nausea: *Graphit.*
Nausea after getting up, with heat, anxiousness and rising of sour water: *Carb. an.*
At 1 A.M. great fear, with alternate heat and nausea: *Arsen.*
Empty eructation, with burning and anxious sweat: *Mezer.*
With chill: *Magn. carb.;* pain in epigastrium: ||*Arsen.*

Chilliness and shuddering; anxious gnawing sensation in epigastrium, with nausea: *Arsen.*

Great nausea, vomiting and retching, with anxiety in epigastrium; heat and chilliness, followed by sweat: *Digit.*

Attacks of cramp in stomach, with anxiety; cold nose, lips, hands and feet, followed by vomiting and belching: *Kali carb.*

Anxiety in epigastrium, with alternate heat and chill: *Sulphur;* with dry heat: *Stramon.;* with gurgling in abdomen and alternate burning and cold feeling: *Lact. vir.*

Anxiousness, with constricting pain in stomach going into chest, with dyspnœa and sweat: *Kali carb.*

Anxious screams about pain in epigastrium, with sweat: *Chamom.*

Anxiety, with burning in stomach and cold body: *Jatroph.*

Burning rising from stomach into chest, with anxiousness and sweat on the forehead and chest: *Phosphor.*

Painful swelling of epigastrium, with great anxiousness: *Arg. nitr.*

Abdomen. Anxious feeling, with fever and thirst: *Arsen.;* with nightly restlessness and hot head and hands: *Nitr. ac.*

Dull, pressing pain, with heat, anxiety and restlessness: *Caustic.*

Pressing pain, followed by sweat and anxiety as if going to die: *Mezer.*

Anxious sensation of heat in abdomen, chest and face: *Bellad.*

Anxiety, with sensation of fullness to bursting in abdomen, the sweat pouring from the head: *Mur. ac.*

Painful distension, with short, anxious breathing, has to undo the clothes; chilliness and shuddering: *Mezer.*

Distension, with bodily heat and anxious feeling in epigastrium: *Arsen.*

Sexual Organs. Pollution, followed by anxious heat in the morning: *Petrol.*

Before catamenia, hot and anxious: *Amm. carb.*

Anxiety and heat, with catamenia: *Nitr. ac.*

Anxiety and faintness, with cold cheeks and inward heat: *Natr. mur.*

Chest. Emaciation, with chilliness on back, flushed cheeks, hoarse, weak voice, anxiety and irritability: *Hepar.*

Anxiousness as if in hot air: *Pulsat.*

Chill, with cold face and hands; anxious constriction of chest: *Pulsat.*

Anxiety, with inward heat and deep breathing: *Phosph. ac.*

Anxious constriction in chest, followed by heat without thirst; bead-like sweat: *Pulsat.*

Anxiety and dyspnœa, with warm sweat on the forehead: *Acon.*

Dyspnœa and anxiousness when standing, with sweat on the chest: *Cina.*

Oppression and anxiousness when walking fast, with sweat on back and chest: *Nitr. ac.*

Short breathing, with anxiety and profuse sweat: *Mangan.*

Dyspnœa and anxiety increasing gradually, from time to time sweat breaks out: *Nux vom.*

Rapid, death-like breathing, with rapid pulse and shuddering: *Pulsat.*

Dry cough in the night, with vomiting and anxious sweat; has to get up: *Silic.*

Heat, with great anxiety as if breath was insufficient; the same anxiety with the sweat: *Coccul.*

Heat in the chest which rises to the mouth, with restlessness and anxiety: *Nux vom.*

Burning in chest, with confusion in head as if he did not know where he is, with anxiety: *Chamom.*

Heat in stomach and chest, with anxiety: *Phosphor.*

Constriction, with anxiety and heat: *Anac.*

Attacks of heat, with anxiety as if the walls of the chest were pressed together: *Mercur.;* as if the chest was too narrow, with inward heat: *Phosph. ac.*

Heat in stomach and chest: *Phosphor.;* warm ebullition: *Carb. veg., Nux vom.*

Ebullition, with anxious dreams, screaming: *Pulsat.;* from the epigastrium to throat-pit: *Platin.*

Ebullition, with anxiousness and heat: *Amm. mur.*

Heart. Anxious feeling at the heart, with dyspnœa and flushes of heat: *Ambra;* internal heat: *Carb. veg.*

Feeling as if the heart would be squeezed off, beside himself with fear, moaning and profuse sweat: *Chamom.;* anxious constriction: *Merc. per.*

Cardiac anxiety and cold sweat: *Phosph. ac.;* anxious sweat: *Plumbum.*

Stitches, with inhalation in hypertrophy: *Plumbum.*

Palpitation, with anxiety and restlessness, constriction of chest, gasping with every exhalation, cold sweat: *Calc. ostr.*

Palpitation, with anxiousness and heat, particularly in the face: *Acon.*

Palpitation, heat and anxiety during catamenia, with trembling of limbs: *Nitr. ac.*

Anxiety, palpitation and sweat from disagreeable reminiscences which excite him: *Sepia.*

Anxiety in the night as if going to die, with cold sweat and audible palpitation: *Amm. carb.*

Outer Chest. Pressure and tension, with anxiety and cold hands: *Ledum;* feels warm about the breast and anxious: *Ol. anim.;* sweat: *Phosphor.*

Back. Shuddering on the back after heat in face, with anxiety: *Pulsat.*

Crawls on the back, with cold sweat on the forehead, anxiousness and shuddering: *Natr. mur.*

Sweat on back at night, followed by heat and uneasiness which prevents her from going to sleep: *Petrol.*

Sweat on back after 3 A.M., with anxious restlessness: ||*Rhus tox.*

Sweat with rash on the back, with dullness of all the senses and anxiety: *Stramon.*

Anxiousness, with trembling of hands and flushes of heat: *Platin.*

Upper Limbs. Crawling on the arms, with anxious fear: *Natr. mur.*

Chilliness running over the arms, with anxiety: *Pulsat.*

Chilliness, real shake, with cold hands and mental depression: *Cinch. off.*

Anxiousness as with a fever; hands are cold and tremble: *Carb. veg.*
Hot hands, with chilliness and anxious weeping: *Ignat.*
Fearful and restless; heat, with inclination to uncover: *Mur. ac.*
Flying heat mostly in hands, as from fear after a fright: *Calc. ostr.*
Anxiousness, with sweat and pain in scapula: *Cimex.*
Sweat on hands, with anxiety: *Chamom., Mercur.*
Cold sweat on hands; stupid: *Coccul.;* in palms of hands, with inability to think: *Calc. phosph.;* with anxious heat: *Lamium.;* with anxiety and irresolution: *Chamom.*
Flushes of heat mostly in hands, with anxiety and sweat: *Calc. ostr.*

Lower Limbs. Awakes about midnight with chill, anxiety and spasmodic drawing in the thighs: *Sepia.*
Restless and anxious, cannot sleep, thighs covered with cold sweat: *Thuya.*
Sudden redness of face, with cold feet and trembling anxiety: *Pulsat.*
When walking in open air trembling of knees, with anxiousness, heat, and burning of soles: *Hepar.*
Twitching of limbs and starting in sleep, with anxious heat: . . . . . .

All the Limbs. Chilliness, with goose-skin mostly on upper arms and outer part of thighs; restless and anxious: *Lam. alb.*
Coldness of limbs, with anxiety and mental derangement: *Stramon.*
Cold limbs, with fearfulness: *Auripig.*
Coldness, with insensibility: *Aethus.;* stupor: *Nux mosch.*
Cold hands and feet, with anguish: *Graphit.;* with anxiety in the evening: *Graphit.;* icy cold, with cold sweat; one cheek red, the other pale; mental and bodily prostration: *Ipec.*
Cold hands and feet from talking: *Moschus;* and hearing conversation: *Amm. carb.;* does not like to be alone: *Calc. ostr.*
When standing cold sweat on the back of hands and feet, with apprehension: *Lil. tigr.*
External coldness of limbs and inward heat, with anxious restlessness: *Arsen.*
Burning of hands and soles of feet, with anxiety: *Copaiv.*
Sudden heat while sitting, with anxiousness: *Graphit.*

Motion. Anxiousness, with sweat all day, worse when in motion: *Magn. carb.*

Nerves. Chilliness before going to bed, wakes with anxiousness and trembling feeling: *Platin.*
Spasmodic attack, with icy coldness and anxiousness: *Caustic.*

Weakness. Weak and prostrated, with anxiousness and sweat: *Mur. ac., Ratanh.*
Anxiety, weeping, palpitation and coldness, with weakness in all the limbs: *Mezer.*
Malarial fevers, with vomiting of mucus and bile, watery discharges, burning sensation in stomach, *great anxiety*, fainting spells, marked prostration, great restlessness and much thirst, particularly during the day; burning heat: *Arsen.*—JOSEPH BÆRTL. *Experience in Intermittents,* p. 101, 1859.

Alum.
Ant. crud.
Arnic.
|| Arsen.
Baryt.
Bryon.
Carb. an.
Graphit.
|| Magn. carb.
Magn. mur.
Merc. subl.
Natr. mur.
Petrol.
Pulsat.
Sepia.
Sulphur.
Zincum.

Heat and Anxiousness at Night. In bed: *Magn. mur.;* does not know what to do: *Baryt., Petrol.*

Anguish all night: *Veratr., Zincum.*

Anxiousness in the night as if from heat: *Pulsat.*

Feels too warm, cannot go to sleep: *Pulsat., Magn. carb.;* lasting until midnight: *Arsen., Graphit.*

Before midnight, afterwards sweat and thirst: *Magn. mur.*

Cannot rest in one place: *Merc. subl.;* tosses about: *Bryon.*

Sleepless and anxious until 2 or 3 A.M.: *Arnic.*

Anxiousness at 3 A.M., with alternate heat and nausea: *Arsen.*

Anxiousness from 3 to 5 A.M.: *Ant. crud.;* from 4 to 5 A.M. and 5 to 6 P.M.: *Sepia.*

Cannot sleep all night on account of heat and restlessness: *Carb. an.*

Awakes in the night, with great anxiety and heat, and a spasmodic feeling: *Sulphur.*

Restless sleep, tosses about, hot and anxious, with jerking of limbs and starting: *Alum.*

Has to uncover: *Natr. mur.;* which she cannot endure long: *Magn. carb.*

Morning. Sweat and anxiety: *Sepia.*

Feeling as if she had done wrong, with cardiac anxiety and sweat: *Aurum.*

Evening. Chilly and anxious: *Phosphor.*

Anxiety, with dry heat: *Hyper.*

Heat after lying down, with anxiousness lasting all night: *Zincum.*

Fear of ghosts, with trembling and flushes of heat, hands and face cold: *Pulsat.*

Warmth and Cold. Heat, like pouring hot water over her, better when uncovering: *Cannab.*

Anxiousness in the night, throws off the covers: *Nux vom.;* after midnight, with inclination to uncover: *Arsen.*

Feels too hot, cannot fall asleep before midnight; inclination to uncover: *Veratr.;* anxious heat, has to uncover: *Mur. ac.*

At 2 A.M. complaining about heat, wants lighter covers: *Ignat.*

Coldness or chilliness not relieved by warmth: *Cuprum.*

Heat, with desire to be covered: *Nux vom.*

Anxious heat when walking in open air, as if the clothes were too tight: *Argent.;* anxiousness and heat when walking out-doors: *Hepar.*

Anxious and hot, with lassitude, getting better in open air: *Gratiol.*

Chill, Heat, Sweat. After eating, chill; anxiousness and sweat in the night: *Ignat.*

Fear, with cold, anxious sweat, from imagining robbers under his bed and in the house: *Arsen.*

Tosses about, with anxiousness and moaning; cold sweat on forehead until 1 A.M.: *Bryon.;* heat, with anxiety: *Stramon.*

Heat as if deluged with hot water, alternating with feeling as if cold water coursed through his veins, with anxiousness: *Rhus tox.*

Sudden attack of anxiousness after going to bed, followed by sweat: *Thuya.*
Sweat in bed, with anxiousness: *Natr. mur.*
Anxious sweat preventing sleep: *Bryon.*
Night sweat, with feeling as if she had done something bad: *Natr. mur.*
Hypochondric restlessness, despondency, anxious sweat and sleeplessness: *Graphit.*
Periodicity. Alternation of chill, with symptoms of the mind: *Crocus, Platin.;* repeated attacks of anxiety, with flushes of heat: *Arnic.*
Attacks of heat, with anxiety: *Sepia, Spongia.*
Sensations. Chills, with pains and anxiety: *Arsen.*
Most symptoms are accompanied by chilliness, shuddering and anxiety: *Acon.*
Fine pricking on the whole body as of pins when getting into a sweat at night in bed, with cardiac anxiety and feeling as if deluged with hot water; better when uncovering: *Cannab.*
Touch and Skin. Chilliness, pale face, goose-skin, sensitive to the touch, with anxiety and restlessness: *Lam. alb.*
Painful vesicles on the left chest and back, with fever and anxiety: *Caustic.*
Children. Continuous anxious screaming, with cold sweat and open fontanelles: *Calc. phosph.*

OTHER UNPLEASANT FEELINGS.

Inconsolable. With attacks as from hot water poured over her: *Calc. ostr.*
With attacks of heat; also during the sweat: *Spongia.*
Morning sweat after grief: *Phosph. ac.*

Acon.	I	II	I
Arsen.	II	II	II
Aurum.	I		I
Bryon.	I		II
Calc. ostr.	I		I
Carb. veg.		I	II
Chamom.	I	I	I
Graphit.	II	I	I
Ignat.	II	I	
Nux vom.	II		II
Rhus tox.	I		I
Sepia.	I	I	I
Stannum.	I		I
Veratr.	II	I	II

Despair. During chill alone: *Ant. tart., Cuprum,* I *Hepar,* I *Mercur.*
During heat: I *Conium,* II *Pulsat.,* I *Spongia,* I *Sulphur.*
Sweat alone: *Lycop.*
Cold shivering and rigor: *Arsen.*
Attacks of anxiety and despair, with weeping; cold body, but little improved by external heat: *Cuprum.*
After the fever hopeless, despairing: *Psorin.*

Arsen.	II	I
Nux vom.	I	II
Pulsat.	II	I
Rhus tox.	II	II
Sepia.	I	II
Spongia.	I	
Thuya.	I	II

Life-weary, Suicidal Disposition. With chilliness: *Kali chlor., Spigel.*
With heat alone: I *Bellad.,* I *Cinch. off.,* I *Laches.,* II *Stramon.,* I *Valer.*
With sweat alone: I *Alum.,* I *Aurum,* II *Calc. ostr.,* II *Hepar,* I *Mercur.,* I *Silic.*
Chilliness; in the evening weary of life, sad: *Kali chlor.;* could commit suicide: *Spigel.*
Heat of body and anxiety, suicidal notions: *Cinch. off.*

Attacks of, anxiety, would like to die on the spot: *Spongia.*
With heat suicidal mania: *Arsen., Bellad., Nux vom.,* **I I***Pulsat., Rhus tox.,* **I I***Stramon.*

Apis.	**II**	**I**	
Arnica.	**I**	**II**	
Cinch. off.	**II**	**I**	**I**
Conium.	**II**		**I**
Caustic.	**I**		**I**
Opium.	**II**	**II**	
Phosphor.	**II**	**II**	**II**
Phosph. ac.	**II**	**I**	**II**
Pulsat.	**I**	**I**	**I**
Selen.	**II**		**II**
Sepia.	**II**	**II**	

Listless, Indifferent. Cold, indolent, unhappy: *Camphor.*
With chill alone: **I I***Ignat.,* **I I***Silic.,* **I***Veratr.*
With heat alone: **I***Viol. tric.*
With sweat alone: **I***Arsen.,* **I I***Bellad.,* **I***Calcar.,* **I***Laches.*
Apathetic: **I***Arnic.,* **I***Arsen.,* **I***Calc. carb.,* **I I***Cinch. off.,* **I***Conium,* **I***Opium,* **I***Phosphor.,* **I***Phosph. ac.,* **I***Pulsat.,* **I***Selen.,* **I***Sepia,* **I I***Stramon.,* **I***Veratr.*

Chilliness and apathy in the evening: *Kali chlor.*
Careless humor: *Veratr.*

FEELINGS AND CONATIONS.

Alum.	**II**	**II**
Ferrum.	**I**	**I**
Ignat.	**I**	**II**
Platin.	**II**	**I**
Valer.	**I**	**II**

Changeable Mood. Chilliness: *Asaf.;* heat alone: **I***Nux mosch.;* sweat alone: **I***Aurum,* **I I***Crocus,* **I***Stramon.,* **I I***Sulph. ac.,* **I***Zincum.*

Crawls over the whole body without heat, wavering mind: *Asaf.*

Apis.	**II**	**I**
Bellad.		**II**
Cinch. off.	**I**	**I**
Conium.	**I**	
Ignat.	**II**	**I**
Lycop.	**I**	**II**
Pulsat.	**II**	**I**
Sepia.	**I**	**II**
Spigel.	**I**	**II**
Sulphur.	**II**	**II**

Faint-hearted, Depressed. With chill: **I***Ant. tart.,* **I***Baryt.,* **I***Calc. ostr.,* **I***Camphor.,* **I***Hepar,* **I***Mercur., Rhus tox.*
With heat: **I I***Acon.,* **I I***Chamom.,* **I***Opium,* **I I***Petrol.,* **I***Stannum.*
With sweat: **I***Spongia.*

Shunning Men. During heat: **I***Conium,* **I I***Hyosc.,* **I***Pulsat.*
During the sweat: **I I***Arsen.,* **I***Bellad.,* **I***Laches.,* **I***Lycop.,* **I I***Pulsat.,* **I I***Sepia.*
When getting among strangers sweat breaks out: **I***Ambra,* **I I***Baryt.,* **I I***Lycop.,* **I***Sepia,* **I***Stramon.*

Acon.	**I**	**I**
Bellad.	**I**	**II**
Bryon.	**II**	**I**
Petrol.	**II**	**II**
Phosph. ac.	**I**	**I**
Rheum.	**I**	**I**
Thuya.	**II**	**II**

Ill Humor, Discontent. With chill: **I***Alum.,* **I I***Anac.,* **I***Calend.,* **I***Capsic.,* **I***Camphor.,* **I***Conium, Kreosot., Magn. carb.,* **I I***Natr. carb.,* **I***Nux vom., Pulsat.,* **I***Rhus tox.,* **I I***Silic.,* **I I***Spigel.*
With sweat: **I***Natr. mur.,* **I I***Thuya.*

Feels indisposed, with inward chilliness and ill humor: *Thuya.*
Alternately hot and chilly, with disgust for everything: *Rheum.*
With a dry cough and evening fever, he torments his family with his bad humor: **I***Psorin.*
Out of spirits, with febrile condition: *Petrol.*
Heat and bad humor in the evening: *Hippom.*
Fever ending with bad humor: *Silic.*
Heat in right hand, with very ill humor: *Pulsat.*

FEELINGS AND CONATIONS.

Ill humor, with pain in throat when swallowing; sour smelling sweat nearly every night: *Thuya.*

Morose. Chilliness, with great moroseness: *Caustic.*
Anxious mood during chill, morose and apprehensive: *Calend.*
Chilly, morose and gloomy: *Pulsat.*
Morose, with flushes of heat: *Angust.*
Sweat, with moroseness: *Angust., Magn. carb.*

Chamom.	I	II	**Hasty, Impetuous.** With heat: *Sepia.*
Coffea.			With sweat: I*Acon.,* I*Arsen.,* I*Bryon.,* I *Carb.*
Nux vom.	II	II	

veg., II *Ferrum,* I*Hepar,* I*Hyosc.,* II*Natr. mur.,* I*Phosphor.,* I*Stramon.,* II*Sulphur,* I*Thuya.*

Acon.	I	I	**Impatience.** With heat: II*Arsen.,* I*Bellad.,*
Apis.	II	I	I*Ipec.,* II*Lycop.,* I*Natr. mur.,* I*Nux vom.,* I*Pulsat.,*
Chamom.	I	I	*Viol. tric.*
Ignat.	II	I	
Mercur.	I	II	
Rhus.	I	II	With sweat: I*Aurum,* I*Sulph. ac.,* I*Zincum.*

General heat, with impatience and sweat: *Mezer.*

Anger. Chill or coldness after anger: *Acon., Arsen., Bryon., Mar. ver., Nux vom.*

Very irritable, inclined to be angry; after getting angry, chilly or a red face and heat in head: *Bryon.*

After anger, chilliness alternating with heat, vomiting of bile and thirst: *Nux vom.*

Gets angry about trifles, with cold hands, hot face and palpitation: *Phosphor.*

Gets hot and beside himself about a trifling vexation: *Phosph. ac.*

Heat after anger: I*Acon.,* I*Chamom.,* I*Nux vom.,* II*Petrol.,* II*Sepia,* I*Staphis.*

General heat; vexed and angry: *Hippom.*

Sweat after anger: I*Acon.,* II*Bryon.,* I*Chamom.,* I*Lycop.,* I*Petrol.,* II*Sepia,* I*Staphis.*

Fretfulness, Irritability. With chill and flying heat: *Arsen.*
Irritability, with heat: *Acon., Carb. veg., Laches., Phosphor., Phosph. ac.*
Hot, sensitive and passionate: *Caustic.*
Chilly, irritable and uncomfortable: *Mezer.*
Chilly and peevish: *Phosphor., Pulsat.*
Cold feet at table, with fretfulness and impatience: *Sulphur.*
Alternately hot and cold, with fretfulness and aversion to speak: II*Borax.*
Inwardly chilly, with fretfulness: *Hepar.*
Right cheek and hand hot, with chilliness of the body and irritability: *Pulsat.*
Chilliness, particularly of the extremities, very irritable and restless: *Thuya.*
Great irritability, everything vexes him, with anxious sweat and flushes of heat: *Angust.*
Fretful, does not know what to begin, with sweat: *Magn. carb.*
Very irritable mood, especially during the chilly stage, the least thing puts him out of humor: *Bellad.*

MIND AND DISPOSITION.

Arsen.	I	I	
Bellad.	I	I	
Bryon.	II		II
Calc. ostr.	II	II	I
Chamom.	I	I	II
Cinch. off.	II		II
Conium.	II	I	II
Hepar.	I		I
Lycop.	II	I	
Mercur.	I		I
Nux vom.	I		I
Pulsat.	I	I)	I
Rheum.	II	I	II
Rhus tox.	II		II
Sabad.	I		I
Sambuc.	I	II	
Sulphur.	I		I
Thuya.	II	I	II

Vexatious Mood. With chilliness: *Cyclam.*
When the chill comes, disposition to tear things, can scarcely suppress her rage: *Cimex.*
With chill alone: I *Arnic.*, II *Capsic.*, I *Caustic.*, II *Ignat.*, II *Kreosot.*, I *Mezer.*, I *Nitr. ac.*, I *Petrol.*, I *Phosphor.*, II *Platin.*, I *Silic.*, I *Spigel.*, I *Sulphur.*
Chill at 7 P.M., with vexatious mood followed by sweat: *Nitrum.*
With heat alone: I *Acon.*, II *Moschus*, II *Natr. carb.*, I.I *Psorin.*, I *Staphis.*
With sweat alone: II *Bryon.*, I *Mercur.*
Chill after vexation: *Mar. ver.*, *Nux vom.*

Chilliness on the back after vexation: *Nux vom.;* with anxiety: *Natr. mur.*
Heat after vexation: I *Petrol.*, I *Sepia;* heat with vexation: *Caustic.*, *Phosphor.*, *Phosph, ac.*
General sweat with vexing ideas: *Sepia.*
Gets into a sweat from suspicion about people in the street: *Baryt.*

ACTIONS.

With cold limbs, inclination to climb: *Stramon.*
With heat, inclination to work: *Opium, Sarsap.*, I *Thuya, Verbasc.*

Bellad.		II	I
Stramon.		I	I
Veratr.		I	I

Singing and Trilling. With heat alone: I *Mar. ver.*, *Sarsap.*

With sweat alone: I *Crocus*, I *Kali carb.*, *Spongia.*
Whistles during the heat: *Capsic.*
Disposed to make fun, with chilliness: *Nux mosch.*
Foolish me.riness with the heat: *Acon.*

Acon.		II	I
Arsen.		I	II
Bryon.		I	II
Chamom.		I	I
Coccul.		I	I
Ignat.		I	I
Ipec.		I	I
Nux vom.		II	I
Rhus tox.		I	II
Sepia.		I	I

Sighing and Groaning. With heat alone: I *Arnic.*, II *Bellad.*, I *Coffea*, II *Pulsat.*, II *Thuya.*
During heat, with anxious breathing: *Pulsat.*
With sweat alone: I *Baryt.*, I *Cinch. off.*, I *Cuprum*, I *Phosphor.*, II *Stramon.*, I *Veratr.*
With a newborn child, recovering after a bath from a fainty, convulsive state: *Millef.*

Acon.		II	I
Bryon.		I	II
Nux vom.		II	I
Veratr.		I	I

Complaining and Lamenting. With sweat alone: II *Ignat.*
Moaning in cold stage: *Eup. perf.*

Wants to be covered during the heat, licks the lips but has no thirst, moaning and groaning: *Pulsat.*
Weeping during the heat: *Spongia;* as if hot water was poured over her: *Calc. ostr.* See Tearfulness, page 304.
Headache gets worse before the chill, with stinging in temples, red eyes, oversensitiveness, complains about dazed feeling in forehead, and becomes passionate and quarrelsome: *Bellad.*—BÆRTL.

DESIRES—AVERSIONS—EXALTATIONS.

Bellad.	I	II	
Chamom.	II	I	
Cuprum.	I	II	
Lycop.	II	I	
Opium.	II	II	
Platin.	II	II	
Stramon.	I		

Crying. With the heat alone: IIAcon., IBryon., ICapsic., IICoffea., IIpec., IPulsat., IVeratr.; with the sweat alone: IArnic., ICalc. ostr., ICamphor., IPhosphor., IIRheum.
Screaming, with cool body: Ipec.
With burning heat: Hyosc., Opium.
Spitting at others during heat: IBellad., IICapsic.

DESIRES.

Inclination to work: IIOpium, ISarsap., IThuya, Verbasc.
Talkative. During the heat and sweat: ILaches.
During heat alone: Coffea, IIMar. ver., IPodoph., IStramon.; sweat alone: IIArsen., IIBellad., ICalad., Coccul., Hyosc., ISelen., IITarax.
After much talking, heat in head and icy cold hands: Phosph. ac.
Shuddering on the head and legs after inclination to laugh: Hura.
During chill, very much out of humor, would like to take his life: Spigel.; suicidal mania: Compare page 313.
Wants to sit alone with closed eyes during heat: Conium.

AVERSIONS.

Aversion to solitude, with coldness of face, hands and feet: Calc. ostr.
Great aversion to the sensation of heat in chest when walking in open air: Rhus tox.; has great aversion to his own sweat: Cimex; all his own exhalations are very offensive to him: Sulphur.

Arnica.	I	II	
Bellad.	I	II	
Ignat.	I	II	
Mur. ac.	I	II	
Opium.	I	II	
Phosphor.	II	II	
Phosph. ac.	I	II	
Veratr.	I	II	

Dislike to Talk. Cold creeps running down the back, vexatious, taciturn: Borax; chilliness and shuddering, with flying heat; aversion to talk: Platin.
During heat alone: IIChamom., IILycop., INux vom., IPulsat.
During sweat alone: IBryon., ICalc. ostr., IICinch. off., IMercur.
Dull and disinterested during the chill: Camphor.; sluggish: Crotal., Laches.

EXALTATIONS.

Acon.	II	II	I
Bellad.	II	II	I
Bryon.	II	I	
Chamom.	II	II	II
Coccul.	II	I	II
Coffea.	II	I	II
Conium.	II	I	
Ignat.	I	I	
Lycop.	II	I	II
Mar. ver.	II	II	II
Nux vom.	II	I	II
Sepia.	I	I	

Excitability. During chill alone: IArsen., IIAurum, IICalc. ostr., ICanthar., IICannab., ICapsic., ICarb. veg., IICaustic., IHepar, ILaches., INatr. mur., IPhosphor., IIPulsat., ISpigel., ISulphur, IVeratr.; chilliness: IICoca.
During heat: IAlum., IApis, IKali carb., IIMagn. carb., IIMoschus, IIOpium, IPetrol., ISarsap., IStramon., IValer.

318   MIND AND DISPOSITION.

During sweat: | *Phosph. ac.*
Excitability, with warmth: *Crocus;* with increased warmth of the body: *Moschus, Mezer.;* with nightly heat: *Apis.*
Increased warmth and agreeable exaltation: *Mar. ver.*
Hot all over, with exaltation: *Opium.*
Chill, with restless sleep and excited brain: *Aloes.*
Chill, followed by burning heat in face and cold feet: *Magn. carb.*
Clairvoyance: *Acon., Cannab., Opium, Phosphor.*
Flighty as at the beginning of a fever: *Lycop.*
Agitation; stinging and cramps in the stomach and extremities; hurry for stool and very liquid diarrhœa, painful and icy coldness over whole body, excessive thirst; pressure and constriction in the epigastrium; spasms; cold perspiration, especially on the head: *Anath.*
Excited fancy: *Bryon.;* heat of head, with excitement: *Mephit.*
Easily excited; hot hands from talking: *Graphit.;* hot hands, with excitement: *Sepia.*
Excitable during sweat: I*Acon.,* I*Bellad.,* II*Chamom.,* I*Coccul.,* II*Coffea,* I*Conium,* II*Lycop.,* II*Mar. ver.,* II*Nux vom.,* I*Phosph. ac.,* I*Sepia.*
Sweat all over; exalted: *Opium;* after excited talking: *Ambra.*

RESTLESSNESS.

Acon.	II	II	II
Amm. carb.	II	I	I
Apis.	I		I
Arnica.	I	I	I
Arsen.	II	I	II
Bellad.	II	II	II
Bovist.	I	I	II
Bryon.		II	II
Calc. ostr.	I	II	I
Chamom.	II	II	I
Cinch. off.	I		II
Coffea.	II	I	
Ignat.		I	I
Ipec.	I	II	
Laches.	I	I	I
Lycop.	I	I	II
Mercur.	I	I	I
Nux vom.	II	I	I
Phosphor.			
Phosph. ac.	I	I	II
Pulsat.	I	II	II
Rhus tox.	I	II	I
Ruta.	I	I	II
Sabad.	II	I	I
Sepia.	II	I	II
Silic.	I	II	II
Stannum.		I	I
Sulphur.		II	II
Veratr.	I	II	I

Restlessness. Coldness: *Phosphor.;* in the night: *Natr. mur.;* through the whole body: *Bovist.*
During chill: II*Anac.,* I*Asaf.,* II*Borax,* II*Cannab.,* II*Capsic.,* I*Carb. veg.,* II*Kreosot.,* I*Mezer.,* I*Natr. carb.,* II*Natr. mur.,* I*Petrol.,* I*Platin.,* I*Spigel.*
Rigor every third day: *Anac.;* waking at night: *Silic.*
During heat: I*Ant. tart.,* I*Baryt.,* I*Conium,* II*Magn. carb.,* II*Magn. mur.,* I*Merc. subl.,* I*Moschus,* I*Mur. ac.,* I*Opium,* I*Rheum,* I*Sabin.,* I*Spongia,* I*Staphis.,* I*Stramon.,* I*Thuya,* I*Valer.*
In the evening in bed restlessness and chill, alternating with heat: *Amm. carb.*
During sweat: *Lachnanth.,* II*Sambuc.;* with nausea: *Graphit.*
Before catamenia chill, followed by heat and restlessness: *Lycop.*
Restlessness and anxiety, with disagreeable heat in abdomen, alternating with general chilliness: *Bovist.*
Restless at night and anxious, cannot sleep; cold legs, covered with cold sweat: *Thuya;* at the beginning of chill restlessness: I*Laches., Phosphor.*
Heat and restlessness in the night, with throbbing in head, preventing sleep: *Arsen.;* with pressing headache and febrile heat: *Ruta.*

RESTLESSNESS.

Unbearable burning heat at night, with restlessness: *Pulsat.*
Great restlessness, with dry burning, hot skin at night: *Rhus ven.*
Heat, with trembling and uneasiness in the limbs: *Calc. ostr.*

Easily Frightened and Startled. Terror and shuddering in the morning: *Calc. ostr., Nux vom.*
Terrified feeling and shuddering: *Carb. an.*
Shuddering, with twitching: *Cerv. bras.*
Easily frightened during the chill: *Veratr.*
Cold sweat and easily frightened: *Card. ben.*
Sometimes cold, sometimes hot after starting in the night: *Bellad.*
Starting, with cold face and hands; or in sleep, with whimpering: *Ignat.*
Coldness, and starting from every noise: *Carb. veg.*
Cold body, starting and trembling: *Opium.*
Starting on falling asleep, with shuddering and stitches through the knee: *Mercur.;* burning heat and starting in sleep: *Lycop.*

Acon.	‖	‖	
Bellad.			**Easily Startled.** During heat: ⎮*Capsic.*,
Calc. ostr.	⎮	⎮	‖‖*Ignat.*, ⎮*Natr. mur.*, ⎮*Opium.*
Nux vom.	⎮	⎮	
Petrol.	‖	⎮	During sweat: ‖⎮*Caustic.*, ⎮*Chamom.*, ⎮*Sabad.*,
Phosphor.	‖	⎮	‖⎮*Sambuc.*, ⎮*Spongia.*
Pulsat.	‖	⎮	
Sepia.	⎮	⎮	Starting in sleep, slight chill, great heat with
Sulphur.	‖	‖	sweat, mental dullness, one cheek flushed: ‖⎮*Chamom.*
Veratr.	⎮	⎮	

Jerking of limbs in typhus: *Apis, Phosphor.*

Acon.	‖	‖‖	
Bellad.	⎮	⎮	**After a Fright.** Chill: ‖⎮*Ignat.*, ⎮*Mercur.*,
Lycop.	⎮	⎮	⎮*Nux vom.*, ⎮*Platin.*, ⎮*Pulsat.*, ⎮*Veratr.*
Opium.	‖	⎮	
Silic.	⎮	⎮	After fright, with icy coldness of the body: *Veratr.*

After fright, alternately chill, heat and sweat: *Lycop.*

Bellad.	⎮	⎮	**Bright Intellect.** Chill alone: ‖⎮*Phosphor.*,
Coffea.	‖	‖	⎮*Spigel.*
Laches.	⎮	⎮	‖
Opium.	⎮	‖	⎮ Heat alone: *Stramon.*
Phosphor.	‖		⎮
Thuya.	⎮	⎮	Sweat alone: *Valer.*, ‖⎮*Viol. od.*

Chill in the morning, with sprightliness: *Spigel.*
When he has no rigor, he knows things quite distinctly and clear: *Rhus tox.*
After chill, heat, with clearness of ideas and good memory: *Opium.*
Increased bodily heat in the evening, with brightness: *Menyanth.*
Agreeable warmth in the whole body, everything seems brighter: *Phosphor.*
Heat with thirst, no chill and cheerful mood: *Thuya.*
Bodily heat, with sweat, great thirst, sparkling eyes and cheerful mood: *Opium.*
Increased power to think, with sweat: *Clemat.*
Morning sweat, with cheerfulness: *Ol. anim.*
After sweat in the evening, cheerful mood: *Hydroph.*

From Thinking, Mental Exertion (Reading or Writing). Whole body cold and moist from thinking: *Aurum.*
Cold feeling at the heart from mental exertion: *Natr. mur.*
Heat from thinking: *Phosphor.*

Morning sweat; chilly with the slightest motion but anxious heat brought on by talking: *Lam. alb.*

Sweat worse from mental exertion (reading or writing): *Bellad.*, *Borax*, **I** *Calc. ostr.*, *Graphit.*, **II** *Hepar*, *Hyosc.*, **I** *Kali carb.*, **II** *Laches.*, *Lycop.*, *Natr. mur.*, **II** *Nux vom.*, **I** *Sepia*, **II** *Silic.*, *Staphis.*, **II** *Sulphur.*

From reading: *Sulphur;* writing: *Borax, Hepar, Sepia, Sulphur.*

Sweat caused by hearing news; cannot collect his thoughts: *Calc. phosph.*

Sweats all over after a serious talk: *Graphit.*

Sweat on outer chest: *Nitr. ac.;* and back: *Cina.*

Sweat better from mental exertion: *Ferrum, Natr. carb.*

Difficult Comprehension. Coldness and thirst: *Capsic.*

Chilliness when getting awake: *Staphis.;* crawling: *Capsic.*

Chill, with difficult comprehension: **II** *Bellad.*, **I** *Bryon.*, *Capsic.*, **I** *Laches.*, *Phosphor.*, *Stannum;* with the chill difficult recognition: *Rhus tox.*

Shaking, with thirst: *Capsic.;* without thirst: *Arsen.*

Great heat of the skin and difficult comprehension: *Chin. sulph.*

Fever heat or sweat, without thirst and difficult comprehension: *Capsic.*

After heat, sweat, with buzzing in ears and difficult comprehension: *Arsen.*

Deprived of power of thinking during the chill: *Cimex.*

Sweat, with lassitude and dullness of senses: *Hyosc.*

Chills, with weakness of intellect: **II** *Bellad.*, *Bryon.*, *Laches.*

Feverish and flushed; weakminded: *Ignat.*

Head hot, body cold, with weak mind: *Stannum.*

Coma and weak mind: *Plumbum.*

Confusion of the Mind. Cold skin; gives disconnected answers: *Laches.*

Beside himself during chill: **I** *Acon.*, **I** *Chamom.*, **I** *Coffea*, **I** *Veratr.*

During heat: **I** *Baptis.*, **I** *Cinch. off.*, **I** *Natr. carb.*

Stupid, as if bound up with heat and sweat: *Magn. sulph.*

Dullness. During chill: **I** *Cicut.*, **I** *Helleb.*, **I** *Ledum*, **II** *Nux mosch.*, **I** *Plumbum.*

During heat: **I** *Argent.*, **I** *Carb. veg.*, **I** *Chamom.*, **I** *Ignat.*, **I** *Pulsat.*, *Silic.*

During sweat: **I** *Cinch. off.*, **I** *Graphit.*, **I** *Sabad.*, **I** *Sulphur*, **II** *Thuya.*

Fever, with gastric trouble, loss of appetite, nausea and vomiting of green, bitter watery fluid; constipation, hard lumps of feces as if burnt; urine scanty and dark, emaciation, dry cough, prostration, apathy and dullness: *Diadem.*—BÆRTL.

Chill in morning, with pain in stomach and left hypochondric region. Thirst begins before the chill and lasts during heat. In apyrexia *dullness in head and loss of appetite;* only cold things taste good: *Nux vom.*—BÆRTL.

INTELLECT.

Arsen.	‖	‖	
Bellad.	ı	‖	ı
Bryon.	ı	ı	‖
Calc. ostr.	ı	‖	‖
Ipec.	ı	‖	‖
Kali carb.	ı	ı	
Lauroc.	ı		ı
Natr. mur.	‖	‖	
Nux vom.	ı		ı
Opium.	‖		‖
Phosphor.	ı	ı	
Phosph. ac.	‖		‖
Pulsat.	‖		‖
Rhus tox.	ı	ı	ı
Veratr.		ı	ı

Muddled. During chill: ı *Capsic.*, ı *Chamom.*, ı ı *Conium*, ı *Hyosc.*
During heat alone: ı *Alum.*
During sweat: ı *Cinch. off.*, ı *Rheum*, ı *Stramon.*
Dull head and stiff neck, with chill: *Cicut.*
Dullness in head and buzzing of ears: *Laches.*
Chill in the afternoon without fever; dazed all day: *Nitr. ac.;* dreaminess, with crawls: *Zincum.*
Dullnesss, with coldness even near the warm stove: *Ruta;* with cold hands and inward heat: *Helleb.*
With great heat of the body and more frequent and violent beats of the temporal artery; muddled; heat, followed by much sweat: *Bellad.*

Acon.	ı	‖	ı
Bellad.	‖	‖	
Laches.	ı	ı	
Opium.	ı	ı	ı
Phosphor.	ı	ı	
Stramon.	ı	‖	

Ecstasy, Excited Fancy. During heat: ı *Cinch. off.*, ı ı *Coffea*, ı ı *Lauroc.*, ı *Pulsat.*, ı *Sabad.*
During sweat: ı ı *Carb. veg.*, ı *Iodium*, ı ı *Nitr. ac.*, ı *Sulphur.*

Thoughts intrude with warmth of body: *Angust.*

Sensitiveness and heat; from reading affecting things emotion, weeping: *Laches.;* feeling as if deluged with hot water when an idea occurs vividly: *Phosphor.*

Lively imagination in the evening; the mere thought of unpleasant things causes shuddering: *Benz. ac.*, *Phosphor.*

Heat and moist skin, with mental derangement: *Stramon.*

Profuse sweating, with quick, erroneous ideas: *Cuprum.*

Bellad.	‖	‖	
Bryon.	ı	‖	
Opium.	ı	ı	
Rhus tox.	‖	ı	

Illusions. During chill: ı *Kali carb.*, *Phosphor.*, *Sulphur;* during heat: ı *Carb. veg.*, ı *Hyosc.*, ı *Magn. mur.*, ı *Mercur.*, ı *Phosphor.*, ı *Sambuc.*, ı ı *Stramon.*

During sweat: None.

In typhoid fever he thinks another person lies alongside of him, or that he is double, or that one limb is double: *Petrol.;* as if he were cut in two: *Platin.*

Believes himself to be three persons; a very troublesome symptom; the patient has dilated pupils: *Nux mosch.*

Imagines herself in pieces and cannot get herself together: ı *Baptis.*

Sees apparitions during chill: *Nitr. ac.*

Crawls when imagining disgusting things: *Phosphor.*

Cold, chilly, and imagining sickness: *Arsen.*

Anxiety, thinks his mind wanders, with chill: *Nitr. ac.*

Cold body, thinks he is not at home: *Veratr.;* not in his house: *Opium.*

When falling asleep, thinks she hears noises above her bed which makes her shudder: *Calc. ostr.*

Sees figures; dullness, followed by heat: *Phosph. ac.*

Voluptuous fancies, with heat: *Ignat.*

Becomes warm after fearful imaginations: *Anac.*

In typhus thinks he is well: *Arnic.*, *Arsen.*

MIND AND DISPOSITION.

Acon.	|	||	||
Arsen.	||	||	|
Bellad.	|	||	||
Bryon.	||	|	||
Calc. ostr.	|	||	|
Carb. veg.	|	|	|
Chamom.	|	|	||.
Cina.	|	|	|
Cinch. off.	|	|	|
Dulcam.	||	||	|
Hyosc.	|	||	||
Ignat.	|	|	|
Iodium.	|	||	|
Kali carb.	|	||	|
Natr. mur.	|	|	|
Nux vom.	||	|	||
Opium.	|	||	||
Phosphor.	||	|	
Phosph. ac.	|	|	|
Platin.	||	||	|
Sambuc.	|	|	||
Spongia.	|	||	
Stramon.	|	||	||
Sulphur.	||	|	|
Veratr.	|	||	|

Delirium. Coldness all over: *Veratr.*
During heat: | *Agn. cast.*, ■ *Ant. crud.*, ■■ *Apis*, | *Canthar.*, || *Capsic.*, | *Coccul.*, ■■ *Coffea*, || *Crocus*, | *Cuprum*, || *Hepar*, | *Laches.*, || *Menyanth.*, ■ *Nitr. ac.*, ■■ *Pulsat.*, ■ *Sabad.*; during sweat: | *Aurum.*

Nightly raving delirium, cannot be kept in bed, profuse morning sweat: *Acon.*

At night delirium, followed by profuse sweat: *Vip. torv.*

During typhoid fevers: || *Agar.*, ■ *Al. p. s.*, *Cuprum*, ■ *Petrol.*, || *Stramon.* (calling bystanders as if absent; talking about business; seems to dream with open eyes); bellowing: || *Cuprum*; with urgent thirst: *Ailanth.*, *Podoph.*; with the greatest exhaustion: *Agar.*

Character. Merry: ■ *Bellad.*, || *Crocus*, | *Cuprum*, ■ *Hyosc.*, | *Spongia*, || *Stramon.*, | *Veratr.*; incoherent: *Atrop.*; anxious: | *Acon.*, || *Bellad.*, || *Crocus*, ■ *Hyosc.*, | *Nux vom.*, ■ *Opium*, | *Pulsat.*, | *Silic.*, *Sepia*, ■ *Stramon.*

Loquacious: | *Bellad.*, | *Cuprum*, || *Laches.*, ■ *Podoph.*, | *Rhus tox.*, ■ *Stramon.*, || *Veratr.*; with spitting: *Bellad.*, *Capsic.*

Taciturn: | *Ant. crud.*, | *Bellad.*, ■ *Hyosc.*, | *Mur. ac.*, || *Veratr.*

Muttering: ■■ *Apis*, *Atrop.*, | *Bellad.*, | *Hyosc.*, || *Mur. ac.*, ■ *Opium*, || *Phosph. ac.*, || *Stramon.*, | *Tarax.*

Imagines herself in pieces and cannot get herself together: *Baptis.*; thinks he is three persons: *Moschus.*

Raving: *Acon.*, || *Bellad.*, ■ *Bryon.*, ■ *Hyosc.*, | *Lycop.*, | *Opium*, ■ *Stramon.*

In the evening: *Laches.*, *Psorin.*; night: *Sepia*; with the pains: *Dulcam.*; from violence of pain: *Veratr.*

With hot skin: *Acon.*, *Dulcam.*, *Opium*, *Stramon.*, *Sanguin.*

With light febrile paroxysms: *Santon.*

With heat; sweat on the head: *Sepia*; tosses about in bed and talks, with open eyes: *Chamom.*

Increased heat and confused talk in intermittent fever: *Menyanth.*

Constant burning heat: *Hyosc.*; with unquenchable thirst: *Hepar.*

Delirium, and feeling as if she would lose her reason: *Psorin.*

Mania, with delirium and sleeplessness, without hallucinations or loss of memory: ■ *Veratr.*; if with it: *Stramon.*—Dr. HERMEL.

Arsen.	|	|	||
Bellad.	||	|	||
Hyosc.	|	||	||
Opium.	|	|	||
Stramon.	||	||	||
Veratr.	|	||	||

Mania. During chilliness: *Calc. ostr.*; chill alone: *Cimex*, | *Platin.*, | *Sulphur.*

During heat alone: | *Ant. crud.*, || *Calc. ostr.*, | *Canthar.*, ■■ *Cicut.*, | *Dulcam.*

Without thirst: | *Cinch. off.*; and wild look: ■ *Cuprum*; burning heat: *Bellad.*; sweat ends the attacks: *Cuprum*, *Sulphur.*

In typhus maniacal delirium, tries to run away, screams, roars, with sunken features, cold feet, very frequent pulse: *Zincum.*

Acon.	||	||
Arsen.	||	**|**
Bellad.	**|**	||
Canthar.			**	**
Lycop.	||	||
Nitr. ac.			||
Nux vom.			||
Stramon.	||		
Veratr.			**||**	**|**

Rage. Chill alone: **|** *Cannab.*, | *Canthar.*
Heat alone: None.
Sweat alone: | *Caustic.*, | *Hyosc.*, **|** *Opium*, | *Sabad.*
Sensitive and inclined to anger; chilly, but easily heated from exercise: *Caustic.*
Burning heat, with rage: *Bellad.*

Heat from anger, with rage: *Chamom.;* heat of the body, with continual fury: *Veratr.*

REPRODUCTIONS.

Vanishing of Thought. With chill: || *Bellad.*, | *Bryon.*, | *Laches.*, | *Rhus tox.;* dullness in head, with shuddering and irregular breathing: *Sepia.*
Coldness; senses leave him: *Camphor.*
Chills, with a loss of feeling: *Spongia.*
Warmth over whole body; senseless: *Stramon.*
Typhoid fever; giddy, vanishing of thought: *Nux mosch.*
Heat, and feeling as if she would lose her senses: *Psorin.*
Cold sweat on forehead; insensibility: *Arsen.*

Acon.		**|**	**|**
Arnica.	||	**|**	
Arsen.	**|**	||	**|**
Bellad.	||	||	||
Camphor.	**|**	**|**	||
Chamom.	**|**	||	
Coccul.	||	**|**	**|**
Helleb.	||		||
Hyosc.	**|**	**|**	**|**
Mur. ac.	||	||	**|**
Natr. mur.	**|**	||	||
Opium.	**|**	||	||
Phosphor.	**|**	**|**	**|**
Phosph. ac.	**|**	||	**|**
Rhus tox.	**|**	||	**|**
Sepia.	**|**	||	**|**
Stramon.	**|**	**|**	||
Veratr.	||	**|**	**|**

Unconsciousness. During chill: || *Capsic.*, | *Cicut.*, **|** *Conium*, | *Kali carb.*
Shaking chills awaken her from unconsciousness: *Cicut.*
During heat: **||** *Apis*, | *Borax*, || *Bryon.*, || *Calc. ostr.*, **|** *Dulcam.*, | *Lauroc.*, || *Nux vom.*, **|** *Pulsat.*, | *Sulphur.*
During sweat: || *Sambuc.*
Chills and warm sweat: *Stramon.*
Cool skin: *Stramon.*
Shuddering, momentary loss of consciousness: *Chelid.;* in typhoid fevers: *Stramon.*
Violent sweat from incessant motion, with unconsciousness: *Stramon.*

Arnica.	**|**	**|**	**|**
Arsen.	**|**	||	**|**
Bellad.	||	**|**	||
Bryon.	**|**	**|**	**|**
Calc. ostr.	**|**	**|**	**|**
Chamom.	**|**	**|**	**|**
Hyosc.	||	||	||
Lauroc.	**|**	**|**	||
Natr. mur.	**|**	||	
Nux vom.	**|**	||	
Opium.	||	**||**	||
Phosphor.	||	**|**	**|**
Phosph. ac.	||	**|**	||
Pulsat.	**|**	||	**|**
Rhus tox.	||	**|**	**|**
Stramon.	**|**	**|**	**|**
Veratr.	**|**	**|**	||

Stupefaction. During chill: || *Borax*, | *Conium* | *Helleb.*
Cool skin, coldness, shuddering: *Stramon.*
During heat: **|** *Apis*, **|** *Camphor.*, || *Sepia.*
In typhoid fevers, after slowness of ideas: *Nux mosch.;* fever beginning, with stupor: *Arsen.*
Heat and stupefaction: *Aethus.*
During hot stage stupidity increases: *Stramon.*
With sweat, sometimes stupor: *Stramon.*
Heat worse after mental exertion: *Ambra*, *Bellad.*, *Nux vom.*, *Oleand.*, *Sepia*, *Silic.*
Heat better after mental exertion: *Ferrum*, *Natr. carb.*
Heat while reading: *Oleand.*

Weakness of Memory. During chill: ||Bellad., |Conium, ||Hyosc., |Rhus tox., Podoph.

Heat in head and cold feet, with forgetfulness: *Sulphur.*
With warmth of body, memory stronger: *Angust.*
During the fever forgetful: *Guarœa.*
After fever forgets all what passed; forgetfulness of words: *Podoph.*
Forgetfulness during fever: *Anac., Guarœa.*
After a typhoid fever the greatest forgetfulness, lasting for a year and making him very morose: *Anac.*
Cold skin, quiet pulse and disconnected answers: *Crotal.*
Shuddering, speech confused, incoherent: *Stramon.*
Chill at 4 P.M., says words he does not want to say: *Chamom.*
Chill and coldness; stupid and awkward: *Capsic.*
Cold body, thinks he talks wrong: *Nitr. ac.*

NOTE.—The mind symptoms in typhoid fevers have been arranged in a specimen number of this work and printed a year ago. They have, therefore, not been wholly reprinted. The volume containing typhoid fevers being one of the last, it may be several years before the plates of the specimen number will be destroyed. Up to that time this number may be obtained from the publishers at a reduced price.

PERIODICITIES, ATTACKS OR SPELLS, INTERMISSIONS.

I Acon.
Aesc. hipp.
Agar.
II Arg. nitr.
Calc. ostr.
Carb. veg.
Cinch. off.
II Conium.
Crocus.
II Cuprum.
Digit.
II Ferrum.
II Graphit.
II Hepar s. c.
I Laches.
II Natr. carb.
Natr. mur.
Nitr. ac.
II Nux vom.
II Phosphor.
Platin.
I Psorin.
Sepia.
Spongia.
II Sulphur.
Thuya.
I Veratr.

Anguish. Lasting for minutes: *Graphit.;* fifteen minutes: *Natr. carb.;* one hour: *Nux vom., Sulphur;* several hours: *Carb. veg., Hepar;* twelve hours: *Caustic.;* returning from time to time: *Acon.;* several attacks every day: *Natr. carb.;* coming and going every five minutes, vertigo and dimness, can only be removed by other thoughts: *Agar.*

Anxiety in attacks: *Acon.,* ||*Nux vom., Veratr.;* with crying: *Cuprum;* frequent attacks: *Graphit.,* ||*Phosphor., Platin.* Compare pages 154, 162, 203, 269.

Spells of anxiety, with sweat in the face, lasting fifteen minutes: *Natr. carb.*

Spells of nausea and faint, anxious feeling, lasting from five to ten minutes: *Nitr. ac.*

Anxiety in spells, with deathly nausea and great depression: *Digit.*

Anxiety, with red cheeks and contraction in the abdomen, coming in spells: *Hepar.*

Pain in chest, with the greatest anxiety in spells: I*Psorin.*

Attacks of cardiac anxiety, with palpitation and heat: *Veratr.*

Great anguish, with severe periodic and frequent palpitation of the heart: *Aesc. hipp.*

Anxious palpitation, without mental anxiety, coming in attacks: *Natr. mur.*

Periodical mania: *Arg. nitr.;* slow thinking: *Cinch. off.;* weak memory: *Carb. veg.*

Sadness at twilight; same hour several days: *Phosphor.*
Spasmodic attacks of mania, changeable mood, rage: *Crocus.*
Moral and nervous disturbances come on in quite regular paroxysms every night, in the morning, or at noon; more particularly after dinner: *Arg. nitr.*
Bodily and mental symptoms alternate: *Platin.*
Alternating states of mind every other evening: *Ferrum.*
Mental symptoms worse every other day: *Laches.*
A painful quivering in the brain on a small spot above the right frontal eminence which intermits; vexatious humor: *Bovist.*
Mental symptoms have an intermitting character: *Conium.*

WORSE DURING THE PHASES OF THE MOON.

According to Bönninghausen and Jahr.

	Full.	New.
Alum.	I	II
Amm. carb.		II
Arg. nitr.	II	
Arsen.		I
Calc. ostr.	I	
Caustic.		II
Cuprum.		I
Cyclam.	II	
Fluor. ac.	I	
Graphit.	II	
Lycop.		II
Mar. ver.	I	
Natr. carb.	I	
Natr. mur.	I	
Sabad.	I	I
Sepia.		I
Silic.	I	II
Sol. mam.	II	
Spongia.	I	
Sulphur.	II	
Thuya.		II

During the increase of moon *Alum.* has I I degree, the same as in the foregoing new moon.

Thuya has I degree; I I in new moon.

During the decrease of the moon *Dulcam.* has I I degree and *Sulphur* I I, the same as in full moon.

With full moon, increasing mania: *Arg. nitr.*

Great anxiety in evening in bed: *Sulphur.*

During high tide, in full moon, difficult comprehension, which is better in low tide: *Sol. mam.*

NOTE.—The great weight such remarks have and the importance for elevating our mere knowledge of things to the rank of a science, ought to make us very careful. The same rule which our master has given us as the highest in getting a true image of the sick, t. i., never to ask questions which can be answered by yes or no, we ought to apply when searching for higher truths; we ought to look to the almanac *after* we have made an observation, not before.—C. HG.

SIDES.

Anxiety, with Symptoms on Right Side. Anxious feeling in chest, with throbbing in lower right side: *Phosphor.*

Anxious feeling in chest, with constriction first in right side, afterwards in whole chest: *Acon.*

Pressing sensation in right side of chest, with great anxiety: *Aurum, Bellad.*

Pressing in right side of chest, near the ensiform cartilage and last true rib, with great anxiety and oppression of breathing: *Hyosc.*

Anxiety, with twitching of right hand: *Pulsat.*

Anxious feeling of weakness in right leg when walking: *Sulphur.*

Anxiety, with Symptoms on Left Side. Pressing in left hypochondriac region, with anxiety and nausea in chest: *Rhus tox.*

Drawing under the left breast, with anxiety; a kind of oppression at the heart, which interferes with breathing: *Nux vom.*

Stitches under left breast, with anxiety: *Phosphor.*

Stitches as from knives into left chest and back, with great anxiety and restlessness: *Caustic.*

Lying on the left side causes anxiety: *Phosphor.;* and palpitation, with dyspnœa: *Pulsat.*

Cannot lie on the left side on account of palpitation and anxiety: *Baryt.*

Feeling of tension in left chest, with palpitation and anxiety: *Cannab.*

Fright, with Symptoms on Right Side. Great fright after a slight surprise, trembles and feels as if paralyzed, right cheek grows hot and purple: *Mercur.*

Startling stitch in right leg after rising from a kneeling posture: *Carb. an.*

Easily frightened; crawling pain in right arm and hand: *Natr. carb.*

Fright, with Symptoms on Left Side. Sharp stitches in the front part of left chest, which startle her: *Graphit.*

Sudden stitches and burning sensation deep in the left side of the chest, frightening her: *Baryt.*

After fright, lameness in left arm and foot: *Stannum.*

Nervous excitement felt in the region of the heart from stinging and unbearable itching in the left eye: *Hura.*

Fretfulness, with Symptoms on Left Side. Fretfulness after a tearing and a stitch in the left big toe, which remains sensitive: *Baryt.*

After vexation stitches in upper part of left chest: *Natr. mur.*

Attacks of anxiety as if coming from under the left breast, trembling and palpitation: *Phosphor.*

Lamenting, with Symptoms on Right Side. With every inhalation a stitch runs from the lowest rib on the right side through to the point of the shoulder-blade, with lamenting: ||*Acon.*

Weeping, with Symptoms on Left Side. Tearing, stinging and swelling of the left wrist, with weeping; is beside himself: *Sabin.*

Screaming, with Symptoms on Right Side. Rapid stitches in the right chest, with desire to scream in the evening: *Baryt.*

A sharp stitch in right chest, has to scream: *Lauroc.*

Itching boring stitch in the dorsum of the right foot while at rest, has to scream: *Spigel.*

Violent tearing in the right big toe, with desire to scream while sitting: *Paris.*

Screaming, with Symptoms on Left Side. Continuous stitches in the left chest, with desire to scream; relieved for a short time by taking a deep breath: *Sulphur.*

Dull stitches in the left chest and abdomen, has to scream: *Clemat.*

A sharp stitch under the left ribs while at dinner, has to scream: *Ratanh.*

Pressing pain in left side and stitch as from a sharp instrument, has to scream: *Hura.*

Tearing stitches in left thigh while at rest, has to scream: *Sepia.*

Left knee feels as if beaten, has to cry out, with anxious heat: *Conium.*

Burning stitch on the inner border of the left foot-sole, has to scream: *Ratanh.*

Difficult Comprehension. With tingling in right arm and hand: *Natr. carb.*

MODEL CURE.

Enlargement and induration of liver; abdomen distended and soft, sore pains all over it, particularly around the navel; hectic fever, unquenchable thirst, when swallowing feels a small, hard lump in throat; sensation as if a worm crept up from the pit of stomach into the throat, which makes him cough; frequent gagging and vomiting of a little bloody phlegm or thin blood, sometimes pus, of a saltish taste; cough worse at night, with shooting in scrobiculum, a kind of weak but very deep cough; has to cough until he raises; *cannot lie on left side;* during the night a dull moaning: *Zincum*^{30}.—C. HG.

PECULIAR SENSATIONS, WITH MENTAL SYMPTOMS.

Fixed. Pressing headache after much talking: *Thuya.*
Fullness, with uncomfortable and anxious feeling: *Phosph. ac.*
Imagines to be larger and uncomfortable: *Platin.;* to be longer: *Pallad.*
Feeling too small, with great discomfort: *Gratiol.*

Steady Motion. Quaking tension felt through the whole body, with fearfulness and ill humor: *Petrol.*
Jerking pains, with anxiousness: *Ant. crud.*
Jerking and dull pecking in the whole body, and sensitive mood: *Natr. carb.*
Tearing pressing pains in forehead: . . . .
Stinging pains worse after vexation: *Rhus tox.*
Pricking in the whole body, with anxiety: *Magn. carb.*

Wave-like Motion. Throbbing all over, hypochondriac mood: *Arg. nitr.*
Prickling in body, electrical uneasiness and anxiety: *Veratr.*
Formication, with anxiety: *Arnic., Borax.*
Unbearable itching: *Sarsap.*

Destructive. As if arms were drawn asunder, with anxiety: *Natr. carb.*
Has to examine his left foot, which turns in when walking, in order to assure himself that it is not twisted: *Psorin.*
Sensation as if beaten, with sadness: *Lauroc., Natr. carb.;* and anxiety: *Borax, Magn. carb.;* and laziness: *Caustic.*
Burning biting pain in the ulcer, with weeping and moaning: *Rhus tox.*

Diminished Activity. Want of bodily sensibility in mania: *Ant. crud.*
Loss of feeling in whole body, with fretfulness: *Cyclam.*
Numb feeling in all nerves, with absentmindedness: *Sepia.*

Feelings. Cheerful, contented mood, with all pains and complaints: *Spigel.*
Increased activity and mobility, with decrease of pains and mental symptoms: *Veratr.*
Feels cross and disagreeable; general malaise: *Uran. nitr.*

OVERSENSITIVENESS TO PAIN.

‖ Acon.
І Agar.
‖ Ant. tart.
‖ Arnica.
І Arsen.
Ars. hydr.
І Asar.
І Aurum.
І Baryt.
Bovist.
І Bryon.
І Canthar.
Caustic.
‖ Cepa.
І Cina.
‖ Chamom.
‖ Cinch. off.
І Coccul.
‖ Coffea.
‖ Colchic.
Crotal.
І Cuprum.
І Graphit.
І Laches.
‖ Magn. carb.
Magn. mur.
І Mangan.
Mezer.,
І Natr. carb.
І Nux vom.
І Phosphor.
Pulsat.
Ruta.
Sabad.
‖ Sarsap.
Sepia.
Silic.
Sulphur.
‖ Veratr.

Terrible pain when discontinuing motion: *Ars. hydr.*
With tolerable pain, constant fear they might become unbearable: *Cepa.*
Pains affect the soul inordinately: *Sarsap.*
His sufferings seem unbearable: *Colchic.*
Unbearable headache: *Sarsap.*
Compare pains with Despair and Madness.
Tearfulness: *Coffea,* ❙*Pulsat.*
Sadness: *Digit., Ignat., Rhus tox.*
Pains cause mental depression: *Sarsap.;* and hopelessness: *Laches.*
With complaints of different kind, the sick are completely hopeless, and insist they never can get well: ‖*Psorin.*
Anxiety: ❙*Arsen., Caustic.,* ❙ *Coffea, Natr. carb., Rhus tox.,* ‖❙*Stramon.;* anguish: *Helleb.;* agony: *Arsen.*
Wakes in the night with great fear and cramp-like pain in the abdomen, then in the mouth, chest and hip-joint, with palpitation: *Sepia.*
Imagines he has pains in his sleep, which cause him great anxiety on awaking: *Alum.*
Anxious pains in the suffering parts while sitting, with whimpering: *Rhus tox.*
Bodily complaints, with anxiety: *Calc. phosph., Caustic.*
Great anxiety and heat with the pains: *Carb. veg.*
Anxiety, trembling and sweat with the pains: ❙*Natr. carb.*
Anxious feeling runs suddenly through the whole body: *Platin.*

Fear. Inexpressible anxiety, with increasing pains; appears as if dying: *Arsen.;* fear the pain may get worse: *Ars. met.*
The pains are bearable, but he fears they may become insufferable: *Cepa.*
Fear of death: *Acon.;* even with slight pains: *Raphan.*
Feels unhappy with every little pain: *Carb. veg.*
Drives to despair: *Acon.,* ❙*Arsen.,* ❙*Chamom., Cinch. off.,* ❙ *Coffea, Colchic., Hyper., Laches., Magn. carb.,* ❙ *Veratr.*
In the evening: *Nux vom.;* at night: ❙*Chamom., Colchic., Magn. carb.*
With rheumatic pains: *Laches.*
The pain is insufferable, would rather take her life than bear it: *Nux vom.*
The pains are worse at night and drive to distraction; constant thirst, heat, redness of one cheek and warm sweat on the head: *Chamom.*
Beside himself: *Coffea, Laches., Nitr. ac.;* inconsolable: *Acon.*
Indifference to pain: *Arnic., Jatroph.*
Changeable mood: *Ignat.*
Want of consideration, with pains: *Hepar, Iodum.*
Faint-heartedness: *Colchic., Hepar s. c., Iodum, Laches., Nux vom.*
Discontented with the pain: *Cinch. off., Hepar.*

Faultfinding: *Nux vom.;* quarrelsome: *Chamom.;* impatient: *Hura.*
Angry about himself: *Aloes.*
Irritability: *Canthar., Daphn. ind.;* fretfulness: *Canthar., Opium;* ill humor: *Canthar., Cinch. off., Hepar, Ignat.*
Irritable, dissatisfied and despondent with the pains: *Hepar.*
Cannot bear being spoken to, it aggravates the pains: *Arsen.*
Weeping: *Chamom., Coffea, Opium, Pulsat.*
Stammers unconnected words, sheds tears and appears as if suffering great pain: *Stramon.*
Attacks of pain cause weeping and laughing: *Hura.*
Lamentations: *Vip. torv.;* and sighing: *Acon.;* quarreling: *Nux vom.*
And complaining about the insupportable pain, in rheumatism: *Laches.*
Weeping and screaming; gets beside himself about trifles: *Ignat.*
Whimpering, complaining, grumbling, scolding, with the pains: *Nux vom.*
Anxious pains in suffering parts, with whimpering: *Rhus tox.*
Pains in the whole body, inducing moaning: *Crotal. casc.*
Great heat from 10 P.M. until after midnight, with short breathing; wants to cough but cannot, talking is very difficult; great restlessness, screams on account of pains in the hands, feet, abdomen and back; stamps her feet and will not allow herself to be touched: *Acon.*
The pains make him scold and swear: *Corall.*
Aversions. During the pain everything is disgusting: *Aloes.*
Disinclined to talk: *Ignat.*
Exaltations. Great nervous excitement with the pains in the eyeballs: *Daphn. ind.*
Restlessness: *Chamom., Cinch. off., Coffea;* starting: *Ignat.*
Intellect. Mental labor increases the pain: *Rhus ven.*
The pains are so violent, patients scratch the wall or the floor with their nails: *Arnic.;* madness: *Veratr.*
The pain in the sore finger drives to distraction: *Cepa.*
The mind fails to return to its usual vigor after great suffering: *Anac.*
Delirium: ||*Dulcam.,* |*Veratr.*
The attacks of pain cause for a short time delirium and mania: *Veratr.*
Talks confusedly, as if tormented by the pain: *Stramon.*
Becomes almost furious about the pain: *Chamom.*
The pains seem unbearable and drive to madness: *Arsen.*
The pains are soon forgotten: *Ars. hydr., Ars. met., Clemat.*
Most pains are felt during a half-conscious condition, and disappear when thinking of them: *Camphor.*
Indescribable violent pain makes her unconscious: *Natr. sulph.;* stupefying pain: *Arsen., Bromum.*
Some Bodily Concomitants. During pains, trembling: *Pulsat.;* and irritability: *Daphn. ind.;* after pains, trembling: *Bryon.*
Fainting, with slight pain: *Hepar, Nux mosch.*
Drowsy with the pains: *Nux mosch.*
With the pains hot and thirsty: *Chamom.*

After mania, pains in stomach, head, jaws, chest and various joints: *Acon.*
Violent, excruciating pains from laceration of nerves: *Hyper.*
The narcotic effect of *Opium* is much diminished by great pain or grief.

TISSUES.

Bones. Bone pain and headache between the attacks of mania or convulsions: *Cuprum.*
Pressing drawing pain in the periosteum, with anxious feeling as at the beginning of an intermittent: *Bryon.*
The bones of the head become so painful when lying down, it makes low-spirited: *Aurum.*

Joints. Pain in joints and muscles, with anxiety: *Caustic.*
Feeling of looseness in his joints, with inconsolable mood: *Stramon.*
Trembling of the joints, with cheerful mood: *Cyclam.*
Joints feel as if beaten; lassitude and ill humor, with sweat: *Phosph. ac.*
Melancholy, with gout: *Helleb.*
Cheerful mood, followed by pain in the joints and anxiety: *Caustic.*

Veins. Stitching in the veins, with anxiety: *Mercur.*
Varices, with nervousness and irritability: *Apis.*
Varicose veins in connection with mental derangement: *Arnic., Arsen.,* ❙*Fluor. ac.*, ❙❙*Laches., Lycop., Sulphur, Zincum.*
Pectoral anxiety, with disappearance of veins from the surface of the skin: *Aloes.*

Loss of Blood. Delirium in consequence of loss of blood: *Arnic., Arsen., Ignat., Laches., Lycop., Phosphor., Phosph. ac., Scilla, Sepia, Sulphur, Veratr.*
Derangement with such who are used to venesections: *Acon.*
Derangement or other mental affections after loss of blood or other fluids: ❙*Carb. veg.*, ❙*Cinch. off., Kreosot., Phosph. ac., Staphis., Veratr.*

Swelling. With confusion: *Bellad.;* of body, with stupor: *Vip. torv.*
Acts better on lax lymphatic, than on thin and firm individuals, the effect on the mind is similar: *Seneg.*—SEIDEL.
In tedious chronic cases where it is desirable to diminish rigidity of fibre: *Acon.*—HAHNEMANN.
With persons of rigid fibre, *Capsic.* is seldom found useful.—HAHNEMANN.

Emaciation. Emaciation after grief: *Phosph. ac.*
Looks dissatisfied, pale, wretched and thin: *Mezer.*
Pale and emaciated; irritable and vexed: *Petrol.*
Emaciated, earthy pale face, blue rings around the eyes, great weakness in all the limbs, no ambition, constant desire to rest: *Arsen.*
Stupor, with vomiting, purging and collapse: *Podoph.*
Mental depression, with beginning atrophy: *Coca.*
Emaciation, with mental derangement: *Anac., Arsen., Calc. ostr., Cinch. off., Graphit., Laches., Lycop., Natr. mur., Nitr. ac., Nux vom., Phosphor., Pulsat., Silic., Sulphur, Veratr.*

TOUCH.

I Acon.	**Better after Mesmerizing.** While being mesmerized, anxiety, trembling and palpitation: *Borax;* desire to be mesmerized: *Phosphor., Silic.*
II Baryt.	
I Bellad.	
I Cinch. off.	
II Conium.	**Fear when others come near.** With faceache the patient holds up his hand if anyone approaches him: *Cinch. off.*
II Cuprum.	
II Graphit.	
I Ignat.	Gout, with the greatest fear of being struck; persons coming across the room have to avoid the straight line: I *Arnic.*
I Iodium.	
I Mar. ver.	
II Natr. carb.	Fear if persons approach him: *Anac., Conium, Ignat., Lycop.;* in delirium: *Cuprum.*
I Nux vom.	
II Phosphor.	
I Sabin.	
II Sepia.	Children cannot bear to have anyone come near them: I *Cina.*
II Silic.	Afraid of pointed things: I *Spigel.;* in delirium: *Silic.;* in dreams: *Mercur.*
I Sulphur.	
II Viol. od.	

Fear of touch: *Arnic., Coffea.*

Fixed idea that the body, especially the limbs are made of glass and will break easily: *Thuya.*

Children cannot bear to be touched: II *Cina;* or looked at: *Ant. crud.*

Great aversion to being looked at: *Ant. tart.*

Taking hold of children offends them: *Ant. tart.,* II *Chamom.,* I *Cina.*

Cries piteously when anyone attempts to take hold of or lead him: *Cina.*

Children are very obstinate during the intervals of fever, and cry when touched or spoken to: *Silic.*

It seems to hurt children to be moved or touched: II *Bryon.*

II Acon.	**Worse from being Touched.** External impressions, strong light, odors, touch, ill behavior of others, bring him beside himself: *Colchic.*
Agar.	
I Ant. crud.	
II Ant. tart.	
II Bryon.	Cries with the slightest touch: *Cuprum.*
II Chamom.	
II Cina.	Cries piteously on being touched: *Cina.*
II Colchic.	After being touched, delirium: *Stramon.*
Cuprum.	
Hepar s. c.	The slightest touch brings him in a rage: *Laches.*
I Kali carb.	
II Laches.	Headache gets worse from the slightest touch: *Mezer.*
Lam. alb.	
II Mezer.	Pressing pain on left temple gets worse from touch or the pressure of the hair: *Agar.*
Ruta.	
Stramon.	
Silic.	Great restlessness, head rolls from side to side; very sensitive to the least touch: *Colchic.*
II Thuya.	

On being touched goose-skin on arms and thighs; feels as if sore and raw, anxiety and restlessness: *Lam. alb.*

Starts from sleep with a scream when touched ever so lightly: *Ruta.*

Starting at the least touch: *Kali carb.*

Stroking and touching the painful foot relieves: *Hepar.*

She is so sensitive, the least touch makes her furious: *Thuya.*

Pressure. Anxiety, has to undo the clothes and seek the open air: *Sulphur.*

Everything is too narrow, with whining: *Platin.*

Leaning hand against anything increases loss of thinking: *Lycop., Ol. anim.*

A feeling as if she would be crazy if she did not hold tightly upon herself: *Lil. tigr.*

Tight shoes make him very irritable: *Kreosot.*

Pressure on sternum worse when sitting bent: *Cinch. off.*

Shaking. Sensitive to the slightest shaking of the floor: ∎*Nux vom.*

Children do not want to step or walk, and cry piteously: *Chamom.*

Uttering sharp cries now and then, especially when shaken: *Stramon.*

Hurts. A prick in the finger with a needle frightens her so, she grows faint and cold, has to lie down: *Calc. ostr.*

When shaving fear of cutting himself: *Calad.*

Will not have the wound touched: *Natr. mur.*

Delirium after a blow or concussion of the brain: *Bellad., Hyosc., Opium, Stramon., Veratr.;* fainting or convulsions: *Hyper.*

Stupor after a blow on the head: *Arnic., Cicut., Conium, Pulsat., Rhus tox.*

MODEL CURE.

Headache after a fall on occiput, in a robust young lady, was combined with a sensation as if being lifted up high into the air; she was tormented by the greatest anxiety, that the slightest touch or motion would make her fall down from this height: *Hyper.*—C. Hg.

PASSIVE MOTIONS.

Ant. crud.
Ant. tart.
Arsen.
Bellad.
∎ Bromium.
∎∎ Chamom.
∎ Cina.
∎∎ Kali carb.
Mercur.
Pulsat.
∎ Rhus tox.
Squilla.
Staphis.
Sulphur.
∎ Veratr.

Children want to be carried, but very slowly: *Pulsat.;* very quickly: *Arsen.;* and even to be shaken: *Veratr.*

Want it quicker and quicker: *Bellad.*

Crying ceases when carried: *Chamom.;* in dysuria: *Staphis.*

The child cannot be quieted unless carried on the arm: *Chamom.;* cannot sleep without it: *Cina.*

Children want to be carried continually: *Ant. tart., Kali carb.*

Restlessness, child wants to be carried: *Sulphur.*

The child grunts and groans when it wants to be carried or when it wants to go to stool: *Pulsat.*

Child wants to be carried, but very quickly; it says, "run," "run," with croup: *Bromium.*—Lippe.

Teething child of twelve months wants to be carried about or at least shaken, all night long, with cough and inclination to bite: *Veratr.*

Dislike to being carried: *Bellad.,* ∎∎*Bryon.;* wants to lie quiet: *Chamom.*

The child cannot bear motion sideways: *Coffea.*

Anxious feeling in epigastrium, as in quick, passive motion, like that in a swing: *Lycop.*

When danced up and down, the child makes an anxious face during the downward motion: *Borax.*

With a quick, downward motion, the child seems afraid to fall: ∎∎*Borax.*

Riding in Carriages. Anxious feeling when driving down hill, as if it would take away his breath: *Borax, Psorin.*

Anxiety from riding in a carriage: *Borax, Laches., Psorin.*

Cardiac anxiety when driving in the morning: *Zinc. cyan.*

Fearful and restless when riding; vertigo and short breathing: *Sepia.*

Apprehension when driving in open air: *Laches.*

When travelling, familiar places appear strange: *Rhus rad.*

When driving, unconsciousness: *Gratiol.;* loss of consciousness for a moment: *Silic.*

When riding out inward mental weakness; thinks he must give up practice: *Osmium.*

Great aversion to all kinds of driving, followed by great desire for it, which cannot be satisfied quickly enough even in bad weather: *Psorin.*

Seasickness. Disgust for everything: *Coccul.;* fear, with contraction of the sphincter muscles: *Bellad.;* wishes to die: *Sepia.*

SKIN.

Itching. Itching pricking all over the body, with great anxiousness: *Petrol.*

Itching causes sadness: *Psorin.*

Itching on going to sleep makes him very impatient: *Osmium.*

General restlessness, with itching: *Cinnab.*

Itching makes him angry: *Apis.*

Tickling all over the body, with irresistible inclination to laugh: *Sulphur, Zincum.*

Itching, with irritability: *Stramon.*

Itching from head to body, with excitement: *Codein.*

Unbearable itching: *Carb. sulph., Psorin.*

Voluptuous itching, like a flea bite, drives to distraction: ❚❚*Psorin.*

Heat in skin, with slow recollection: *Chin. sulph.*

Anxiousness, with red spots on hands, which are not hot but tremble: *Pulsat.*

Dark red spots, with strong memory: *Bellad.*

Anxiety, with breaking out of black spots: *Laches.*

Jaundice, with quiet manner: *Cuprum.*

Gets very sad about the eruption: *Psorin.*

Timid and shy, with measles: *Stramon.*

Anxiety before a rash, or dullness: *Stramon.*

Sad and dejected after nettle rash: *Natr. mur.*

Burning eruption, with great anxiety: *Arsen.*

Vesicular eruption, causing moaning and weeping: *Bellad.*

Dry itching tetter, with anxiousness: *Ledum.*

Afraid of falling into delirium, with scarlatina: *Cuprum.*

Lectrophobie, will not stay in bed, with scarlatina: *Cuprum.*

Violent delirium in suppressed scarlatina: *Apis.*

MIND AND DISPOSITION.

Delirium in neglected measles : *Cuprum.*

Mania after suppressed erysipelas : *Cuprum.*

Mania after suppressed eruption : *Arsen., Bellad.*

Delirium, with itching vesicles which exude a yellow fluid; scales from under which exudes offensive ichor : *Plumbum.*

An ulcer gets worse from a fright : *Laches.; Silic.* cured it.

Cardiac anxiety, pain in the wounded foot and lameness in right arm each year, when the time comes round in which she was bitten : *Laches.*

Yellow skin, with indifference : *Laches.*

Phagadenic ulcers are very painful to touch, with impatience : *Mercur.*

TEMPERAMENTS AND CONSTITUTIONS.

NOTE.—Fashions have no reasons. After Galen had become the sole ruler during the downfall of the sciences, his four temperaments were generally adopted and the Arabians adorned them with their astrological nonsense. After the awful crush by Hohenheim of the worshipped system and after the arabesques of astrology had been demolished by Copernicus, the four temperaments were kept up like the four seasons, and used as very convenient boxes, around which some later writers made pigeon-holes. In this way the classification is kept up and highly esteemed by non-observers.

At the beginning of our collection we will put what Hahnemann said, who was too great an observer to adopt corrupt doctrines.

HAHNEMANN'S REMARKS.

Persons of careful, zealous, fiery, passionate temperament, or deceitful, malicious and quarrelsome disposition : *Nux vom.*

Changeable mood, from cheerfulness to weeping; tender-hearted, sensitive disposition : *Ignat.*

Disposition to hide grievances : *Ignat.*

Timid, tearful disposition; inclined to brood over grievances and vexations in silence : *Pulsat.*

Mild, yielding disposition : *Pulsat.*

Good-natured, mild; sometimes light-hearted, careless, kind, good-hearted and mischievous : *Pulsat.*

Slow, phlegmatic temperament : *Pulsat.*

Inclined to be angry and irritable; fever, with hot face, unquenchable thirst, bitter taste, nausea, anxiety and restlessness : *Chamom.*

CONTRADICTORY SYMPTOMS.

Hahnemann was the first who introduced the doctrine of counterindications, which is one of the most important, as he was the first not only to establish the main rule, but also all the important sub-rules of therapeutics.

In his lectures at Leipzig, 1818–20, he dictated to his class the following negative symptoms :

Rarely or never we can expect a quick or lasting effect from *Acon.* in quick, eventempered, calm and placid individuals; from *Nux vom.* in a mild, phlegmatic mood; from *Pulsat.* in gay and cheerful or obstinate dispositions; or from *Ignat.* in unchangeable characters, who are not subject to fright or vexation.

Remarks by Others.

Anxious, fearful, often desponding, unmanageable, imagines horrible things; wanton, his mind cannot be quieted; great nervous excitement and illusions: *Valer.*—Franz.

Mental excitement; gets beside himself, with howling and screaming about the least bodily or mental suffering: *Coffea.*—Stapf.

Restless temperament: *Acon., Arnic., Asar. can., Ignat.*

Nervous persons: *Pulsat., Veratr.*

Irritable disposition, nervous temperament, dry, meager, bilious, dark complexion, black or brown hair and eyes: *Bryon.*

For very particular, careful, zealous persons, inclined to get excited and angry, or of a spiteful, malicious disposition: *Nux vom.*

Malicious persons: *Anac., Nux vom.*

Sallow people, with cold limbs, haughty disposition when sick, mistrustful, slow comprehension, weak memory: *Lycop.*

Venous constitution, disposed to hemorrhoids and peevishness: *Sulphur.*

Mild persons who are easily offended: *Ignat.*—Bute.

Gentle disposition: *Bellad., Lycop., Pulsat.*

Sandy hair and inclination to great submissiveness: *Pulsat.*

Affectionate, blue eyed women: *Pulsat.*

Mild temperament, with children and women with blue eyes, light hair, fair complexion, delicate skin: *Bellad., Bromum.*

Mild, gentle disposition, inclined to be sad, desponding and tearful: *Pulsat.*

Yielding mind, inclined to be faint-hearted; anxious mood: *Silic.*

Mind and mood more or less affected in weak constitutions, with a delicate, tender skin: *Sepia.*

Thin skin, fair complexion, hemorrhages from the surface: *Coca.*

Thin, scrawny, cachectic subjects: *Sec. corn.*

Tall, slender, lean people, with fair skin, black hair, bright black eyes: *Phosphor.*

Emaciated; dirty white or brownish complexion: *Calc. phosph.*

Dwarfish people, children who do not grow, especially when caused by eating ice cream: *Baryt.*

Scrofulous constitution, large belly, weak ankles, head sweat, worse from uncovering: *Silic.*

Beginning of atrophy, with depression of mind: *Coca.*

Temperaments and Constitutions
According to Jahr, H. Gross, in his Comparative Materia Medica, and Others.

Lymphatic constitutions: *Arnic., Bellad., Iodium, Lycop., Mercur., Nux vom., Pulsat., Spongia, Sulphur.*

Leucophlegmatic constitutions: *Cinch. off., Lycop., Mercur., Plumbum, Sulphur.*

Lymphatic temperament; lean persons with a stooping gait: *Sulphur.*

Lymphatic and plethoric temperaments: *Bellad.*

MIND AND DISPOSITION.

Phlegmatic : **|** *Aurum*, **||** *Bellad.*, **|** *Capsic.*, **||** *Caustic.*, **|** *Chelid.*, **||** *Cyclam.*, **||** *Iodum*, *Laches.*, **||** *Mercur.*, **||** *Mezer.*, *Natr. mur.*, **||** *Pulsat.*, **|** *Seneg.*

Phlegmatic temperament, with an obstinate, irritable, faultfinding disposition : *Cyclam.*

Phlegmatic temperament, with mild, yielding, good-natured disposition : *Pulsat.*

Sluggish and morose, particularly phlegmatic constitutions : *Laches.*

Phlegmatic sanguine : *Arnic.*, *Nux vom.*, **||** *Opium*, **|** *Pulsat.*

Sanguine : *Acon.*, *Arnic.*, *Bromum*, *Ignat.*

Sanguine temperament in young girls who lead a sedentary life : *Acon.*

Sanguine nervous temperament, with a sensitive disposition, quick and lively perceptions : *Phosphor.*

Sanguine choleric : **|** *Coffea*, **||** *Ferrum*, *Nux vom.*, **||** *Phosphor.;* choleric sanguine temperament; malicious and irritable; dark hair : *Nux vom.*

Impulsive, sanguine temperament : **||** *Cicut.*

Choleric : *Acon.*, **|** *Arsen.*, *Bryon.*, *Caustic.*, *Chamom.*, *Coccul.*, **|** *Coloc.*, *Phosphor.*, *Sulphur.*

Choleric melancholic : *Arsen.*, *Laches.*, *Nux vom.*

Melancholic : *Ant. tart.*, **|** *Laches.*, **||** *Lycop.*, *Mercur.*

Melancholic phlegmatic (but cheerfully disposed) : *Pulsat.*

Melancholic, meager, weak people : *Laches.*

CHILDREN.

Compare Passive Motions, page 332.

NOTE.—The large collection which had been made, was much increased by adding the remarks from Guernsey's Obstetrics.

Feelings. Oversensitiveness: **|** *Acon.*, *Ant. crud.*, **||** *Ant. tart.*, **||** *Bellad.*, *Calc. ostr.*, **|** *Chamom.*, **||** *Mar. ver.;* with whooping cough : *Cuprum.*

Very sensitive to the least impression, mental or physical : *Staphis.*

Sadness. Inexplicable : *Calc. ostr.*, *Caustic.;* awaken in unhappy mood or distressed condition : *Laches.*

The least thing makes the child cry : *Caustic.*

Children suddenly become peevish, sad and disposed to cry, and vomit easily : *Pulsat.*

Crying, with restlessness, wants this thing and that, which, when offered, is pushed away : *Chamom.*

Melancholy and ill-natured, with drawing stitching pains along the spine : *Rhus tox.*

Fear : *Acon.*, *Bellad.*, *Caustic.;* of spectres : *Pulsat.;* at night of ghosts : *Carb. veg.*

Afraid of every one who approaches him : *Cuprum.*

Shrinking from every one : *Cuprum.*

Complains that it is falling : *Borax*, *Cuprum*, *Gelsem.*

Clings to something : *Borax;* with every attempt to lower the child from the arms of the nurse, even during sleep, it cries out and throws up its hands as from fear: *Borax.*

Great fear at the onset of cerebro spinal meningitis: *Acon.*

Fearful, restless and distressed; in brain diseases: *Acon.;* or afraid of something, starts as if in affright: *Opium.*

Fears the cough, avoids it as long as possible; in bronchial catarrh: *Phosphor.*

Seems frightened at its own starting: *Bellad.*

Afraid to go to bed: *Acon.*

Fear of sleeping on account of the frightful dreams: *Nux vom.*

Will not stay in bed but wants to lie on the lap: *Cuprum.*

Fright awakening, with starting eyes: *Bellad.*

Fear on awakening; in brain diseases: *Zincum.*

Fear on wakening, red face; in delayed small-pox: *Stramon.*

Shrinks from everything; measles do not come out: ▮*Stramon.*

Expression of fear; with a rash on the skin: *Acon.*

Diarrhœa from a fright: *Opium;* chorea: *Natr. mur.*

After fright, children weep and move arms and hands about: *Sambuc.;* convulsions, with starts: *Opium.*

Anxiousness: *Borax, Calc. ostr., Kali carb.*

Towards evening feverish heat, with anxiety, which lasts the greater part of the night; threatening hydrocephalus; *Zincum.*

Anxiety, with colic: *Aurum, Calc. phosph., Chamom.*

And oppression, as if the lungs were giving out; in scarlatina: *Calc. ostr.*

Anguish. Infants awake at night, with anguish; they are able to inhale but not to exhale: *Sambuc.*

Anguish in spasms: *Acon.*

Great anguish, with red or purplish streaks on the neck, back, etc.; meningitis: *Bufo sahit.*

Anguish in face, lies stretched out in semi-comatose condition; in brain diseases: *Aethus.*

In paroxysms day and night, during which it strikes its face or head with its hands, as though that afforded relief: *Arsen.*

Despondency; in chorea: *Nux vom.*

Distress. Awakening in distress; in diarrhœa: *Laches.;* after sleep, as if dying; in croup: *Laches.*

In breathing, until head and shoulders are raised to a sitting position: *Acon., Hyosc.,* ▮*Spongia.*

Great distress, with much cough; in pneumonia: *Mercur.*

Grief. Convulsions, if the child had been punished or reprimanded, and brought to bed immediately: ▮*Ignat.*

Jealous and much depressed, after a new baby takes the attention of the family away: *Ignat.,* ||*Hyosc.*

Indifference. Wishes to be kept quiet, seems to dread being moved: *Bryon.*

Sullen, unwilling to play during the day: *Cina.*

Nothing pleases the child for a moment: *Cina.*
Very listless, wants nothing and cares for nothing: *Phosph. ac.*
Indifference to everything; all the senses except hearing become dull: *Calc. ostr.*
Loses its accustomed brightness, and becomes quiet and inactive: *Lycop.*
Does not laugh, is not inclined to play or to amuse itself in any way: *Hepar.*
Lazy, unwilling to play or be active: *Baryt., Laches.*, a.m.m.

Apathy. The child lies in an apathetic condition, now and then sighing, and reaching with the trembling hands to the head: *Helleb.*
Apathetic, wants nothing and cares for nothing, but is restless; after scarlatina disappears suddenly: *Phosphor.*
In erysipelas: *Phosph. ac.;* with stupor; in brain disease: *Gelsem*

Feelings and Conations. Ill-humored: **I**Ant. tart., **II**Arsen., *Borax, Graphit., Pulsat., Silic.*
Very unamiable when getting awake: *Laches., Lycop.;* kicks off its coverings and behaves in an angry manner: *Kali carb.,* **I***Lycop.*
Awakens with ill humor: *Arsen.,* **II***Kali carb., Laches.,* **I***Lycop.*
Ill-natured and disagreeable, particularly after the siesta and towards evening; flightiness in sleep; hydrocephalus: *Zincum.*
Irritable and peevish on awakening: *Lycop.*
Child wants many things, which are rejected after being offered; choicest playthings or food are repelled with violence: *Cina.*
Ill humor, cry for things, which, after getting, they petulantly throw away; worse early in the morning: *Staphis.*
Want now this thing, now that: *Kali carb.;* even when in a cheerful mood: *Pulsat.*
Very unamiable, nothing pleases nor satisfies it, picks the nose; in bronchial catarrh: **I** *Cina.*
Gets very cross with the sniffles: *Chamom.*

Irritable, Fretful. Irritable disposition: *Apis;* peevish and fretful all the time: *Calc. phosph.;* irritable and fretful: *Chamom.;* irritable like hypochondriacs: *Nux vom.;* peevish, do not like to be looked at, spoken to, or even touched: *Cina.*
Fretful peevish, cries when looked at or touched; in summer complaint: *Ant. crud.*
Will not be looked at, wants to be alone; gets out of humor: **I***Ant. crud.,* **II***Arsen.,* **I***Chamom., Cina.*
Dislike to be spoken to: *Arsen., Chamom., Gelsem., Natr. mur., Natr. sulph., Nux vom., Rhus tox.;* weeps if spoken to: *Natr. mur.;* coughs: *Arsen.*
Will not be quieted, petting and caressing are of no use: *Cina;* worse from friendly persuasion. See page 89.
Irritable, wants to be alone; in brain diseases: *Nux vom.;* wrinkled forehead, screaming spells: *Helleb.*
Very irritable and fretful, distress after nursing: *Chamom.;* milk does not agree, vomits it up: *Aethus.*

Fretful, with alternate constipation and diarrhœa: *Nux vom.*

Very cross and fretful, with bloody mucous stools: ❙❙ *Chamom.*; one cheek red the other pale, must be carried to be appeased; in bronchial catarrh: ❙❙ *Chamom.*

Cross and troublesome as long as it does not sleep: *Cina.*

Frets and worries, not cross but sleepless: *Coffea.*

Irritable, sensitive, weeping and wakeful; in measles: ❙❙ *Coffea.*

Irritability early part of night, and very worrying and sleepless: *Podoph.*

Irritability almost amounting to mania: *Mar. ver.*

Perverse and Refractory. The child becomes disagreeable, hasty and hard to be managed: *Sulphur;* perverseness: *Calc. phosph.*

Extremely obstinate, throw themselves angrily on the floor when in the least opposed and cannot get their breath: *Thuya.*

When getting angry the coughing spell comes on: *Ant. tart.*

Peevish wrathfulness; wishes to vent itself in rage; it strikes, kicks, bites, etc.: *Carb. veg.*

Irritable when waking; scream, strike about them, do not wish to be spoken to: ❙ *Lycop.*, ❙ *Kali carb.*

The child stiffens its body, with peevishness: *Pulsat.*

Little children are very self-willed, inclined to fatten and have dilated pupils: *Calc. ostr.*

Mischievous, reckless and wanton: *Anac.*

Disobedient behavior: ❙❙ *Cinch. off.*

Disobedient without being in a bad humor: *Lycop.*

Supplicative mood, pleading for help, or very irritable, with raving and disposition to strike, bite and injure others; in chorea: *Stramon.*

Seems violent and destructive in its motions, speech indistinct, gets angry if not understood; in chorea: *Lauroc.*

Strikes its head or face with fists for relief; in brain disease: *Arsen.*; the head against the walls or on the floor: *Rhus tox.*

Disposed to bite everything: *Secal.*

Biting at the glass or spoon when drinking: *Cuprum;* striking and biting: *Carb. veg., Stramon.*; and tearing things: *Bellad.*; bites its fists: *Acon.*

Biting or grinding the teeth; in meningitis: *Bellad.*

Easily offended, worse from gentle persuasion, strikes about and at the attendants: *Helleb.*

ACTIONS AND EXALTATIONS.

Loquacity; staring, distorted eyes: *Hyosc., Stramon.*

After excessive laughing and playing, an attack of convulsions: *Coffea.*

Hasty and eager in drinking: *Bryon.*; hurried in all its motions: *Acon.*; hurried manner in taking food: *Caustic., Hepar.*

Nervous excitability, much crying; sleepless; seems as if it could not sleep at all: *Coffea.*

MIND AND DISPOSITION.

Excitement of nerves greater than that of the circulation; before scarlet fever: *Coffea.*
Excitability and fear, with worm diseases: *Stannum.*
Laughs one moment and cries the next: *Coffea.*
Quiet mood and sighing, alternating suddenly with weeping, timidity and anxiety: *Pulsat.*
Cross and irritable or indifferent and dull; in brain affections: *Cuprum.*
Now in a vexed, then in a laughing mood: I I *Borax.*

Sighing. Compare page 191.
Sighing, sobbing and crying; in brain diseases: *Ignat.*
Much sighing and groaning; excoriating nose and lips: I *Arum triph.*, I I *Mur. ac.*
The child grunts frequently during restless sleep: *Lycop.*
The child weeps and laments a great deal: *Cina.*
Sighing or moaning on second day of pneumonia: *Cuprum.*
Sighing and moaning, frightful visions, tottering gait, the knees give way: *Pulsat.*

Moaning. Moans a great deal, as though the moaning caused partial relief of suffering, with drowsiness; in brain diseases; half sleeping, half waking, with jerking of limbs; in dysentery; with every breath a hoarse cough, mucous rales large or crepitous; in pneumonia; drowsiness, sore throat; in measles; with whimpering and crying; in scarlet fever; grinding teeth in a stupid state; in dropsy; all this mostly with precocious children, blue eyes, fair skin: I I *Bellad.*
Moaning in sleep with half closed eyes, rolling the head in summer-complaint: I *Podoph.*
Moans at 3 A.M.: *Kali carb.*; latter part of night: *Rhus tox.*

Weeping and Whining: *Arsen., Bellad.,* I I *Borax, Camphor.,* I *Chamom.,* I *Cina,* I *Coffea, Graphit.,* I I *Hyosc.,* I I *Ignat.,* I I *Kali carb.,* I I *Lycop., Nitr. ac., Pulsat.,* I *Rheum,* I *Seneg., Silic.* Compare page 127 and page 304.
The boy gets involuntarily into a fit of weeping: I I *Alum.*
Crying and putting its hands to the back of the head, or boring the head into the pillow: *Bryon.*
Gets into a fit of crying and restlessness with the cough at night: *Sulphur.*
If you take the child by the hand to lead it, it cries terribly: *Cina.*
Sucklings refuse the breast, weep, start from sleep, grow pale and wilted: *Borax.*
Weep and toss about in sleep: *Kali carb.*; getting awake from sleep: *Bellad.*
Starting and jumping in sleep, with muttering, lamenting and whining: *Sulphur.*
Whining and crying, seems afraid to breathe: *Bellad.*

Crying. Cries and is unamiable: *Cina;* long continued: *Calc. ostr.;* hard: *Coloc.;* constant, with moaning: *Pulsat.*
Cries as if from being frightened by seeing hideous objects: *Stramon.*
Hides in corners, cries, feels hurt, and takes everything amiss: *Camphor.*
Cries pitifully when refused the least thing: *Chamom.*

ACTIONS AND EXALTATIONS. 341

Suddenly and ceasing suddenly, appearing as if nothing had been the matter: *Bellad.*

Whines, frets, gnaws at its fingers or fists, or something else during dentition: *Acon.;* worrying and grinding teeth: *Podoph.*

During and after nursing, or as soon as the child begins to take food: *Arsen.*

As from colic: *Aethus.;* and calling for water frequently: *Cina.*

Writhes and curls up double with colic: *Coloc.;* better when pressing hand on belly: *Coloc.*

With bellyache: *Cuprum.*

Cries horribly, turns blue all over; seems full of incarcerated flatus: *Senna.*

Crying with colic; relief is obtained by carrying it with belly resting on the nurses shoulder or pressing firmly against it: *Stannum.*

Cries and screams before passing water, relieved immediately afterwards: *Lycop.*

When crying, without being angry, breathing ceases: I I *Cuprum.*

Cries every time it coughs or even before, as though it dreaded it: *Arnic.*

Constant crying, with anxious countenance and great uneasiness; in pneumonia: *Acon.*

Cries at the attempt to put it down in cradle, taking hold of things near, as if afraid of falling: *Borax.*

If moved; in fever: *Bryon.*

Cries or laughs wih spasms: *Ignat.*

Cries, starts, jumps during sleep, rolls head from side to side; or after being cross and irritable, cries out during sleep, and if awakened, expression of fear; in brain diseases: *Zincum.*

Cries of discomfort whilst awaking from sleep or soon after: *Acon.*

Screaming and Weeping. When refused the least thing, if kindly spoken to it makes it worse, pupils easily dilated or contracted: *Bellad.*

The more they try by persuasion to quiet it, the worse it gets: *Calc. phosph.*

Cessation, puts its fists into its mouth; face pale, body cool: *Ipec.*

From agonizing pain in rectum and anus; with dysentery: *Colchic.*

Just previous to passing water: *Lycop.*

Day and night; with whooping cough: *Stramon.*

And violent trembling all over: *Ignat.*

And grasping with hands: *Calc. phosph.*

With the most curious and frightful contortion of limbs; in chorea: *Cicut.*

Turns and twists after a spasm until another occurs: *Cuprum.*

With the jerks during sleep: *Zincum.*

Before or during the spasm: *Opium.*

When "good" all day, screaming and restless all night: *Jalap.*

Awakening with screams as if in affright, clinging to something as if afraid: *Borax;* and starting in sleep: *Bellad.*

When getting awake: *Sulphur.*

And sleeplessness; in erysipelas: *Apis.*

In spells, loss of speech, unconscious, motionless; scarlatina struck in: *Zincum.*

Shrieks. Piercing cries, screams out suddenly and sharply during sleep, as from a stabbing, occurring more at night; when asked what hurts it, the reply is "nothing:" *Apis.*

Violent shrieking and screaming spells, at longer or shorter intervals: *Apis.*

"Cry cerebrale," sudden sharp outcries; in scarlatina: **I***Apis.*

Piercing shrieks: *Cuprum.*

Piercing cries awake the child from sleep, trembling all over: *Ignat.*

Shrieking out during sleep: *Cina.*

Restlessness: *Arsen., Chamom., Cina, Kali carb.;* irritable and whining: *Arsen.;* tosses about restlessly even when awake: *Cina.*

And anxiety, cries much, reaches for this thing and that, without taking anything: *Kali carb.*

Hot head, sore, as if bruised; in meningitis: *Arnic.*

Wants to be kept in motion almost constantly, to be rocked or carried about; in brain disease: *Cina.*

Gnaws its fist; stools hard and difficult: *Acon.*

Constant from a distress, which no change of posture seems to relieve; during dentition: *Acon.*

A little more comfortable during the day; but from 6 P.M. till 6 A.M. by rubbing, patting and tossing and worrying with the child, only a few short naps are obtained; during dentition: **I***Kreosot.*

Excitable, watery, dark stools: *Acon.*

Tossing too and fro, and very weak, worse after midnight; summer complaint: **II***Arsen.*

And sleeplessness, aversion to heat and covering, involuntary stools: *Secal.*

And distress; in dysentery: **II***Acon.*

The latter part of night; screaming spells; in dysentery: *Apis.*

And screaming in sleep, bright red pimples and constipation: *Apis.*

Sleeplessness and irritation from thread-worms: *Mar. ver.*

At night itching, stinging and burning of anus, nose and other parts: *Urt. ur.;* and tossing, which affords no relief: **I***Apis.*

Change of position affords temporary relief; in chorea: *Rhus tox.*

Before every attack of convulsions: *Arg. nitr.*

After midnight: *Arsen.;* from 4 P.M. till 8 P.M.: *Lycop.* Both in dropsy.

In-doors, wants to go into the air; in dropsy: *Pulsat.*

Before and with measles: **II***Acon.*

Cannot sleep, measles do not come out: *Apis.*

And uneasiness; in scarlet fever: *Apis.*

Restlessness and anxiety, every breath seems to be the last; in small-pox it seems to be retrogressing: *Apis.*

And tossing about; preceding convulsions in scarlet fever: *Arg. nitr.*

Worse after midnight; if measles disappear: *Arsen.*

And marked exhaustion after every movement; in scarlatina: *Arsen.*

And exhaustion; in black small-pox: *Arsen.*

And fever increasing about 3 A.M.; in scarlet fever: *Kali carb.*

At night, parotid glands swollen, suppurating: *Rhus tox.*

Tossing about; sordes on teeth and lips, shrinking eruption in confluent small-pox: *Rhus tox.*

Delirium. Calls for papa and mamma, although they are present and consoling: *Stramon.;* vision of dogs and cats: *Aethus.;* fears bed-clothes will catch fire: *Cuprum;* wild fancies; in brain diseases: *Act. rac.;* wild, strange look, red face, muttering, picking bed-covers; in brain diseases: *Hyosc.;* tossing and anguish; in meningitis: *Arsen.;* merry; in brain disease: *Stramon.;* starting and twitching; in summer complaint: *Bellad.;* unconsciousness in scarlet fever, with hot skin, sordes on lips and teeth, black crusts, glands swollen and hard as a stone: *Conium;* with very hot fever all night: *Bellad.;* with scarlet fever: *Ailanth.;* with jerks, twitching and moaning; in erysipelas: *Bellad.;* talking on going to sleep; erysipelas turns bluish: *Laches.;* say words they do not want to say; in scarlatina: *Cuprum.*

Rage. Bellowing in delirium: *Cuprum.*

Indomitable rage, horrible anguish, complain of having been poisoned: *Hyosc.;* and fury in paroxysms, suffering expression in face; cerebro spinal meningitis: *Canthar.;* anguish, delirium in paroxysms, wants to get out of bed and be uncovered; retarded small-pox: *Hyosc.*

The best, if children get angry and have spells of rage, is *Acon.*—G. BUTE.
Behave like maniacs from itching: *Platin.*

Stupor. With brain affections: *Cuprum;* ceases to make its wants known except by motions: *Stramon.;* stupid after waking; brain disease: *Opium;* stupor, constant involuntary motion of one leg and arm: *Apoc. can.;* does not notice surrrounding objects; in brain disease: *Stramon.;* when questioned loudly opens eyes, gazes stupidly and steadily, answers slowly: *Phosph. ac.;* with brown miliary patches; in scarlet fever: *Ailanth.;* eyes fixed: *Opium;* simile to *Opium,* which failed to relieve in scarlet fever: *Zincum;* drowsy, scarlet rash faintly developed: *Amm. carb.;* and delirium, restless tossing, turning and twitching: *Cuprum;* vacant staring, drowsy, answers no questions; in scarlet fever: *Hyosc.;* nervous excitability, illusion of the imagination, indistinct muttering; in scarlet fever: *Hyosc.;* dull and stupid, cares for nothing, wants nothing, notices nothing; retarded small-pox: *Phosph. ac.;* dull and drowsy in suppressed small-pox: *Ant. tart.*

NOTE.—The first thing a new born child does, is, it screams, and, as we can clearly hear, in a burst of anger and displeasure at the unwelcome change.

It is the first sign that there is a human soul within. No animals scream when born, not even monkeys, neither mother nor child.

A well-trained ear will know by the sound what the child means by its cry, also when it is older. In sleep the face shows the state of mind. We should avoid wakening a child or making it scream.

In our endeavors to find out even the slightest traces of a true image of the case before us, we must avoid all rough handling as much as the case will allow. Children will never afterwards trust; they cannot forget or forgive a stranger. Let the mother do as much as possible. We gain very little, if anything, by forcing their mouths open to see what we can just as well hear. Does it ever tell us what to give?

Hohenheim, the greatest master of the healing art before Hahnemann, says in the pledge, he proposes for young men before allowing them to go and heal the sick: Never leave a woman in the hour of her need, and never use force with a child.

In America the first was realized, may it be the land where the second also is acknowledged.

Young children who can talk, tell their ailments better than older persons, but we must warn the mother before hand never to resort to such suggestive queries, as: Does it not this or that to you? Do you not feel such or such a thing? As Hahnemannians, we ought to know that such inquiries never give us a true image of the case. See Introduction, p. 23.

WOMEN AND OLD PEOPLE.

Young fullblooded girls of lively disposition and placid complexion, inclined to blush: *Acon.*

Women get a dislike to their usual housework: *Citr. ac.*

Flies from her own children: *Lycop.*

In climacteric years great and anxious solicitude about her health; apprehension: *Silic.*

Mental derangement during climacteric years: *Aster., Laches., Pulsat., Therid.*

Old People. Premature old age, imbecility: *Coca.*

Send nurses away without whom they cannot do: *Fluor. ac.*

Elderly men find it more difficult to think in the morning: *Ambra.*

Great weakness of mind and body of old men: *Baryt.*

Weakly and nervous, with gastric complaints: *Coca.*

Crossness like that of children; cannot bear the weight of their arms lying on either side in bed, it awakens them: *Chamom.*

Aged persons get very fleshy: *Kali carb.*

OTHER DRUGS.
Some Remarks by Hahnemann.

Oversensitiveness after Nux vom.: *Acon.*

Oversensitiveness, anxious sensibility, overhastiness from Ignat.: *Coffea.*

Anxious beside himself, with coldness; a burning in brain after Veratr.: *Acon.*

Grief, with despair after Graphit.: *Arsen.*

Ill humor or fretfulness after Nux vom.: *Chamom.*

Ill humor, offended, suspicious, inclined to reproach after Lycop.: *Caustic.*

Anger or impetuosity after Anac.: *Coffea.*

Tearfulness, with chilliness or headache from Bellad.: *Pulsat.*

In drunkenness from Bellad.: *Wine.*

Muddledness from Stramon.: *Tabac.*

Stupor, madness or rage from Bellad.: *Hyosc.*

All acids cause anxiety; they do not agree: *Sulphur.*

Remarks of Others.

Dyers in blue become melancholy; dyers in red passionate.

After abuse of mercury excessive nervousness: *Nitr. ac.*

From smoking, internal uneasiness and discomfort: *Calad.*

After stopping the use of tea inability to make resolutions, especially in making choice of a remedy: *Thea*, high, has relieved.

The mind is enfeebled by liquor, although the patient knows what he is about: *Act. rac.*

Hears voices and sees animals after having taken alcohol often in small doses: *Arsen.*

Note.—Delirium tremens will be analyzed more fully in another volume.

APPENDIX.

CHAPTER I.

FRIGHT AND FEAR.
(See page 72.)

Ears. Starting with every noise: *Stramon.*
Paralysis caused by fright: *Natr. mur.*

SHOCK OF INJURY.
(See page 76.)

Great nervous depression: *Hyperic.*

GRIEF AND SORROW.
(See page 86.)

Face. Emaciation: *Phosphor.*
Appetite. Disgust for coffee or tea and no appetite for food: *Phosphor.*

EMOTIONS AND EXCITEMENT.
(See page 97.)

After hearing unpleasant news: ❙❙*Gelsem.*, ❙*Calc. phos.* (numbness).

CHAPTER VIII.

FACE.
(See page 135.)

Flushed face and hot head, with delirium and moaning: *Bellad.*

APPENDIX.

CHAPTER XV.

EATING.
(See page 148.)

After eating. Anxiety, with cold sweat on head and forehead, has to go into open air, dyspnœa, and stitches in r. side: *Merc.;* irritability after dinner: *Chamom;* pectoral anxiety, one and a half hours after dinner: *Phelland.*

CHAPTER XVII.

ANXIETY IN SCROBICULUM.
(See page 158.)

Abdomen distended, cold limbs, cold sweat, stupor with vomiting and purging: *Stramon.*

CHAPTER XX.

DIARRHŒA.
(See page 166.)

Hurried feeling; if an appointment is made patient becomes uneasy long before the time fixed and gets an attack of diarrhœa: *Arg. nitr.*

CHAPTER XXIV.

PARTURITION.
(See page 185.)

Fear of death during labor: **I** *Acon., Coffea.*
Childbed. Laughing mania with retained placenta: *Secale.*
Puerperal fever; enormous distension of abdomen: *Coffea.*

CHAPTER XXVI.

IMPEDED BREATHING WITH ANXIETY.
(See page 201.)

With every breath a loud noise as if it would be the last: *Calc. ostr.*

CHAPTER XXVII.

COUGH.
(See page 205.)

Singing, with bronchitis: *Alumin.*

CHAPTER XXXVI.

NERVES.

(See page 244.)

Slight tremor in all the joints, with a happy mind: *Cyclam.*
Forgetfulness with subsultus tendinum: *Camphor.*
Convulsions (see page 247). Gets angry if not understood, yet talks incoherently before spasms: *Bufo.*
Delirium and stupor with the spasms: *Æthusa.*
Oversensitive to pains (see page 328). *Colocyn.*

CHAPTER XXXVII.

SLEEP.

(See page 266.)

Heavy languid sleep after suppression of the menses: *Helonias.*
On awaking (see page 273).
Ant. tart.,
Argent.,
Arsen.,
|Caustic.,
Cina,
|Ignat.,
|Ipecac.,
|Nitr. ac.,
|Nux vom.,
|Petrol.,
|Phosphor.,
Plumbum,
|Pulsat.,
|Rhus tox.,
|Scilla,
Thuja.
After awaking (see page 277).
Jacea.
|Lachesis.
||Lycopod.
Pulsat.

When waking in the morning (see page 277). Palpitation, with anxiety, after getting up: *Spigel.*

After loss of sleep (see page 279). Mentally tired, with bad taste, nausea, and languor: *Colchic.*

CHAPTER XL.

CHILL, HEAT, SWEAT.

(See page 303.)

Violent chill, toward evening, lasting several minutes, must lie down; followed by nausea and vomiting and spasmodic pain in chest lasting all night, with short breath and inward anxiety with profuse sweat on the head: *Kal.*

CHAPTER XLVI.

ERUPTIONS.

(See page 333.)

Threatens his family, wants to kill them, to set fire to the house, can be managed with difficulty; sits silent and motionless in the corner of the room; involuntary passage of urine and fæces; itch-like eruption on body breaking into open sores here and there: *Hepar.*

CHAPTER XLVII.

TEMPERAMENTS.

(See page 385.)

Hydrogenoid constitution: *Arg. nitr., Manganum.*

Very tender and sensitive disposition: *Ignat.*

Melancholic choleric temperament, occasionally in phlegmatic bloated persons (young men) with dark eyes, inclined to moodiness and inactivity; seldom indicated in persons with florid complexion and fine, soft, easily indented skin, nor in sanguine temperaments, excepting when melancholic or choleric, in which case it has acted well on women with freckles and red hair: *Lachesis.*

Hypochondriasis, with studious men, sitting too much at home, suffering with abdominal complaints and costiveness: *Nux vomica.*

Plump and full-blooded people: *Acon.*

Children (see page 336). Hasty drinking: *Bellad.*

Hasty eating: *Calad., Coffea.*

Talkative, with heavy tongue: *Dulcam.*

If crossed, pupils dilate: *Stramon.*

INDEX TO MODEL CURES.

NOTE.—These "Model Cures" were especially intended to fill up such spaces as otherwise would have remained blank, for it was considered desirable not to break the margin lists.

Some cures being such good illustrations were placed at the end of the paragraph to which they belong or even inserted in the middle of a page, but this exceptionally.

Many select cures had to be laid aside for want of suitable space. Some of these may be printed further on, and after the work is done a collection of cases made to be used as illustrations in a little book containing our practical rules.

Author.	Remedy.	Page.	Author.	Remedy.	Page.
Aegidi,	*Sabin.*,	237	Gross, Wm.,	*Ignat.*,	223
Attomyr,	*Ignat.*,	91	"	"	246
	Pulsat.,	91		*Psorin.*,	84
J. Bærtl,	*Arsen.*,	311	Haden,	*Colchic.*,	134
	Bellad.,	316	Hahnemann, 1840,	*Nux mosch.*,	109
	Nux vom.,	320	1796,	*Veratr.*,	164
Becker,	*Stramon.*,	272	Hartlaub, G.,	*Nux vom.*,	109
Bell, J. B.,	*Badiag.*,	214		*Rhus tox.*,	76
	Spongia,	214		*Stramon.*,	292
Berridge,	*Conium*,	109	Haynel,	*Arsen.*,	292
	"	171		*Nitr. ac.*,	108
	Laches.,	109		*Petrol.*,	292
Bethmann,	*Hyosc.*,	192		*Sepia*,	177
	Pulsat.,	179		*Thuya*,	226
	"	184	Helbig,	*Secal.*,	185
	Stramon.,	143	Hering,	*Coccul.*,	279
Bicking,	*Bellad.*,	98		*Laches.*,	208
	"	247		"	217
Bluff,	*Nux mosch.*,	250		"	266
Bönninghausen,	*Hyosc.*,	109		*Hyper.*,	332
Brennfleck,	*Psorin.*,	294		*Ox. ac.*,	222
Bute,	*Mancin.*,	251		*Zincum.*,	327
Caspar,	*Atrop.*,	262	Hermel,	*Platin.*,	296
Elwert,	*Conium*,	132	Jeanes,	*Lob. coer.*,	159
Engelhardt,	*Bellad.*,	169	Joussell,	*Merc. sol.*,	179
Farrington,	*Nux vom.*,	167	Kiesselbach,	*Bellad.*,	181
Finch,	*Laches.*,	252	Knorre,	*Petrol.*,	115
Goullon, Sr.,	*Caustic.*,	186	Lembke,	*Cuprum*,	264
Gross, Wm.,	*Acon.*,	226	Liedbeck,	*Osmium*,	197
	Arsen.,	212	Lippe,	*Calc. phosph.*,	90
	Cuprum,	200		*Gelsem.*,	302
	Ignat.,	178	Lorbacher,	*Nux mosch.*,	241

INDEX TO REMEDIES.

Author.	Remedy.	Page.	Author.	Remedy.	Page.
Malaise,	Pulsat.,	226	Schelling,	Arsen.,	161
Marcy,	Zizia,	132	Schmid,	Cupr. ac.,	108
Martin,	Borax,	276		Phosphor.,	181
J. C. M., an Austrian,	Veratr.,	181		Zincum,	96
Morgan, J. C.,	Acon.,	76	Schueler,	Opium,	169
	Amm. caust.,	109		Veratr.,	107
	Arnic.,	109	Seidel,	Aurum,	269
	Camphor.,	109	Sonnenberg,	Bellad.,	122
	Caustic.,	109	Stapf,	Hyosc.,	86
	Coffea,	109		Hyosc.,	109
	Cuprum,	188	Stens, Jr.,	Arsen.,	216
	Gelsem.,	76	Sztarovezky,	Pulsat.,	124
Müller, G. F.,	Hyper.,	134		Stramon.,	125
Müller, M.,	Platin.,	135	Tafft,	Ant. crud.,	192
N. N.,	Caustic.,	247	Thorer,	Hyosc..	119
	Lithium,	95	Tietze, Sr.,	Psorin.,	248
	Secal,	256	Trinks,	Stramon.,	292
	Xanthox.,	129	Von Tagen,	Chamom.,	266
Nankivell,	Digit.,	216		Eup. purp.,	266
Neumann,	Al. p. s.,	219	Wells, P. P.,	Spongia,	223
	Arsen.,	155	Wesselhœft, C.	Sambucus,	276
Nithak,	Sepia,	212	" W.,	Laches.,	216
Norton, C. R.,	Aethus.,	168	Whitting, C.,	Arsen.,	204
Raue,	Opium,	248	Williamson, W.,	Acon.,	208
Rentsch,	Calc. ostr.,	129		Podoph.,	159
Ruckert, Th.,	Pulsat.,	139		Thuya,	178
Schellhammer,	Stramon.,	264	Woost,	Veratr.,	226

INDEX TO REMEDIES.

Remedy.	Author.	Page.	Remedy.	Author.	Page.
Acon.,	Gross,	226	Arsen.,	Stens, Jr.,	216
	J. C. Morgan,	76		Whitting,	204
	Williamson,	208	Atrop.,	Casper,	262
Aethus.,	Norton,	168	Aurum,	Seidel,	269
Al. p. s.,	Neumann,	219	Badiag.,	J. B. Bell,	214
Amm. caust.,	J. C. Morgan,	109	Bellad.,	J. Bærtl,	316
Ant. crud.,	Tafft,	192		Bicking,	98
Arnic.,	J. C. Morgan,	109		"	247
Arsen.,	J. Bærtl,	311		Engelhardt,	169
	W. Gross,	212		Kiesselbach,	181
	Haynel,	292		Lindner,	224
	Neumann,	155		Sonnenberg,	122
	Schelling,	161	Borax,	Martin,	276

INDEX TO REMEDIES. 351

Remedy.	Author.	Page.	Remedy.	Author.	Page.
Calc. ostr.,	Rentsch,	129		Farrington,	167
Calc. phosph.,	Lippe,	90		G. Hartlaub,	109
Camphor.,	J. C. Morgan,	109	Opium,	J. C. Morgan,	109
Caustic.,	Goullon,	186		Raue,	248
	J. C. Morgan,	247		Schüler,	169
	N. N.,	109	Osmium,	Liedbeck,	197
Chamom.,	Von Tagen,	103	Ox. ac.,	C. Hg.,	222
Coccul.,	C. Hg.,	279	Petrol.,	Haynel,	292
Coffea,	J. C. Morgan,	109		Knorre,	115
Colchic.,	Haden,	134	Phosphor.,	Schmidt,	181
Conium,	Berridge,	104	Platin.,	Hermel,	296
	"	109		M. Müller,	135
	"	171		N. N.,	169
	Elwert,	132	Podoph.,	Williamson,	159
Cuprum,	W. Gross,	200	Psorin.,	Brennfleck,	294
	Lembke,	264		Wm. Gross,	84
	Morgan,	188		Tietze, Sr.,	248
	Schmid,	108	Pulsat.,	Attomyr,	91
Digit.,	Nankivell,	216		Bethmann,	179
Eup. purp.,	Von Tagen,	104		"	184
Gelsem.,	Lippe,	302		Malaise,	226
	Morgan,	76		Th. Rückert,	139
Hyosc.,	Bethmann,	192		Sztarovcszky,	124
	Bönninghausen,	109	Rhus tox.,	Hartlaub,	76
	E. Stapf,	86	Sabin.,	Aegidi,	237
	"	109	Sambuc.,	C. Wesselhöft,	276
	Thorer,	119	Secal.,	Helbig,	185
Hyper.,	C. Hg.,	332		N. N.,	256
	Müller, G. F.,	134	Sepia,	Haynel,	177
Ignat.,	Attomyr,	91		Nithak,	212
	W. Gross,	178	Spongia,	J. B. Bell,	214
	"	223		P. P. Wells,	223
	"	246	Stramon.,	Becker,	272
Laches.,	Berridge,	109		Bethmann,	143
	Finch,	252		Hartlaub,	292
	C. Hg.,	208		Schellhammer,	264
	"	217		Sztarovcszky,	175
	"	266		Trinks,	292
	W. Wesselhöft,	216	Thuya,	Haynel,	226
Lithium,	N. N.,	95		Williamson,	178
Lobel. coer.,	Jeanes,	159	Veratr.,	Hahnemann,	164
Mancin.,	Bute,	251		J. C. M.,	181
Mercur.,	Joussel,	179		Schüler,	197
Nitr. ac.,	Haynel,	108		Woost,	226
Nux mosch.,	Bluff,	250	Xanthox.,	N. N.,	129
	Hahnemann,	109	Zincum,	C. Hg.,	327
	Lorbacher,	241	Zinc. ox.,	Schmid,	96
Nux vom.,	J. Bærtl,	320	Zizia,	Marcy,	132

INDEX.

Abbreviations, 67.
Abdomen, chapt. 19, p. 34.
    pendulous, 185.
Abdominal complaints with anxiety and other concomitants, 160.
    diseased states, 165.
    diseases, sensations, with mental concomitants, 165.
Abridgment of names, 56.
Actions, of children, 339.
    during fever, 316.
Afternoon, 287.
    anxiety in, 288.
    desires and aversions in, 289.
    exaltations in, 290.
    feelings in, 287.
    feelings and conations in, 288.
    intellect in, 290.
After pains, 185.
Agitation, 240.
Ailments, better while thinking of, 100.
    from emotions and exertions of the mind, 71.
    from overexertion of mind and body, 108.
    owing to fear, 82.
All day, 286.
Alone, complaints when, 87.
Amenorrhœa, 178.
Anger, complaints after, 95.
Anguish during fever, 305.
    of heart, 213.
    with nausea, 153.
    during and after stool, 170.
Anus, 172.
Anxiety, 153, 306.
    with abdominal complaints, 160.
    in afternoon, 288.
    ailments after, 82.

Anxiety, on awakening, 273.
    with orgasm of blood, 224.
    bodily conditions with, 307.
    with impeded breathing, 201, 346.
    before, during and after catamenia, 179.
    with pain in chest, 209.
    with other sensations in chest, 210.
    chill, heat and sweat with, 312.
    with colic, 162.
    with constriction and oppression, 209.
    with cough, 205.
    with dreams, 269.
    in evening, 293.
    with fever, 306.
    with gastric symptoms, 157.
    with headache, 113.
    heat and cold with, 307.
    heat and sweat with, 306.
    after midnight, 267.
    with nausea, 153.
    nightly, 267.
    with pains, 328.
    pectoral, 208.
    præcordial, 160.
    in scrobiculum, 158, 346.
    and sleep, 267.
    preventing sleep, 260.
    with sleeplessness, 263.
    when speaking, 142.
    during and after stool, 170.
    with toothache, 141.
    vomiting, 156.
    with weakness, 252.
Anxiousness, see anxiety.
Anxious face, 139.
Apathy, 252.
Appearance of eyes, 125.
Appetite, diminished, 147.

INDEX.

Apprehensions during fever, 305.
Arrangement, 26.
Attacks or spells, 324.
Autumn, 302.
Aversions during fever, 317.
    to food or drink, 147.
Awakening or being woke, 273, 347.
    after, 277, 347.
    anxiety on, 273.
    apprehension on, 273.
    exaltations on, 275.
    fear and fearfulness on, 273.
    feelings on, 273.
    feelings and conations on, 275.
    intellect on, 275.
    in morning, feelings on, 277.
Back and neck, 227.
    coldness of, 228.
Bed, driving out of, 243.
    covering, effects of, 298.
Bearing down pains, 175.
Black before eyes, 124.
Blindness, 124.
Blood, loss of, 330.
Body, complaints after over-exertion of, 108.
    and mind weak, 249.
Bodily symptoms connected with the mind, 70, 91.
Bones, 330.
    of skull, 120.
Book, how to use this, 23.
Breakfast, complaints after, 149.
Breasts, 186.
Breathing difficult, 203.
    impeded, with anxiety, 201, 346.
    quick, 199.
    short, 199.
    slow, labored, panting, 200.
Bowels, looseness of, 167.
    aversions, with, 168.
    conations, with, 168.
    exaltations, with, 168.
    feelings neutral, with, 167.
    feelings painful, with, 167.
    feelings pleasurable, with, 167.
    feelings unpleasant, with, 167.
    irritability, with, 168.
    productions, with, 168.
Cancer of mammæ, 186.
Cardiac anxiety, 213.
Carotids throbbing, 227.
Carriages, complaints from riding in, 333.

Catamenia, anguish of heart during, 214.
    with anxiety, anguish, apprehension, 179.
    conations during, 180.
    too copious, 177.
    delirium during, 181.
    depression during, 181.
    exaltations during, 180.
    ill humor during, 180.
    insanity during, 181.
    irritability during, 180.
    with mental concomitants, 179.
    rage during, 181.
    sadness during, 179.
    vexation during, 180.
    weeping during, 196.
Changes according to time, chapt. 41, p. 43.
Cheeks, hot, 135.
    hot and red, 136.
    red, 137.
Chest, diseases of, 212.
    inner, and lungs, chapt. 28, p. 37
    pain, with anxiety, 209.
    outer, chapt. 30, p. 38, 226.
    sensations in, with anxiety, 210.
Childbed, 186.
    after, 186.
Children, 336, 348.
    actions and exaltations of, 339.
    anguish of, 337.
    anxiousness of, 337.
    apathy of, 338.
    conations and feelings of, 338.
    crying of, 340.
    delirium of, 343.
    distress of, 337.
    fear of, 336.
    feelings of, 336.
    grief of, 337.
    indifference of, 337.
    irritability of, 338.
    moaning of, 340.
    rage of, 343.
    restlessness of, 342.
    sadness of, 336.
    screaming and weeping of, 341
    shrieking of, 342.
    sighing of, 340.
    stupor of, 343.
    weeping of, 340.
Chill, heat, sweat, 303, 347.
    actions during, 316.

354 INDEX.

Chill, heat, sweat, anger during, 315.
    anxiety during, 306.
    aversions during, 317.
    changeable mood during, 314.
    character during, 322.
    complaining and lamenting during, 316.
    confusion of mind during, 320.
    crying during, 317.
    delirium during, 322.
    depression during, 314.
    desires during, 317.
    desire to talk during, 317.
    despair during, 313.
    difficult comprehension during, 320.
    dislike to talk during, 317.
    dullness during, 320.
    ecstasy during, 321.
    exaltations during, 317.
    excitability during, 317.
    feelings and conations during, 314.
    unpleasant feelings with, 313.
    fright during, 319.
    ill-humor during, 314.
    illusions during, 321.
    impatience during, 315.
    intellect during, 321.
    bright intellect during, 319.
    irritability during, 315.
    listlessness during, 314.
    mania during, 322.
    moroseness during, 315.
    rage during, 323.
    reproductions during, 323.
    restlessness during, 318.
    shunning men during, 314.
    sighing and groaning during, 316.
    singing during, 316.
    stupefaction during, 323.
    suicidal disposition during, 313.
    thinking, mental exertion during, 319.
    unconsciousness during, 323.
    vanishing of thought during, 323.
    vexatious mood during, 316.
    weakness of memory during, 324.
Clairvoyance, 239.
Coition, after, 174.
Cold, heat and sweat, feelings during, 303.
    anguish and fear during, 305.
    apprehension during, 305.
    dejection during, 304.
    fear of death during, 305.
    melancholy during, 305.

Cold, sadness during, 304.
    tearful mood during, 304.
Coldness of head, 119.
Colic with anxiety, 162.
    other mental concomitants, 163.
Coma, 265.
Company, better in, 87.
Complaints after laughing, 71.
    after mental exertion, study, meditating, etc., 104.
    after talking, speaking, conversing, 101.
    before, during and after urination, 173.
Conclusion, 68.
Conditions and concomitants of pain, chapt, 43, p. 50.
    mental, of cough, 297.
Congestion of heart, 223.
    to head, 117.
Constipation, 169.
Constitutions, 334, 335.
Constriction and oppression, with anxiety, 209.
Conversation, complaints after, 101.
    of others increases suffering, 90.
Convulsions, 247, 346.
    actions during, 248.
    with or without consciousness, 247.
    depression during, 248.
    desires during, 248.
    with feelings, 247.
    after fright or fear, 247.
    productions during, 248.
    reproductions during, 248.
    after shock of injury, 247.
Coryza, 132.
Costiveness and constipation, 169.
Cough, chapt. 27, p. 37, 205, 346.
    with anxiety, 205.
    conations with, 206.
    causes and conditions, 207.
    from emotions, 207.
    exaltations with, 207.
    feelings with, 205.
Countenance, 133.
Covering, 298.
Crying and screaming, 198.
    of children, 340.
Dark, worse in the, 121.
Day, all, 286.
    times of, 281.
Daylight, better from, 121.
Dejected during fever, 304.

INDEX. 355

Delirium, before sleep, 261.
   of children, 343.
Depression, 251.
   during fever, 304.
Deranged mind during fever, 317.
   with headache, 116.
Desire for food and drink, chapt. 14, p. 33, 147.
   for light, 121.
   for open air, 298.
Desires during fever, 317.
Diarrhœa, 167, 346.
Difficult breathing, 203.
Digestion, complaints during, 152.
Dilated pupils, 124.
Discomfort, indisposition, 254.
Diseases of chest, 212.
   of heart, 214.
Dislike to be spoken to, 89.
Dreams, with anxiety, 269.
Drink, aversion to, 147.
   desire for, 147.
Drinking, before, while and after, 148.
   complaints after, 152.
Drugs, 344.
Dysmenorrhœa, 178.
Dysphagia, 145.
Ear, outer, 131.
Earache, 131.
Eating and drinking, before, during and after, chapt. 15, p. 33, 148, 345.
   better while, 148.
Eating, anxiety after, 150, 345.
   better after, 148.
   complaints after eating too much, 149.
   complaints while, 148.
   particular food, 152.
   ill humor after, 150.
   indifference after, 150.
   mental states after, 149.
   sadness after, 149.
   worse before, 148.
Ebullition of blood, 223.
Ecstasy, 239.
Emaciation, 330.
Emissions, seminal, 174.
   of wind, 166.
Emotions, complaints after, 97, 345.
   looseness after, 166.
   palpitation from, 222.
   trembling after, 244, 346.
Epigastric region, chapt. 17, p. 34.

Epileptic spasms, 247.
Eructations, 153.
Eruptions, 333, 347.
Evening, 291.
   actions in, 296.
   anguish in, 294.
   anxiety in, 293.
   apprehension in, 292.
   bodily conditions in, 293.
   care and sorrow in, 291.
   delirium in, 298.
   desires and aversions in, 296.
   fear in, 294.
   feelings in, 291.
   ill humor in, 295.
   intellect in, 297.
   irritable, fretful and peevish in, 295.
   restlessness in, 297.
   weeping in, 296.
Exaltations on awakening, 275.
   during fever, 317.
   before sleep, 261.
   and sleeplessness, 262.
Excitable, agitated, 240.
Excitement, after, 97, 345.
Exertion, worse after, 236.
   of eyes, 123.
   headache from, 102.
   of mind, followed by looseness, 166.
Exhalation, 199.
External head, chapt. 4, p. 29.
Eyes, 124.
   appearance of, 125.
   better with closed, 122.
   black before, 124.
   after closing, 121.
   dark around, 128.
   exertion of, 123.
   fixed, 125.
   movements of, 127.
   on opening, 122.
   pain in, 126.
   pupils of, 124.
   red, 127.
   staring, 125.
Eyebrows, 128.
Eyelids, 127.
Face, chapt. 8, p. 32, 135, 345.
   anxious, 139.
   earthy pale, 139.
   flushed, 137.
   flushes of heat of, 135.

356   INDEX.

Face, hippocratic, 139.
    hot and red, 136.
    lower part of, chapt. 9, p. 32.
    motions of, 134.
    paleness of, 138.
    red, with mania, 138.
    skin of, 140.
    sweat of, 136.
    swelling of, 140.
Faceache, 133.
Faint-heartedness, 252.
Falling, 256.
Fatigue, 254.
Fear, 72, 345.
    ailments owing to, 82.
    in dark, 121.
    of death, 305.
    during fever, 305.
    when others come near, 331.
Features, 133.
Feeble, mind and body, 249.
Feelings, pleasant during fever, 303.
    unpleasant during fever, 313.
    and conations during fever, 314.
Feet, 232.
    coldness of, 233.
    heaviness of, 232.
    sensations in, 232.
    soles of, 233.
Female organs, chapt. 23, p. 35.
    inner organs, 175.
    outer parts, 182.
Fever, chapt. 40, p. 43, 303.
    actions during, 316.
    aversions during, 317.
    desires during, 317.
    exaltations during, 317.
    intellect during, 321.
    reproductions during, 323.
    restlessness during, 318.
Fingers, 230.
Fixed eyes, 125.
Flatulency, 165.
Flatus, emission of, 166.
Flightiness, 265.
Flushes of heat, 135.
Flushed face, 137.
Food, aversion to, 147.
    desire for, 147.
    and drink, desire for, chapt. 14, p. 33.
Forenoon, 284.
    actions in, 285.

Forenoon, conations in, 285.
    desires and aversions in, 285.
    feelings in, 284.
    intellect in, 285.
Fright, spasms from, 246.
    starting from, 246.
    twitching from, 246.
Fright and fear, 72, 345.
    convulsions after, 75.
    debility after, 75.
    diarrhœa after, 74.
    sleep after, 75.
    suffocation after, 75.
    trembling after, 75.
    twitchings after, 75.
Fullness of head, 117.
Gaping and yawning, 257.
Gastric symptoms, chapt. 16, p. 33, 153.
    with anxiety, 157.
Grief and gloom, 251.
    and sorrow, 86, 345.
Groaning, 192.
Hæmorrhoids, 172.
Hands, 229.
    coldness of, 230.
    heat of, 230.
    motions of, 229.
    outside of, 230.
    sensations in, 229.
    sweat of, 230.
    trembling of, 229.
    weakness of, 230.
Happy surprise, 71.
Head, coldness of, 119.
    heat in, 117.
    heat of, 119.
    movements of, 119.
    outer, 118.
    positions of, 119.
    rush of blood to, 117.
    sensation of fullness, 117
    sweat of, 119.
    whole outer, 121.
Head symptoms, 110.
    with headache, 112.
    according to locality, 110.
    according to sensations, 111.
Headache and affections of inner head, chapt.
    3, p. 29.
    with anxiety, 113.
    external, chapt. 4, p. 29.
    with ill humor, 114.

INDEX. 357

Headache, with diminished intellect, 115.
    with deranged mind, 116.
    from exertions of mind, 102.
    with restlessness, 115.
Hearing and ears, chapt. 6, p. 31, 128.
    diminished sense of, 130.
Heart and circulation, chapt. 29, p. 38.
    diseases of, 214.
    anguish of, 213.
    palpitation of, 218.
    palpitation of, with bodily symptoms, 219.
    rush of blood to, 223.
    sensations in, 217.
Heartache, 215.
Heat, effects of, 298.
    flushes of, 135.
    in head, 117.
    of head, 119.
    and mental symptoms, 303, 347.
Heaviness of mind and body, 255.
Hiccough, 153.
Hippocratic face, 139.
Hoarseness, 187.
Homesickness, 84.
Hot cheeks, 135.
How to use this book, 23.
Howling, 197.
Hunger, 146.
Hurts, 332.
Hypochondriac regions, chapt. 18, p. 34, 159.
    during fever, 305.
Idle, worse from being, 239.
Ill humor, worse from friendly persuasion, 89.
    with headache, 114.
    and weakness, 253.
Immovable pupils, 124.
Impeded breathing, 201, 346.
Index to chapt. 43, p. 48.
Indifference, 252.
Indolence, 255.
In-doors, better, 300.
    worse, 299.
Inhalation and exhalation, 199.
Inhalation, deep, 200.
Injuries, shock of, 76, 345.
Inner chest and lungs, chapt. 28, p. 37.
Intellect, during fever, 321.
    headache with diminished, 115.
Intellectual work, headache from, 102.
Intermissions, 324.

Introduction, 11.
Involuntary stool, 171.
Irritability with weakness, 250.
Itching, 333.
Jaws, 140.
Jealousy, 86.
Joints, 330.
Joy, 71.
Knees, 231.
Labor pains, 185.
Lameness, 256.
Laughing, 189.
    complaints after, 71.
    spasmodic, 190.
    alternating with weeping, 197.
Larynx, chapt. 25, p. 37.
Larynx and windpipe, 187.
Lectrophilie, 89, 239. Add Veratr.
Lectrophobia, 89, 239. Add Cupr., Acon.
Legs and calves, 232.
Leucorrhœa, 182.
Light, desire for, 121.
    shunning, 122.
Lightness, 239.
Limbs, upper, chapt. 32, p. 39, 228.
    motions of, 228.
    sensations in, 228.
Limbs, lower, chapt. 33, p. 39, 231.
    motions of, 231.
    sensations and conditions of, 231.
Limbs, all the, chapt. 34, p. 39, 233.
    cold, heat, sweat of, 234.
    heaviness in, 234.
    lameness, 234.
    pain in, 233.
    sensations in, 233.
    trembling in, 234.
    twitching in, 234.
    want of strength in, 234.
Limitation, 56.
Lips, 140.
List of names and their abridgments, 57.
Liver, region of, 159.
Locality of head and mental symptoms, 110.
Loins, 166.
Looked at, will not be, 89.
Loss of sleep, after, 279.
Looseness following emotion and exertion, 166, 167.
Love, ailments after, 85.
Malacie, 176.

Male functions and organs, chapt. 22, p. 35.
Marks and signs, 67.
Meditating, complaints after, 104.
Melancholy during fever, 305.
Menorrhagia, 177.
Mental causes and conditions, 207.
    causes of cough, 201.
    states after eating, 149.
    complaints at night, 270.
    complaints before, during and after stool, 170.
    concomitants, 205.
    concomitants, with weakness of body, 251.
    exertion, better from, 103.
    complaints after, 104.
Mesmerizing, 331.
Metritis. 176.
Metrorrhagia, 177.
Mind and disposition, chapt. 1, p. 29, 69.
    complaints from over-exertion of, 108.
    headache with deranged, 116.
    headache from exertions of, 102.
    and body, loss of control of, 256.
    and body weak, feeble, relaxed, 249.
    symptoms during pregnancy, 182.
Moaning and groaning, 192.
Moon, phases of, 325.
Morning, 281.
    aversions in, 282.
    awakening in, 277.
    depressions in, 283.
    exaltations in, 283.
    feelings on awakening in, 277.
    feelings in, 281.
    feelings and conations in, 282.
    intellect in, 283.
    on rising in, 283.
Mortification, complaints after, 90.
Motion, better from, 235.
    passive, 332.
    worse after, 236.
Mouth, inner, chapt. 12, p. 33, 143.
    froth about, 143.
    roof of, 144.
Movements, 235.
    of head, 119.
Music unbearable, 128.
Names, abridgment of, 56.
    list of, 57.
    notes to list of, 65.
Nausea, with anxiety, 153.

Neck and back, chapt. 31, p. 38, 227.
Nerves, chapt. 36, p. 41, 346.
Night, apprehension at, 270.
    delirium at, 272.
    dreams at, 271.
    excitability at, 270.
    fearfulness at, 270.
    ill humor at, 270.
    intellect at, 272.
    mental complaints at, 270.
    merriment at, 270.
    restlessness at, 271.
    sadness at, 270.
    sorrow at, 270.
    talking at, 272.
    weeping at, 270.
    whimpering at, 271.
Night walking, 266.
Noises, subjective, 130.
    unbearable, 129.
Nomenclature, our, 53.
Noon, 285.
Nose, 131.
    outer, 132.
Nosebleed, 131.
Nosodes, 66.
Nostalgia, 84.
Notes to list of names, 65.
Nursing, 186.
Old people, 344.
Open air, better in, 299.
    desire for, 298.
    walking in, 299.
Ophthalmia, 127.
Oppression with anxiety, 209.
Orgasm, with anxiety, 224.
Os uteri, rigid, 185.
Our nomenclature, 53.
Out-doors, better, 299.
    worse, 300.
Outer chest, 226.
    ear, 131.
    head, 118.
    whole, 121.
    nose, 132.
Overexcitability, 240.
Overexertion of mind and body, ailments from, 108.
Oversensitiveness, in fevers, 303.
    of hearing, 303.
    to pain. 328.
Overstudy, complaints after, 104.

Oxyopia, 121.
Pain, anxiety with, 328.
    aversions during, 329.
    bodily concomitants during, 329.
    in chest with anxiety, 209.
    exaltations during, 329.
    in eyes, 126.
    fear with, 328.
    intellect during, 329.
    oversensitiveness to, 328, 346.
    sadness with, 328.
    weeping with, 329.
Palate and throat, chapt. 13, p. 33. 144.
Paleness, 138.
Palpitation, 218.
    with bodily symptoms, 219.
    from emotions, 222.
    after emotions or exertions, 219.
    after mental exertions, 223.
Panting breathing, 200.
Parturition, during, 185, 346.
    fainting during, 185.
Passive motions and touch, chapt. 45, p. 52, 332.
Pectoral anxiety, 208.
Periodicities, chapt. 41, 324.
Persuasion, friendly, increases ill humor, 89.
Perverted vision, 123.
Phases of moon, 325.
Place, change of, 242.
Placenta retained, 185.
Positions, 237.
Position, change of, 242.
    kneeling, 238.
    leaning, 238.
    lying, 238.
    sitting, 237.
    standing, 237.
Præcordial anxiety, 160.
Pregnancy and parturition, chapt. 24, p. 36, 182.
    threatening abortion during, 184.
    chorea during, 184.
    conations during, 183.
    diarrhœa during, 184.
    feelings during, 182.
    gastric complaints during, 184.
    hæmorrhoids during, 184.
    pain in lumbar and pelvic regions during, 184.
    productions during, 183.
    toothache during, 183.

Pressure, complaints from, 331.
Prostata, 175.
Puerperal convulsions, 185.
Pulse, frequent, 224.
    full, 224.
    hard, strong, 225.
    irritable, 225.
    and mental states, 224.
    quick, 225.
    tense, 225.
    weak, small, 225.
Pupils, dilated, 124.
    immovable, 124.
Rage of children, 343.
Reading, when, 123.
Rectum and anus, chapt. 20, p. 34, 172.
Redness of face, 137.
Relations to space, chapt. 42, p. 44.
    to warmth, air and water, wind and weather; seasons, chapt. 39, p. 42, 298.
Relationship with other drugs, chapt. 48, p. 52.
Relaxed, mind and body, 249.
Remarks, 67.
Reproductions of mind during fever, 323.
Respiration, chapt. 26, p. 37.
Rest, position, motion, chapt. 35, p. 39.
    inclined to, 239.
    worse from, 239.
Restlessness, 242.
    of children, 342.
    during fever, 318.
    with headache, 115.
Riding in carriage, 333.
Rising, 236.
    on or after, 283.
Roof of mouth, 144.
Room, better in, 300.
    coming in, 300.
    worse in, 300.
Run away, desire to, 243.
Rush of blood to head, 117.
    to heart, 223.
Sacrum, 227.
Saliva, 144.
Scalp, 120.
Screaming, 198.
    of children, 341.
Scrobiculum, anxiety in, 158, 346.
Seasickness, 333.
Seasons, 302.
Sensations classified, chapt. 43, p. 44.

Sensations, in chest, with anxiety, 210.
  in chest, with other mental symptoms, 211.
  of fullness of head, 117.
  in head, 111.
  in heart, 217.
  in heartache, 215.
  peculiar, 327.
Sensorium, chapt. 2, p. 29.
Sexual desire, 173.
  decreased, 174.
  increased, 173.
Sexual organs, female, 175.
  female, outer, 182.
Shaking, complaints from, 332.
Shock after injuries, 76, 345.
Shoulder and other joints, 228.
Shrieks of children, 342.
Shunning light, 122.
Sides of body, 325.
  anxiety, with symptoms on l., 325.
  anxiety, with symptoms on r., 325.
  fretfulness, with symptoms on l., 326.
  fright, with symptoms on l., 326.
  fright, with symptoms on r., 326.
  screaming, with symptoms on l., 326.
  screaming, with symptoms on r., 326.
Siesta, worse after the, 280.
Sight and eyes, chapt. 5, p. 30; 121.
Sighing, 191.
Singing, 188.
Skin, chapt. 46, p. 52; 333.
  itching of, 333.
  of face, 140.
Skull, bones of, 120.
Sleep, chapt. 37, p. 41, 257, 347.
  and anxiety, 267.
  anxiety and bodily conditions during, 260.
  anxiety preventing, 260.
  before, 259.
  cold and heat during, 269.
  conditions after, 280.
  exaltations and delirium before, 261.
  fear before, 260.
  after loss of, 279, 347.
  skin during, 269.
  disturbed by restlessness, 263.
Sleepiness, 257.
  feelings with, 257.
Sleeplessness with anxiety, 263.
  with exaltation, 262.

Sleeplessness with grief, fear, vexation, 263.
Slumber, 265.
Smell and nose, chapt. 7, p. 31, 131.
Sobbing, 193.
Society, dislike to, 89.
Solitude, complaints with love of, 88.
  dislike to, 87.
  love of, 88.
Somnambulism, 239.
Sorrow, ailments after, 86, 345.
Space, chapt. 42, p. 44.
Spasms, 247.
Speak, inability to, 143.
Speaking, anxiety when, 143.
  complaints after, 101.
Speechlessness, 143.
Spleen, region of, 159.
Spoken to, dislike to be, 89.
Spring, 302.
Stages of life, chapt. 47, p. 52.
Staggering, tottering, 256.
Staring, 125.
Starting from fright, 246.
Stiffness of body, 256.
Stimulants, after taking, 152.
Stomach symptoms, with anxiety, 157.
Stooping, 236.
Stool, anguish, during and after, 170.
  anxiety, during and after, 170.
  before, during and after, 170.
  during and after, 170.
  involuntary, 171.
Stretching, 236.
Stupor of children, 343.
Subsultus tendinum, 246.
Suffocation, threatening, 204.
  after emotions and exertion, 204.
Sunlight, effects of, 298.
Supper, complaints after, 149.
Surprise, 71.
Sweat, 303, 347.
  of head, 119.
  of face, 136.
Swelling, 330.
  of face, 140.
Symptoms appear when thinking of them, 99.
Talk of others increases sufferings, 90.
Talking, 142, 187.
  complaints after, 101.
Taste, talk, tongue, chapt. 11, p. 32.
Taste, 142.
  bitter, 142.

INDEX.

Tears, 126.
Tearful mood during fever, 304.
Teeth and gums, chapt. 10, p. 32, 141.
    chattering of, 141.
    grinding of, 141.
Temperaments and constitutions, 334, 348.
Tenesmus, 171.
Thighs, 231.
Thinking of ailments makes them appear, 99.
    of something else, betters, 100.
    of ailments betters them, 100.
Thirst, 146.
Throat, 144.
    constriction in, 145.
    dryness of, 144.
    sensations in, 144.
    swelling of, 145.
Thunder-storms, feelings during, 302.
Times of day, chapt. 38, p. 42, 281.
Tissues, chapt. 44, p. 51, 330.
Toes, 233.
Tongue, 143.
Toothache, 141.
    with anxiety, 141.
    during pregnancy, 183.
Touch, 331.
Touched, fear of being, 331.
    worse from being, 331.
Trembling, 244.
    after emotions, 244.
    feelings with, 244.
    of parts or whole body, 245.
Unpleasant feelings during chill and fever, 303.
    feelings during fever, 313.
Upper limbs, 228.
Uterus, hourglass contraction of, 175.
Uterine symptoms, 176.
    congestion, 176.
Urinary organs, chapt. 21, p. 35.
Urination, before, during and after, 173.
Urine, copious, 173.
    scanty, 173.
Uropoetic organs, 172.

Use of this book, 23.
Vagina, induration of, 182.
Vaginal growths, 182.
Veins, 330.
Vexation, complaints after, 92.
    with indignation, 92.
Vision, perverted, 123.
    while reading perverted, 123.
    when writing perverted, 124.
Voice, 187.
Vomiting, with anxiety, 156.
Walking, better from, 235.
    worse while, 235.
    in open air, better, 299.
    out doors, worse, 301.
Warmth, air and water, seasons, chapt. 39, p. 42, 298.
Weak and sad, 251.
    mind and body, 249.
Weakness, 251.
    with anxiety, 252.
    intellect with, 253.
    with irritability, 250, 253.
    with mental and bodily concomitants, 254.
    nervous, 254.
Weather, effects of, 302.
Weeping, 126, 194.
    alternating with laughing, 197.
    better after, 127.
    better from, 197.
    during sleep, 196,
When awaking in morning, 277.
Whimpering during fever, 304.
Whining, 194.
Wind, emission of, 166.
Windpipe, 187.
Winter, 302.
Woke, being, 273.
Women and old people, 344.
Working, when, 237.
Writing, when, 123.
Yawning, 257.

HOMOEOPATHIC PHARMACY - HAHNEMANN'S WAY

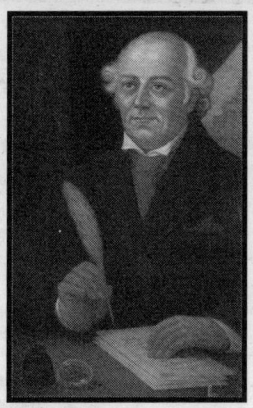

MASTER HAHNEMANN was a person who envisioned an entire system of medicine and then fully developed it into a powerful and practical tool within the span of a single life. This system of medicine he named it as Homoeopathy. In his books at various places he tells us about the various important facts and his observations which he found were important and gave us the cardinal principles of homoeopathy.

§ 1 Mission of Physician
§ 1(a)
THE physician's high and only mission is to restore the sick to health, to cure, as it is termed.

§ 4 Physician as Preserver of health
§ 4
He is likewise a preserver of health if he knows the things that derange health and cause disease, and how to remove them from persons in health.(a)

§ 6 Unprejudiced observed
§ 6
The unprejudiced observer—well aware of the futility of transcendental speculations which can receive no confirmation from experience—be his powers of penetration ever so great, takes note of nothing in every individual disease, except the changes

§ 3 Knowledge of Physician
§ 3
If the physician clearly perceives what is to be cured in diseases, that is to say, in every individual case of disease (*knowledge of disease, indication*), if he clearly perceives what is curative in medicines, that is to say, in each individual medicine (*knowledge of medicinal powers*), and if he knows how to adapt, according to clearly defined principles, what is curative in medicines to what he has discovered to be undoubtedly morbid in the patient, so that the recovery must ensue—to adapt it, as well in respect to the suitability of the medicine most appropriate according to its mode of action to the case before him (*choice of the remedy, the medicine indicated*), as also in respect to the exact mode of preparation and quantity of a required (*proper dose*), and the proper period for repeating the dose;—if, finally, he knows the obstacles to recovery in each case and is aware how to remove them, so that the restoration may be permanent, *then he understands how to treat judiciously and rationally, and he is a true practitioner of the healing art*.(a)

Doctor Hahnemann's say on

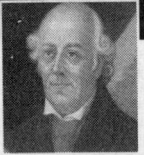

§ 123 Unadulterated Herbs

§ 123

Each of these medicines must be taken in a perfectly simple, unadulterated form; the indigenous plants in the form of freshly expressed juice, mixed with a little alcohol to prevent it spoiling; exotic vegetable substances, however, in the form of powder, or

§ 268 Quality Control to Check Genuinity of Herb

§ 268

The other exotic plants, barks, seeds and roots that cannot be obtained in the fresh state the sensible practitioner will never take in the pulverized form on trust, but will first convince himself of their genuineness in their crude, entire state before making any medicinal employment of them.[1]

[1] In order to preserve them in the form of powder, a precaution is requisite that has hitherto been usually neglected by druggists, and hence powders

B.Jain assures herbs from original source of cultivation or reliable vendors.

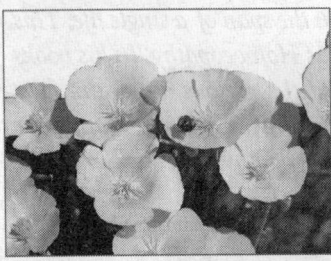

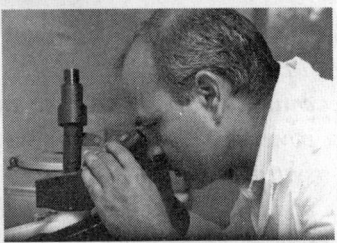

B.Jain QC Department checks variousparameters like TLC,UV, Infrared assuring genuinity of herbs and 100% accurate Mother Tincture.

§ 264 Genuine Medicine

§ 264

The true physician must be provided with *genuine medicines of unimpaired strength*, so that he may be able to rely upon their therapeutic powers; he must be able, *himself*, to judge of their genuineness.

At B.Jain we guarantee accurate herb and thus 100% accurate & pure Mother Tincture.

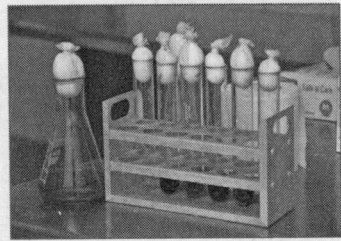

Mother Tincture and Dilutions

§ 269 Dynamization/Potentization

in the **Sixth Edition**, as follows:

[This remarkable change in the qualities of natural bodies develops the latent, hitherto unperceived, as if slumbering² hidden, dynamic (§ 11) powers which influence the life principle, change the well-being of animal life³. This is effected by mechanical action upon their smallest particles by means of rubbing and shaking *and through the addition of an indifferent substance, dry or fluid are separated from each other*. This process is called dynamizing, potentizing (development of medicinal power) and the products are dynamizations⁴ or potencies in different degrees.⁵]

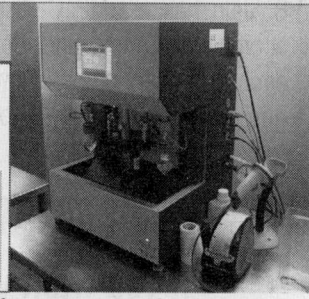

B. Jain latest K-Tronic potentiser for accuracy of potency (99.6% accuracy) of B. Jain Liquid Dilutions

§ 270 Pure Alcohol

§ 270

millionth part in powder form. For reasons given below (b) one grain of this powder is dissolved in 500 drops of a mixture of one part of alcohol and four parts of distilled water, of which *one drop* is put in a vial. To this are added 100 drops of pure alcohol³ and given one hundred strong succussions with the hand against a hard but elastic body⁴. This is the medicine in the *first* degree of dynamization with which small sugar globules⁵ may then be

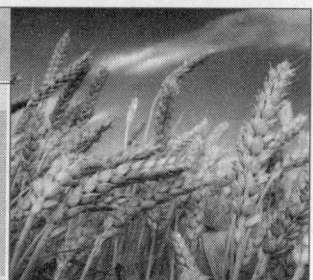

B. Jain uses Grain based ENA for MT and Dilutions which is purest form of alcohol is less bitter thus assuring pure vehicle.

§ 270 Highest Quality Globules

§ 270

ᵃ The vial used for potentizing is filled two-thirds full.
ᵇ Perhaps on a leather – bound book.
ᶜ They are prepared, under supervision by the confectioner, from starch and sugar and the small globules freed from fine dusty parts by passing them through a sieve. Then they are put through a strainer that will permit only 100 to pass through weighing one grain, the most serviceable size for the needs of a homoeopathic physician.

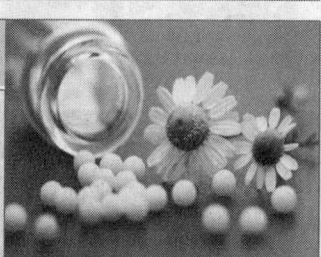

B. Jain uses pharma grade sugar for preparation of globules to assure unadulterated vehicle for you.

§ 271 Medicine preparation method should be reliable

['If the physician prepares his homoeopathic medicines himself, as he should reasonably do in order to save men from sickness,[2],

[2] 'Until the State, in the future, after having attained insight into the indispensability of perfectly prepared homoeopathic medicines, will have them manufactured by a competent impartial person.

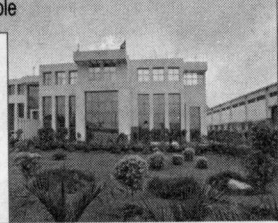

B. Jain has a GMP Certified manufacturing plant with two accrediation (India and Health Canada). B.Jain documents each and every steps followed in preparation of medicine to guarantee the reliability a homeopath needs

Do You Have Access to all above?

If you want your medicines to comply to above standards

Ask for B. Jain Medicines

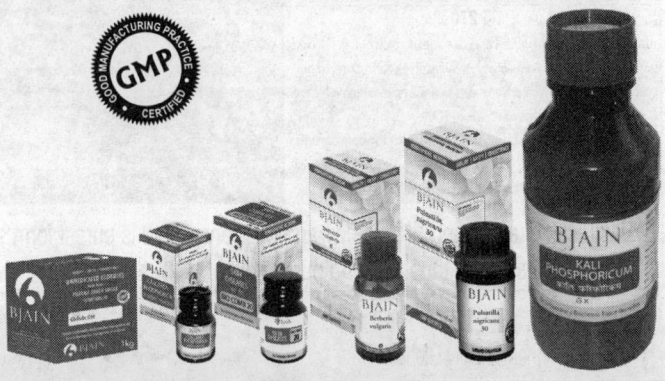

BJAIN Pharmaceuticals (P) Ltd.
Corporate Office: 1921/10, Chuna Mandi, Paharganj, New Delhi - 110055 (INDIA)
Factory Office: E-41/F, RIICO Industrial Area, Khushkhera, District Alwar, Bhiwadi - 301707 Raj. (India) Tel. +91-11-45671000 Fax: +91-11-45671010
Email: pharma@bjain.com | www.pharma.bjain.com